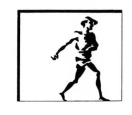

GLAMOUR'S HEALTH & BEAUTY BOOK

A COMPLETE SHAPE-UP PROGRAM

BY THE EDITORS OF GLAMOUR MAGAZINE

Simon and Schuster • New York

Published by Simon and Schuster
A Division of Gulf & Western Corporation
Simon & Schuster Building
Rockefeller Center
1230 Avenue of the Americas
New York, New York 10020

Manufactured in the United States of America
1   2   3   4   5   6   7   8   9   10

Library of Congress Cataloging in Publication Data

Main entry under title:
Glamour's Health & beauty book.
    Includes index.
    1. Beauty, Personal.   2. Women—Health and
hygiene.   I. Coffey, Barbara.   II. Glamour.
III. Title: Health & beauty book.
RA778.G563   1978   646.7'2   78-5426
ISBN 0-671-23089-1

Edited by
Barbara Coffey
Designed by
George Hartman

Photographs
Tito Barberis
Patrice Casanova
William Connors
Patrick DeMarchelier
Frank Horvat
David McCabe
Tony Moussoulides
Rico Puhlman
Mike Reinhardt
John Stember

Drawings
Margaret Brown
Sheila Camera
Loring Eutemey
Durell Godfrey
Mariah Graham
Barbara Hanlon
Tom Huffman
Marie Michel

CONTENTS

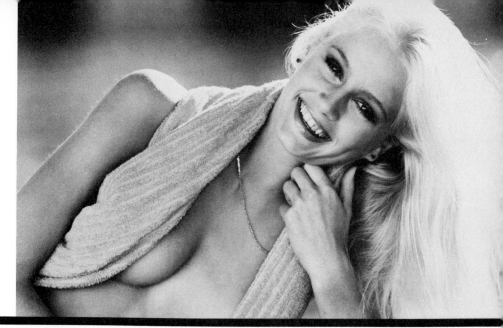

INTRODUCTION

HEALTH

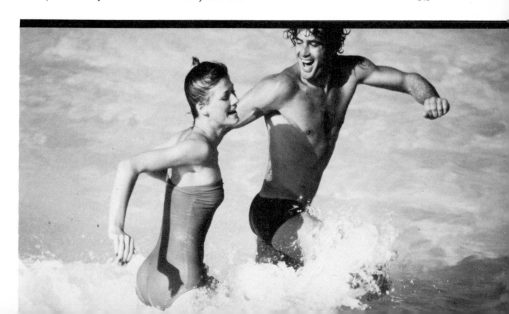

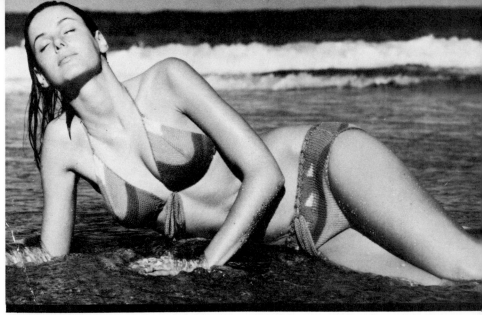

BODY

HAIR

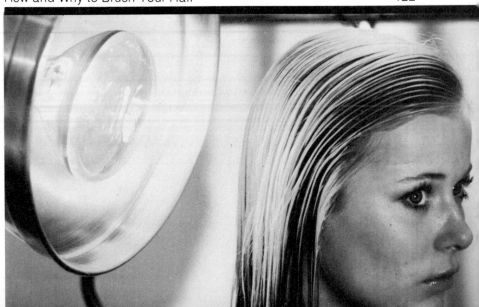

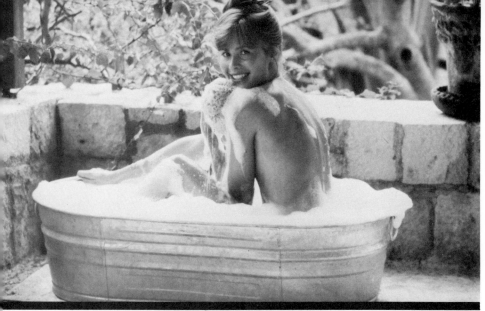

SKIN

COSMETIC SURGERY

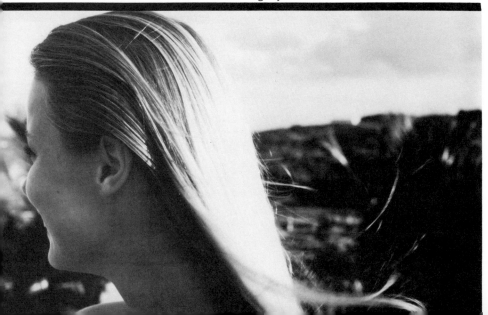

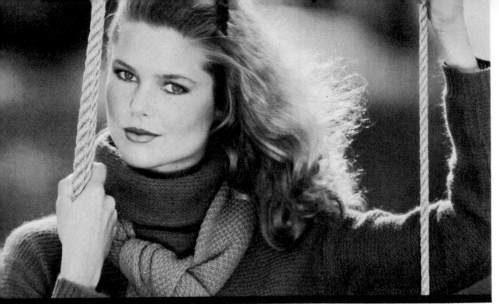

MAKEUP

BEAUTY ON-THE-GO

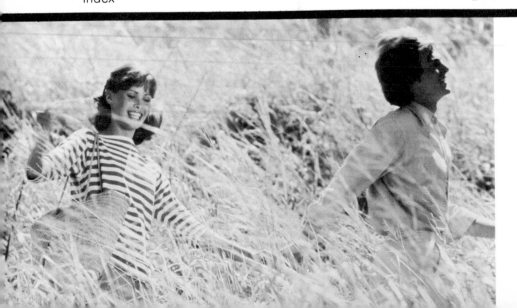

GLAMOUR'S
HEALTH
& BEAUTY
BOOK
A COMPLETE SHAPE-UP PROGRAM

A DIF

KIND

FERENT
OF
BEAUTY

This is a different kind of beauty book for a different kind of woman, one who knows that some of her most important beauty options have as much to do with health as they do with beauty. It's a book for the woman who's as interested in whether she needs to take vitamin supplements as she is in new makeup techniques. She's concerned about safe birth control options, healthful weight reduction diets and new hairstyles. It's for the woman who demands a lot of her looks and doesn't have a lot of time to work with them. She lives a time-prioritied life and wants it to run as smoothly as possible.

If you're like her, this book is made for you. You'll find that it has all the hair, makeup and skin advice you want, some of it divided into seasonal help to make it even more useful. You'll also find that some of the most important comprehensive chapters have to do with your health options. You'll find a chapter of Beauty-on-the-Go—it's almost a mini beauty book within this book and it's full of ideas on how to get more beauty in less time. There's a special diet section here for people who lead active lives but insist on healthful, low-calorie eating. You'll also find that many of the chapters start with some sort of quiz to help you locate yourself in terms of hair type, body type, skin type and so forth, so that you can immediately pinpoint the information that will be most useful. With that idea in mind, start right now with the quiz here to see how well you have been taking care of yourself and how much work you might want to do on your looks now, with the help of this book.

How much have you been getting from your looks?

Don't guess. Take this quiz and find out. Remember that getting the most from your looks means living up to your own personal beauty potential—being open-minded enough to consider what's new, yet knowing yourself well enough to reject what's not right for you, even though it may be the newest thing going. It means valuing yourself enough to take time to care for your face and body and especially your health without letting it become an obsessive preoccupation.

In each case, check the description that sounds *most* like you.

HEALTH

About health information, I:
★ Try to keep informed and up-to-date and assimilate what's relevant for me.
● Figure I'm young so why worry.
■ Try to keep up when there's time.

About my doctor, I:
● Haven't seen him/her in ages.
■ Go only when I'm really feeling sick.
★ Have a good rapport and go when I feel the need out of sickness or just for sound emotional or physical advice.

My weight is:
★ Great, I watch my diet and exercise.
● A mess, I can't diet and I don't like to exercise.
■ It has its good and bad times, but more good than bad.

BODY

I use body lotion:
■ In winter or after sunning only.
● Never.
★ After every bath or shower and whenever else I can slather it on.

My legs are:
● Never shaved or waxed.
★ Always shaved or waxed.
■ Shaved or waxed carefully in summer only or for special occasions.

MAKEUP

Blusher for me is:
★ Indispensable.
● For winter only.
■ Never worn.

I use foundation:
★ Everyday.
■ When I want special polish.
● Hardly ever.

About the combination lipstick/lipgloss:
★ I've got one.
■ I'm considering trying one.
● Never heard of them.

SKIN CARE

I use moisturizer:
● Never.
■ Usually.
★ Always.

My cleansing routine:
■ Is geared to my skin type.
● Takes advantage of what's handy.
★ Changes frequently according to what I've read that makes sense for me.

I use a facial mask:
● Never.
★ Faithfully once a week.
■ When I think of it.

HAIR

I have my hair cut:
■ When I think of it.
★ Every 4 to 8 weeks.
● I can't remember when I cut it last.

About the use of heat lamps for hair drying:
★ I've tried it and do it frequently.
● I can live with my old way of drying my hair.
■ I'm considering giving the idea a try.

I've worn my present hair-style:
● Forever.
★ Not long, I change it a lot.
■ For as long as it has looked contemporary and right for me.

scoring

Give yourself 10 points for each ★.
Give yourself 7 points for each ■.
Subtract 2 points for each ●.

Below 86: You're saying NO to your looks and health. Paying a little more attention to yourself would get you a lot more for your looks.

86-97: You're a MAYBE type. You care, but sometimes not quite enough to get the most from yourself.

98-131: You're saying YES to yourself. If you keep up the good work, you'll continue to reap the benefits.

132-140: Stop overdoing it. There is such a thing as being a slave to yourself.

How to make
MORE TIME
for yourself

No beauty guide will make sense unless you first make the time to follow it through. That's why we start off with this how-to exercise to prove you have as much time for yourself as you want! If you don't believe it, we're going to change your mind. The secret is in the word "want."

If you haven't complained about not having enough time, you're not human. Everyone feels pressured now and again, but there really is enough time to go around if you concentrate on important things. You probably think that's what you're doing, but try this little experiment. It's suggested by time expert Alan Lakein in his book *How to Get Control of Your Time and Your Life.** Sit down and make a "priority list" of the things you really consider important now—improving your looks, losing ten pounds, whatever it is. Number the things on your list in order of their importance. Now put your list away and don't think about it. In the meantime, check out how you spend your time on a typical day. Do it for several days running. You don't have to keep track of every minute, but get an idea of how you spend the hours in your day. Now pull out your priority list and compare how you'd like to spend your time with how you *do* spend it. Pretty surprising, isn't it? If you're like most of us, you're probably doing a lot of low-priority things, or things not on your list at all.

To make more beauty time, start by eliminating the activities not on your list at all. You can probably eliminate a big chunk of your low-priority activities without anything drastic happening. For example, if you *always* drive the neighborhood kids to school, it's time for another mother to help. If you cook *and* clean up every night, ask your husband to at least clean up a couple of nights a week. Don't waste your lunch hour everyday running silly errands. Instead join an exercise class. Actually, you'll probably be so shocked at how you "waste" time, you won't have trouble cutting out the wasteful activities. Make it a point to make at least one half hour extra every day to spend on yourself. By decreasing or eliminating the time you spend on low-priority things, you'll find you've increased time in any area of your life where you *want* to spend more time. Right now, what you want is to make more time to make yourself better-looking!

* Alan Lakein, *How to Get Control of Your Time and Your Life*, David McKay Co., Inc., New York, 1973.

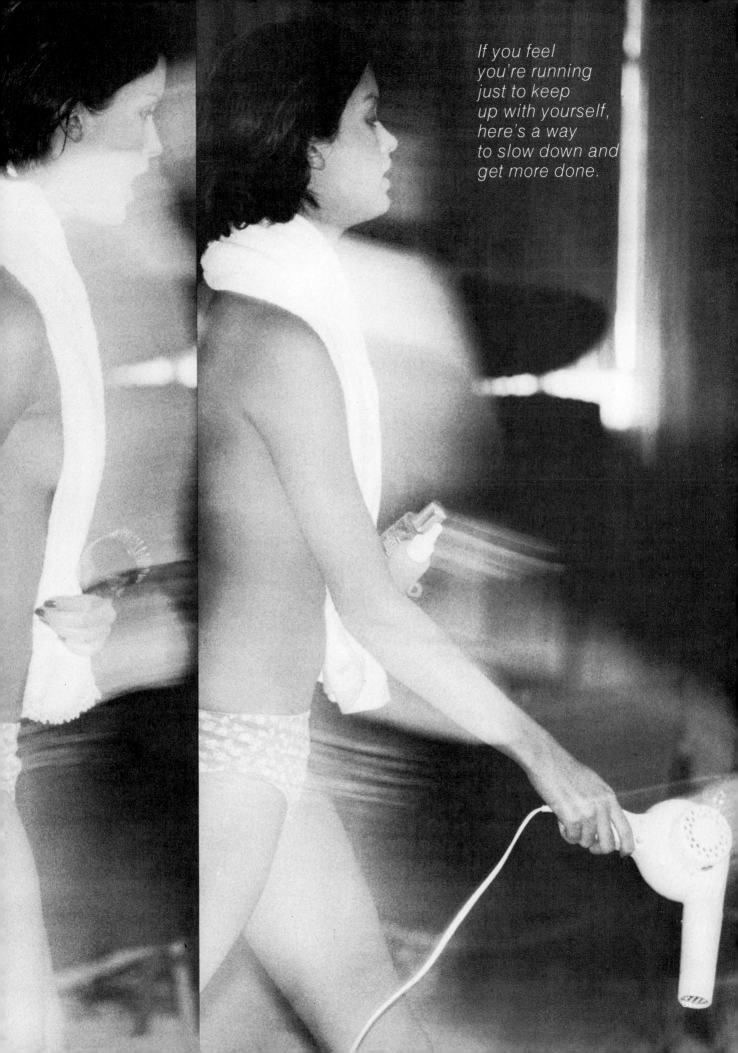

If you feel you're running just to keep up with yourself, here's a way to slow down and get more done.

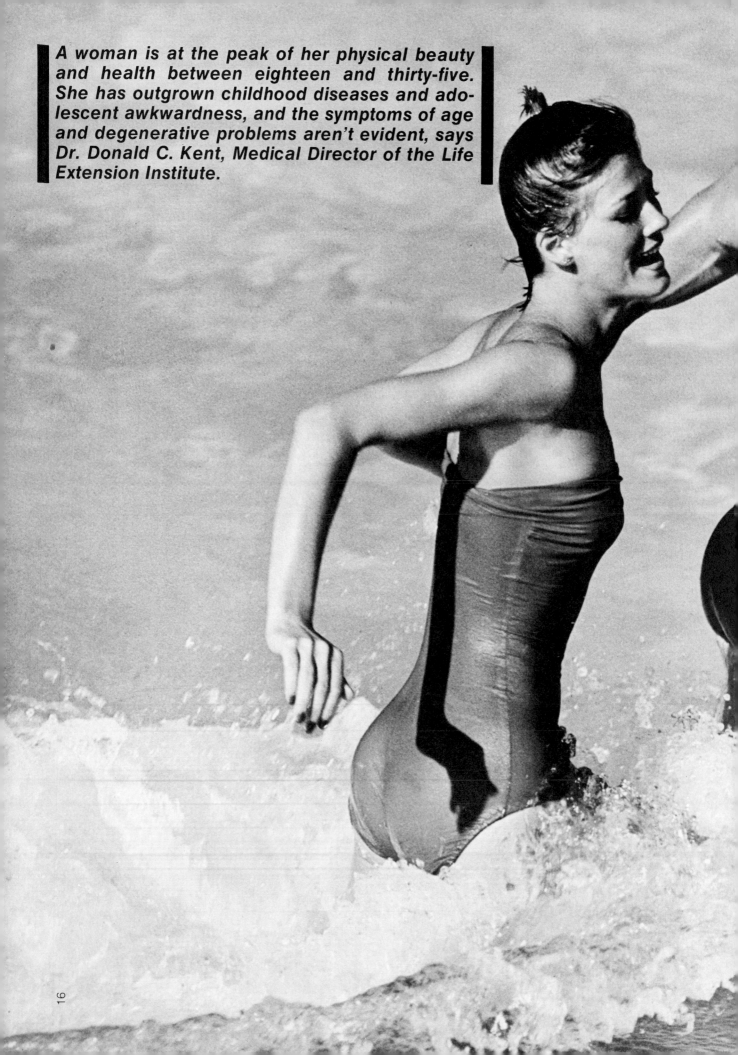

A woman is at the peak of her physical beauty and health between eighteen and thirty-five. She has outgrown childhood diseases and adolescent awkwardness, and the symptoms of age and degenerative problems aren't evident, says Dr. Donald C. Kent, Medical Director of the Life Extension Institute.

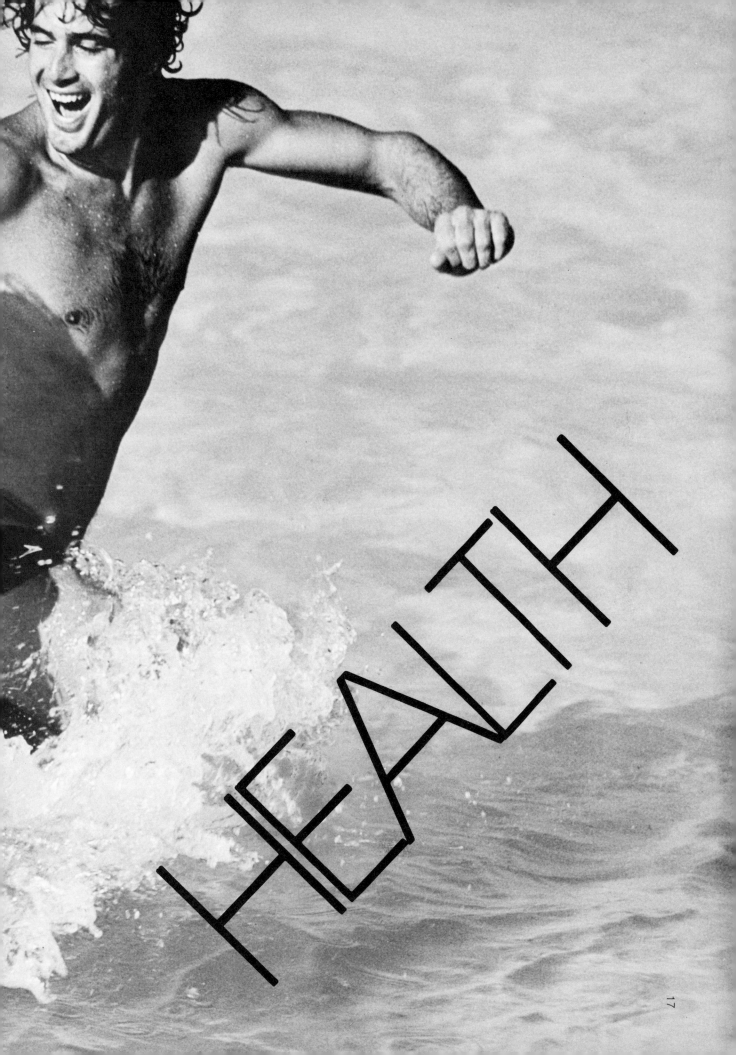

HEALTH

YOUR TOP BEAUTY AND HEALTH PRIORITIES FROM AGE 18 TO 35

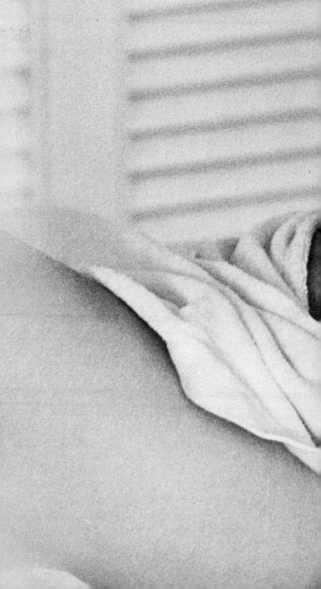

Since the years between eighteen and thirty-five are likely to give you the fewest health problems in your lifetime, they are the best years for establishing preventive health habits to keep you fit for all the years to follow. Here are what many experts believe are the three most important areas to work on.

1. EXERCISE

Get enough of it, soon enough. It is not only a prime factor from childhood on in maintaining a firm, sleek body, but lack of it will start producing physical symptoms of degeneration early in life. You'll learn in the following pages not only what can happen to a woman's body from eighteen to thirty-five—the stresses and strains put on it—but why and what to do about it. Looks, however, are only one significant part of the whole picture; an exercise deficiency can affect how well your heart, lungs, back and other vital health organs function and how soon you may have problems relating to them.

2. WEIGHT

Watch it. Being really fat isn't just unacceptable in terms of what this society considers good-looking and desirable; it's unhealthful. Overweight is associated not only with psychological problems but with problems such as heart and artery disease, diabetes, varicose veins and even such a seemingly unrelated condition as asthma. All the information you need for changing bad eating habits to good ones, for losing weight and gaining confidence in your body and yourself is contained in this chapter, and throughout the book.

3. BODY AWARENESS

Pay attention to what your body tells you. The signals that each part of it from head to toes sends out are listed following. Get to know not only the cyclical highs and lows of your own body but also of your own moods, since they affect your physical and emotional performance. You can find out how in the article "Misconceptions We All Have About Our Mental Health," later in this chapter.

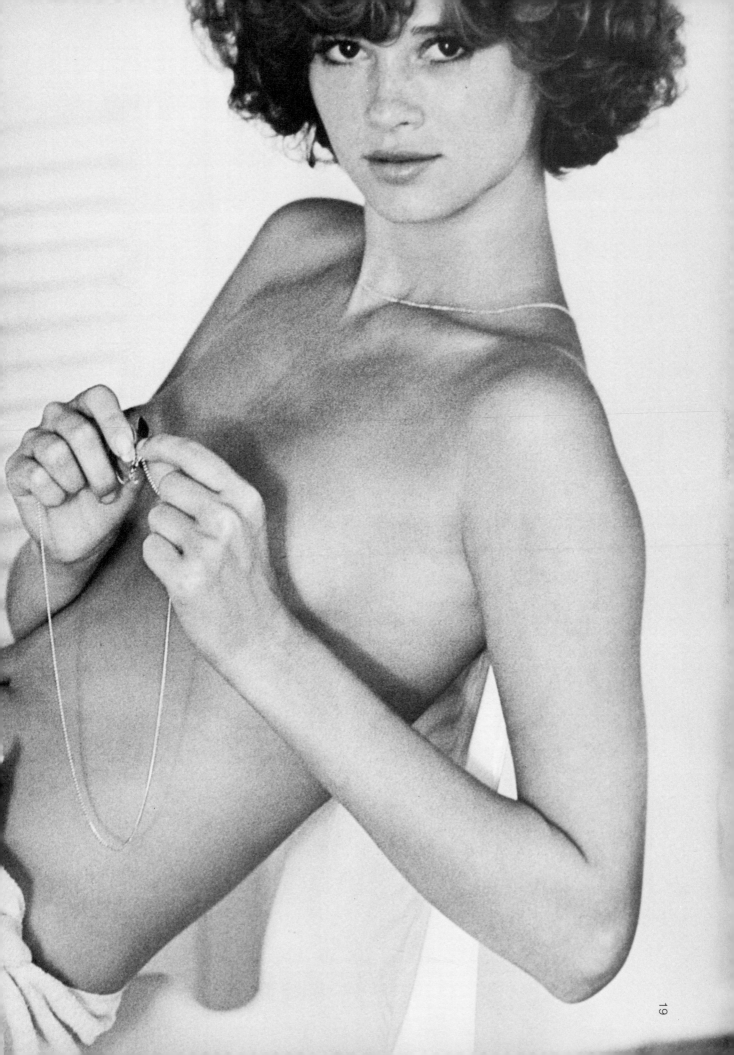

BODY AWARENESS CLUES

*Head-to-toe clues to the most
common beauty and health problems
of women eighteen to thirty-five*

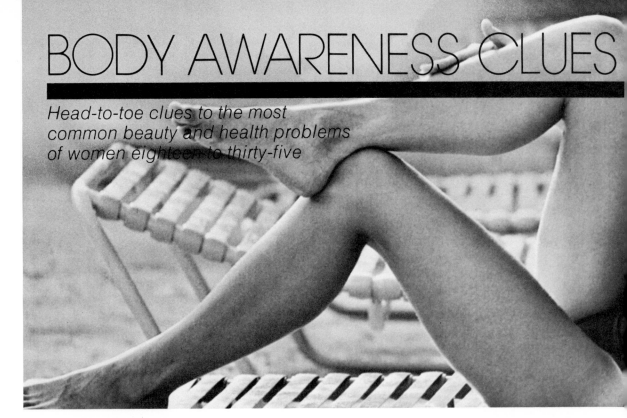

Many women ignore the signals their bodies are sending them in terms of physical changes like suddenly drier, more lifeless hair, even pain that could be alleviated. All these are a drain on your looks as well as the smooth performance of your body. Other women panic at the slightest body change—a rash, sag or discoloration of skin—or rush to a doctor for a common cold. Knowing something about the function and appearance of your body can provide a better balanced view of what it is telling you, and can help you take better care of it, as well as relieve panic reactions. That's why we've prepared this brief rundown of some of the more usual physical problems that directly affect your looks during the eighteen to thirty-five-year-old period—what they mean, what to do or not to do about them. This is not however a comprehensive do-it-yourself medical guide. Any drastic change in body appearance or function should be checked by a physician.

HAIR

Sudden dryness and lifelessness can be an indication of thyroid problems. . . . Abnormal loss of hair—that's anything over a hundred or so hairs a day—can indicate a nutritional deficiency or scalp disease such as severe dandruff (frequently accompanied by acne). A dermatologist can help both. . . . Don't worry about temporary hair loss that often follows childbirth or stopping the birth control pill.

FACE

For any rash (anywhere on the body) that lasts for more than a day or two, consult a dermatologist. . . . Acne is the physical manifestation of hormonal changes, especially during adoles-

cence. To avoid the emotional problems and scarring that severe acne cause, put yourself in the care of a dermatologist.

SKIN

Freckles are hereditary. Sun exposure brings them out. Some peeling agents administered by a dermatologist can minimize them, but that is considered drastic therapy. . . . Most moles can be removed by a doctor. . . . Large pores react very little to help; astringents can have a slight temporary tightening effect on them. . . . The drier your skin, the greater its tendency to wrinkle. There's no prevention, but emollient cosmetics soften the skin, help to eliminate some of the finer wrinkling. Use emollients from your teens on. . . . The fairer your skin, the more sun protection it needs to prevent solar keratosis and skin cancers later in life. Skin that burns in patches, while other patches don't, may be undergoing a photosensitive reaction to certain drugs, especially certain tranquilizers and tetracycline, an antibiotic commonly given to women with acne. Always ask your doctor about possible side effects of any medication before you take it.

EYES

Dark circles under eyes usually have no medical importance and are hereditary. Illness, exhaustion or great weight loss can make the darkness more prominent. . . . Swelling of lids can be attributed to kidney disease, allergic reactions, overactive thyroid gland, sinusitis, hay fever or chronic dermatitis. . . . Red or itchy and/or swollen lids could be conjunctivitis or an allergy. Yellow-tinged whites can signal hepatitis. All require medical attention.

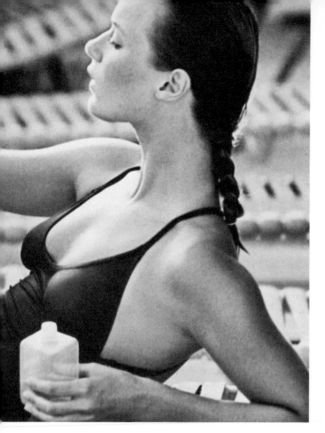

NOSE

A constantly runny nose or one that is always stopped up may indicate an allergy and is definitely a beauty spoiler. Regular cold remedies sold over the counter seldom work for it; a disfigured or disproportionate nose doesn't have to be endured; talk over your possibilities for a new one with a plastic surgeon.

MOUTH

Keep tartar off your teeth now—its buildup contributes greatly to periodontal disease, the leading cause of Americans losing their teeth as they get older. Tartar shows up as irregular yellow spots behind or between teeth and is a combination of food particles that have been allowed to remain in the mouth, bacteria, and the product that results when the bacteria works on leftover food. When still soft, it's called plaque and can be removed with a toothbrush and dental floss. Allowed to harden, it must be removed by a dentist or dental assistant with professional tools. Bleeding gums need dental attention too. Fever blisters, cold sores, or herpes simplex are all the same, and while they can appear anywhere on the body, they often appear on lips. Sun, wind, a cold, gastrointestinal upsets, fever or emotional stress can bring them out. Zinc ointments or special medicated lipsticks can protect against sun and wind; once blisters break out, spirits of camphor, drying lotions or tincture of benzoin can help dry them up. They usually go away within a week to ten days. If they become infected, see your doctor.

NECK

Swollen glands in the neck area are the principal symtom of mononucleosis and also signal other infections, all of which need a doctor's care.

HANDS

Any sudden swelling—for instance, your watch strap or rings don't fit from one week to another—should be reported to your doctor. You may be retaining fluid or having a severe allergic reaction. Particularly if you are pregnant, call your doctor, since the swelling could indicate a condition that, unless treated promptly, may be dangerous to you as well as your unborn child. . . . Nails that turn brittle may be telling you that you need more protein in your diet, but check it out with a doctor. Some people are just born with soft or brittle nails.

BREASTS

The threat of breast cancer is very rare between the ages of eighteen and thirty, but that is no reason for a woman twenty or younger not to begin the sound health practice of examining her own breasts regularly for lumps right after each menstrual period. . . . Many young women develop breast cysts, which are usually benign but should be reported to a doctor. Some women develop a condition known as cystic mastitis, which consists of a number of small cysts that reoccur regularly in a specific period of the menstrual cycle; these, too, are harmless but should be diagnosed by a doctor. . . . A discharge from the nipples, unless you're pregnant, needs medical investigation; it does not necessarily mean cancer. . . . Red or inflamed breasts accompanied by a fever often means mastitis, an infection of the breast ducts, which can occur following childbirth and in nursing mothers but can also occur for other reasons. Your doctor will probably treat it with antibiotics. . . . One breast somewhat larger than the other is a common occurrence and no sign of medical trouble unless the size suddenly changes.

LEGS

With younger women, probably the most common leg problem is varicose veins, which can result because of pregnancy or obesity; later in life there are other causes. If pregnancy is the cause, they usually go away by themselves once the baby is born. If obesity is the cause, loss of weight helps. Anyone not pregnant and on the pill should report varicose veins to her doctor who will probably want to switch her to some other method of contraception.

FEET

Flat feet aren't really much of a beauty problem, but they can make you uncomfortable, even more so when you're older. Some women are born with them, others develop them. Excessive weight or the wrong kind of shoes contribute to the development of this condition and the discomfort. A doctor can help by recommending the right shoe or arch support for your feet.

DO YOU KNOW?

To keep you up on offbeat and not-so-offbeat areas of scientific research that could influence your life, we've put together this collection of items. Some are news items you might not have heard about, others are misconceptions that you might not have the clear facts on.

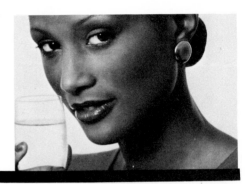

Does alcohol affect your looks?

For one thing, it can make you fat. It's one of the quicker putters-on of pounds around. A couple of drinks before dinner every night can add as many as 500 calories to your daily intake, depending on what kind of drink you have. For another, the persistent overuse of alcohol has also been associated with a skin condition called seborrhea (a cousin of the "heartbreak of psoriasis"). Seborrhea is characterized by brownish-gray skin scales on the face and on the scalp; it can lead to thinning of the hair. Eventually, alcohol affects skin tone and muscles, too.

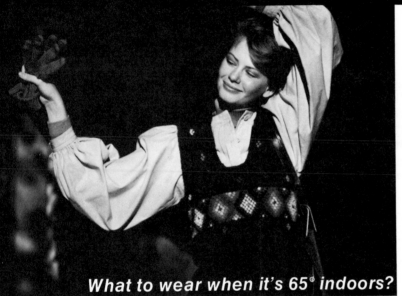

What to wear when it's 65° indoors?

The best way to keep warm in a house or office when the temperature is only sixty-five degrees to conserve energy is to dress like a British gentleman—even if you're an American woman. British men tend to wear layers of clothing (i.e., shirts, vests, sweaters, jackets, often long johns, rather than one heavy suit or heavy sweater and pants). According to the *ASHRAE Journal* (The American Society of Heating, Refrigerating and Air Conditioning Engineers, Inc.), this is the most effective method of combating not only a cold body, but also cold hands and feet. Incidentally, cold hands are not necessarily *best* warmed by wearing woolen gloves. Physiologically, the body attempts to maintain the temperature of the brain and the internal organs at about a constant ninety-nine degrees. If, in a cool environment, the internal body temperature drops, the blood supply to hands and feet will be diminished. In a moderately low indoor temperature, i.e., sixty-five degrees, cold hands and feet can indicate you are not dressed warmly enough all over. The remedy, according to ASHRAE, is to add extra clothing, which will help warm your internal organs and brain, thus your cold hands and feet.

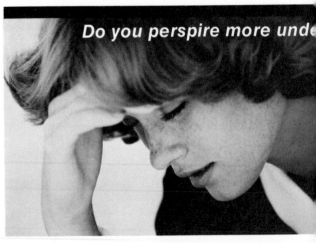

Do you perspire more unde

It may seem like a paradox, but you perspire *more* skiing downhill in freezing weather than stretched out in the sun. The reason—you're likely to be frightened, or at least emotionally keyed up while racing downhill and you're probably quite relaxed on the beach. Whenever your emotions are stirred, the sweat glands all over your body are stimulated, especially the apocrine sweat glands in the armpits. Actually, all of us have two kinds of perspiration. One is apocrine, which is chiefly responsible for underarm odor and which responds primarily to emotional stimuli. The other is eccrine, which acts as the body's cooling system by reacting to external temperature changes. Emotional

These facts might change your mind and your health habits

stimuli can also cause eccrine sweat glands to react, especially on palms of the hands and soles of the feet. So much has been learned recently about the connection between perspiration and emotions that behavioral scientists now see "skin talk," as the skin's response to emotional stimuli is called, as a new and important tool in discovering the real and hidden feelings of people. So, next time you find yourself "breaking into a sweat," you might look to the emotional reason for a change instead of adjusting the temperature.

Does smoking cause wrinkles?

Smoking, along with the sun, is being considered by some authorities as a prime enemy of smooth skin. Research done by Dr. H. W. Daniell in California and reported on by the *Journal of the American Medical Association* was able to establish a correlation between the amount of skin wrinkling and smoking. Dr. Daniell suggests that smoking may cause wrinkling because nicotine makes the small blood vessels contract and over a period of time causes deterioration of skin tissue.

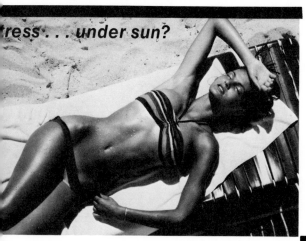

...ress . . . under sun?

Can sex cure insomnia?

You have probably heard that there is nothing like good sex to produce a good night's sleep. So have many sleep researchers who are scientifically pursuing the idea in their attempts to find a remedy for insomnia. A very promising area of sleep research concerns itself with the use of certain sex hormones as the "perfect" sleep-inducing drug that has so far eluded chemists and doctors. (Almost all prescription drugs now on the market are either addictive or habit-forming and, what's more, actually interfere with REM sleep, which represents our deepest periods of relaxation.) Almost every woman who has ever been pregnant has no-

ticed that in the early stages of pregnancy she tends to become drowsy easily. The hormone that a woman excretes in more than usual amounts in early pregnancy is progesterone. Researchers are now using injections of this drug to induce sleep in cats. Unlike other chemicals, it seems to produce natural sleep, not the disturbed sleep patterns that barbiturates and tranquilizers do. But to date, the experiments have been done on animals, and researchers warn that no one should try taking birth control pills that contain progesterone for insomnia. Although some women on the pill have reported they become drowsy, others have complained of sleeplessness. It is paradoxically the same with sexual fulfillment, which apparently acts as a sedative for some, while a great many others make love in the morning and go off to work, drive cars, take care of children with ease, which they couldn't do if they were very sleepy.

Is there a two-minute pregnancy test?

Several new pregnancy tests have been developed in the last decade, two of which will eliminate the usual two-day wait the old rabbit test required before a woman could have her pregnancy confirmed. (They also eliminate the need for a rabbit.) The fastest of the tests produces results in two minutes. A tiny amount of the woman's urine is combined on a slide with a special solution and studied for a chemical reaction. Another test that is more reliable requires about two hours and uses urine mixed with a solution containing a hormone produced during pregnancy. If a woman is pregnant, an antibody reaction can be observed in the solution in two hours. Both tests can be used from four weeks after conception.

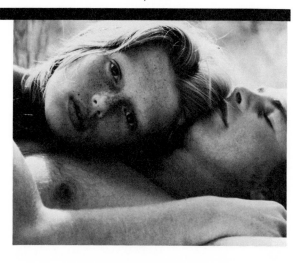

MISCONCEPTIONS

WE ALL HAVE ABOUT OUR MENTAL HEALTH

By M. Dorothea Kerr, M.D.

Psychology is now a common freshman course in college. We are inundated with books and articles about mental health. We constantly evaluate the behavior of our friends and loved ones as to what is "sick" and what is "normal"—out loud if we're feeling hostile; otherwise, silently and subconsciously. We all feel we are experts on mental health, but with all our intelligence and sophistication we have many misconceptions about mental health that can taint our lives and render our judgments invalid.

1. If you're mentally healthy one day, you're the same the next

We tend to think of mental health as a fixed state in which a person is always emotionally and mentally healthy or emotionally and mentally sick. But mental health is not static; it is a continuing balance with individual variations of mood, thought and energy, which color our personality and make up our characteristic emotional and mental patterns.

We vary from day to day, waking up one morning depressed and staying that way all day, whereas the next day we arise inexplicably cheerful with energy to spare. Each one of us has his/her own pattern with marked variations of mood, energy and concentration. Our negative variations, especially those influenced by depressing situations, can fit within the category of mild emotional or mental sickness, just as our positive variations can reach a temporary too-high mood.

Part of knowing oneself means knowing one's emotional and mental patterns. This is probably best done by rapidly recording one's moods, energy and thinking levels each day on a calendar like the one opposite, in a range from 1 to 5. If you do this fairly conscientiously for three to six months and then chart a rough graph, your highs and lows become apparent. Everyone's mood, energy and thought-ability patterns are cyclical. Knowing your highs and lows can help you judge yourself so you can appreciate the limits of your variations in these areas. It also enables you to plan events in your life to coincide with your inner self (your feeling and thinking self) so that you will be successful and become a more integrated and whole person, i.e., you would not schedule a challenging event at a time you might be at your lowest ebb.

2. Mental health is happiness

Confusing mental health with life satisfaction is a great misconception. Life satisfaction may re-

Opposite: This sample calendar is for charting your ups and downs so that you will know what to expect of yourself and when—in terms of mood, energy and concentration. We all have a cyclical pattern for these, and finding it can help you to schedule important events at times when you are at your peak rather than at your worst. Keep a calendar like this for three to six months, rating yourself in each category from 1 to 5. Then graph your highs and lows and you'll see a very revealing pattern about yourself.

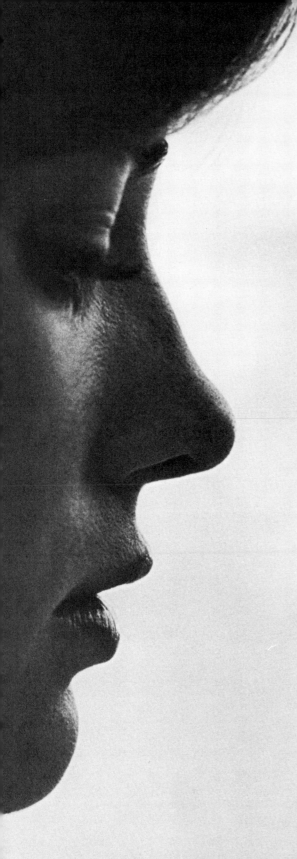

quire one to be successful in a job or marriage, thus adhering to group values, or it may mean learning to do one's thing, following a different drummer. But we can be extremely dissatisfied with life and yet be mentally happy. And vice versa, we can be very satisfied with ourselves and life as it is, yet be psychotic. To be satisfied in life, to feel you have not missed out, does not require sampling every pleasure and adventure the world has to offer. It does require finding a self-identity, a path of one's own. We make the decisions of our life essentially alone. We live up to the responsibility of possible failure instead of escaping. We know somehow intuitively where we are going day by day.

Mental health means that one is functioning as a whole with one's emotional, logical and intellectual selves and with the world; that we are not torn apart by conflict between desires, or between desires and conscience or between fears and what the world tells us to do. Mentally healthy people recognize feelings of dissatisfaction with all their many disguises. They not only recognize the feelings, but identify the problem and go on to solve it in some self-constructive or at least nonself-destructive fashion. Mentally or emotionally ill people may be satisfied only because they do not recognize the deep wellsprings of feeling and thinking within. They have little insight, meaning they are not conscious of feelings of self-dissatisfaction, not aware of problems. We see this unawareness easily in the many compulsive ways people escape: drugs, alcohol, sex, work.

Mental, emotional and psychosomatic symptoms all have a meaning. In physical illness, fever is a symptom warning of something wrong with the body. Emotional overreaction and mental confusion are similar warnings of something wrong with our thinking and feeling body.

Emotional and psychosomatic symptoms are not just proof of being sick; they are trying to tell us we have a conflict within ourselves, that we are not *emotionally ready* for our present life even though we may be intellectually and physically ready. For example, people with stage fright or exam jitters: the fear (anxiety) means they do not feel emotionally ready for the task at hand though they know they have the knowledge for the exam or the talent for the stage performance. Not being emotionally ready may be because of being in a situation we do not want or about which we have conflicting feelings.

We have at least three selves: physical, intel-

chart your pattern of ups and downs

	1	2	3	4	5	6	7	8	9	10	11	12	13	14	15	16	17	18	19	20	21	22	23	24	25	26	27	28	29	30	31
Mood																															
Energy																															
ntration																															

lectual, and emotional. The intellectual self and physical self—our thinking and our outside appearance—are what the world sees and from which we form our "image" for others. The emotional self is our inner self: our feeling, unconscious self; our self-image.

The rules by which our emotional self operates are different from our logical and intellectual selves. It is our emotional self that decides if we are "ready" for a task whether the task is tennis or becoming a rock star.

This concept of emotional readiness is tested in many areas today. For example, reading readiness tests are given in early grade school to determine if a child is emotionally ready for the physical and intellectual task of learning to read. It is part of good aptitude testing to see whether a candidate is emotionally ready for the job or career he/she wants as well as inherently talented and motivated.

There are several clues that determine your emotional readiness in daily life. 1. Ability to talk freely, openly and spontaneously to anyone about the task at hand without marked feelings of apprehension. 2. Ability to do the task without marked feelings of fear or worry. 3. Enjoyment of what you're doing; not a heady feeling of excitement that may mask anxiety, but a deeper quieter feeling of enjoyment. 4. Postmortem satisfaction; to think, feel and talk about it afterward with satisfaction, not a heady feeling of triumph or a feeling of "ashes-in-the-mouth" after a looked-for success. Understanding and cooperating with these rules of "emotional readiness" will help us succeed consistently at a task instead of frustrating ourselves by starting and stopping.

Anyone who begins a journey of self-discovery, either alone or with the help of a therapist, will be less encumbered with baggage if he/she gets rid of some of the common misconceptions about what mental health is and is not. Identifying the problem and becoming more objective about one's own prejudices will help make the trip faster. The results of all inner discovery can be very gratifying, an exploration of the unknown, going someplace no one has ever been before. It is a learning-through experience that seems to remain with us, to be used every day of our life and savored through memory.

3. No one denies that we are a product of our past but . . .

The accepted cause or causes of mental illness are very much in flux among professionals at present, and this has given rise to many misunderstandings and misconceptions. The theoretical causes that are most popular fall into three categories: psychological, biochemical and sociocultural. Each theory has its adherents who tend to believe in a single cause, but fortunately most therapists are open to multiforms of treatment, based upon their experience, and tailor their therapy to each patient's needs. The multiphased approach may operate by changing the biochemical milieu of the cell and/or relieving psychic pain by food and drugs, as well as changing patterns of thought and feeling by understanding and reconditioning present and past personality mechanisms.

During the 1930s and 1940s, psychoanalysis was the vogue in intellectual and educational circles with its emphasis on past history and rearing as the cause of current personality difficulties. As a result, every one of us with difficulties has a vague feeling that somehow it is our fault. We have become a nation of guilty patients as well as guilty parents. This guilt in turn adds to our indecisiveness and self-blaming so that we are on a confused not-so-merry-go-round of "What am I doing?" "How can I do better?" No one denies that we are a product of our past but research of the last ten years has focused on biochemical body mechanisms as causes of mental and mood illnesses. Psychoactive drugs and nutrition of the body have become important in overall treatment. Therapeutic drug use varies from very mild tranquilizers for overreaction in everyday situations to the tranquilizers and antidepressants used in the treatment of psychotic breaks.

4. Psychoactive drugs are a crutch

A popular misconception is that psychoactive drugs are a crutch. Believers of this feel that willpower should be used to overcome personal difficulties, and understanding to comprehend and solve them. Determination and persistence combined with gradual understanding is a more permanent way of solving the conflicting attitudes and feelings that give rise to symptoms, but it is not necessary to deprive yourself of the help that a drug can give in the process. Emotional and mental symptoms result in psychic pain, which causes more and deeper suffering than physical pain. We do not hesitate to use painkillers from aspirin to narcotics for the temporary relief of physical pain while we seek a permanent cure through treating the cause. Why then deny responsible use of medication to ourselves when emotionally ill?

5. Mental illness is culturally caused

Community psychiatry sees mental illness as culturally caused and attempts to cure large numbers of people by changing society itself. It is an approach that appeals to the idealism of the younger generation with its promise of group change and "total cure" through prevention. However, anthropological data and world health projects point out that the mental and emotional values of a culture change very slowly. Consequently, we cannot expect to see any rapid improvement from the worthwhile work currently being done by those in community psychiatry.

6. People who have had psychotherapy are undependable

Many people still regard psychotherapy as a stigma. These people feel no one could seek this help voluntarily for his/her betterment but only if compelled because of symptoms or unusual behavior. Psychiatry and psychology have gradually evolved, however, from emphasis on diagnosis and symptoms to a focus on the individual's personal, social and spiritual growth. As people have taken advantage of this primarily educational opportunity for personal growth, psychotherapy in practice has become an individual tutoring-learning process even more than a treatment.

The misconception of psychiatric treatment as a stigma poses a problem for anyone who feels a desire or need for help. It holds many people back from achieving, in this way, an understanding of their personality, emotional reactions and behavior. The public still feels there is an aura of undependability about anyone who admits having had psychiatric or psychological treatment. The fear of stigma makes us hesitate to admit having undergone psychotherapy to a man we love or when applying for a job. This moral dilemma is best solved by our inner feelings. Those with a strong conscience may need to take the risk of disclosure; otherwise, the conflict between their requirement for honesty and their fear of being found out will keep them miserable. A person with a strong practical sense realizes it is often wise not to admit a potentially damaging fact until one is sure of the attitude of the recipient.

7. Being normal guarantees mental health

Our misconceptions of normality and the pressures in our lives to "be normal" can often interfere with our growth as individuals. Mental health consists of developing one's own identity, expanding one's consciousness of self. Group social health may require conformity to an average, a norm. Failure to measure up to or surpass the norm may produce feelings of inadequacy that threaten mental stability, while at the same time conformity to the norm does not guarantee mental health.

A definition of normality is hard to come by in terms of mental health. Committees of experts have struggled for days to define this common word without acceptable results. Yet we all think we know who is abnormal and who is not. Our definitions and judgments reflect not only our own prejudices but also our objectivity in terms of what our cultural group calls normal.

Still, each of us is unique. We have a number of selves that alone and in combination are totally unlike any other person's. Like our fingerprints, each line is conventional, but the pattern is unique. Developing individuality is a difficult task as we have no experience to follow. There are guidelines in the books written by those who have traveled the path before us. But they can only tell of that individual's experience, not ours. So each of us starts out in his or her own uncharted ocean. It is a lonely voyage as uniqueness means none of us will be exactly like another. We can find compatible companions but not total togetherness, which is no longer individuality. A compatible companion gives the security of standing beside you and sharing, not the identical gluing and smothering of togetherness. The norms of any society tend to evolve and change. Women today have several new norms to live up to such as being active in sex and competitive in work. Female liberation emphasizes one's own choice, one's own identity thus enhancing personal mental and emotional health.

But to many women, sexual liberation means the pressure, not the freedom, to be active, even aggressive, in sex, taking the active positions in sexual relations, having multiple orgasms. This new norm mistakenly says that since science has demonstrated that women are sexual beings with more constant sexual desire and response than men, they should take over the active role in sex to be truly female and allow the male to change his role and be the passive recipient. Is this perhaps not the same old pressure of conforming to a male expectation, a male fantasy of the woman who always wants him sexually? Sex is at best a sharing, a partnership, in which each partner does what comes naturally, responding to desires and inner urges, not simply pleasing the other. Sex is a desire, an urge, an appetite to be satisfied. We do not eat to please our dinner partner; he or she can derive pleasure from seeing us enjoy. Sex is a similar body drive.

Most of us have been taught not to even stroke our body, not to feel a sensual pleasure in its softness and warmth, much less to produce genital pleasure. As we attempt to learn, we feel self-centered and narcissistic. But we cannot truly feel pleasure in another's body until we have first learned to like our own. Learn to like your own body in any way you can. Any movement that gives you pleasure will help. Try belly dancing, not to be the favorite in a harem, but for exercise, and because moving and accentuating separate parts of the body in rhythm provides a very sensual experience. Depending solely on a man's body for pleasure, women remain forever prisoners of the search for permission from the male. Learning self-pleasure first means we can then share our pleasure with others and blend our mutual pleasures in our bodies and can tell our partners what gives us pleasure so our partner does not have to learn by stumbling, blind trial and error. "Knowing thyself" applies to our bodies, our senses, as well as our minds.

Editor's Note: M. Dorothea Kerr, M.D., is a clinical assistant professor of psychiatry at Cornell University Medical College.

MISCONCEPTIONS

WE ALL HAVE ABOUT OUR PHYSICA HEALTH

By Barbara Coffey

Serious physical illness is rare between the ages of eighteen and thirty-five. This happy fact alone could calm the nerves of the thousands of young people who sit in doctors' offices across the country convinced they have some terrible disease. Dr. Jack Richard, practicing internist and clinical associate professor of medicine at Cornell University Medical College points out that these years can be very stressful and that society generally pressures the young adult to deny this stress, encouraging him or her to think of life as easy and carefree. The young people themselves, often because of a pressured lifestyle, develop health habits that will cause them considerable physical problems now and perhaps more serious ones later on. Understanding just how stress and health habits can affect how well we feel now and later, can help us to get rid of some of the major health misconceptions many of us have. Let's take a look at some of them.

1. Young people don't suffer from stress

Dr. Richard ranks stress as number one in sending young people to their doctor with physical symptoms. This doesn't mean that the physical symptoms or illnesses are not real, but that emotional stress may well be contributing to the problem, as with migraine headaches or peptic ulcers. Recognition of the stress factor as part of the physical problems won't make them go away automatically, but it can relieve the disturbing misconception many young people have that something is terribly wrong with them. Such anxiety cannot only aggravate the physical condition, but in some cases can keep people from seeking the treatment that could help. After having passed through the emotional traumas of adolescence, young adults

have to face the pressures of college and a first job, perhaps adjustment to marriage, children or coping with city life and the singles scene— all highly stressful situations that work in a number of ways against their health.

2. Malnutrition exists only among the poor

One unnecessary physical stress we put on our body stems from a common nutritional misconception. Dr. Richard feels that poor nutrition is second only to stress in causing physical problems in young women. The misconception so many of us have is that living in a country of plentiful food, nutritional deficiencies don't exist. We tend to think of malnutrition as some shadowy condition that exists only in overpopulated, poorly fed areas of the world. Severe malnutrition is indeed rare in this country, but mild malnutrition, or "snack malnutrition" as it is sometimes called, causes thousands of young women to experience illnesses they could avoid.

Dr. Erwin Di Cyan in his book *Vitamins in Your Life* makes the point that many Americans don't get enough vitamin A. One reason may be that some of the foods richest in vitamin A are fattening (cream and other rich dairy products, sweet potatoes) or disliked (liver and spinach). Vitamin C is another one a surprising number of people don't get enough of, perhaps because of their lifestyle, says Dr. Richard. A young secretary, for example, probably grabs coffee and

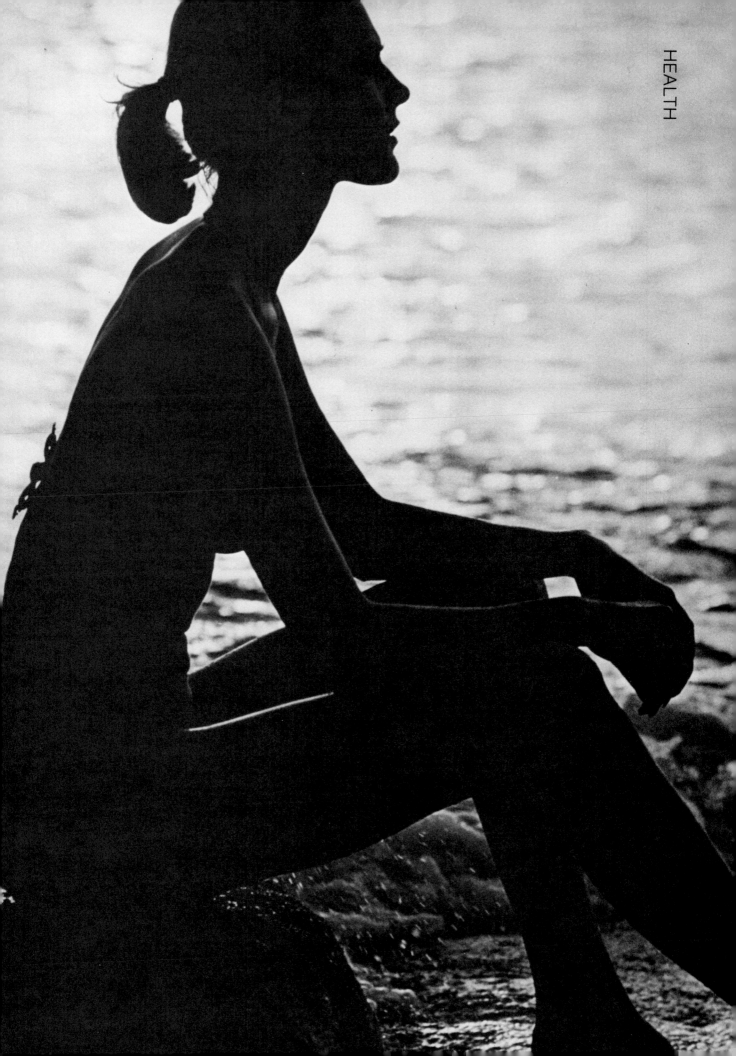

a sweet roll in a local coffee shop on the way to work or eats the same thing at her desk. Lunch is usually a sandwich, and supper, if she isn't going out, is whatever she can throw together. This not only shortchanges her on vitamins, it puts her into a high carbohydrate and high-fat eating pattern that can cause her to be overweight even though she may not actually be eating that much. Too many of us just don't take the time to open that can of orange juice in the morning to get some vitamin C, nor do we usually take the trouble to eat a nonfattening source of vitamin A in a daily portion of eggs, carrots or green leafy vegetables.

The fact that so many women are taking birth control pills also enters into the vitamin picture. There is strong evidence that the pills can produce a shortage of folacin, one of the B vitamins, and many doctors prescribe supplements of this vitamin for their patients on the pill.

Most doctors agree that it's unwise to take vitamins *in place of food.* Food, after all, is our body's natural fuel, and we function best when our nutrition comes from natural sources. But if you can't or won't eat correctly, it's certainly better to get what your body needs through vitamin supplements prescribed by a doctor than not to get the vitamins at all.

Another commonly held food misconception is that malnutrition means only vitamin deficiencies. It includes mineral deficiencies, particularly those of iron and calcium. The best source of iron is meat, and the young woman who eats primarily high carbohydrate and high-fat snack foods may not be replacing the iron she loses every month through menstruation. As a consequence, iron-deficiency anemia, with its chronic fatigue, is one of the most common problems of young women. Poor calcium intake, as it occurs in one who takes little milk or milk products, produces no immediate effects. It may, however, show up years later in the form of weak and brittle bones, which constitute a major problem in women after menopause.

3. Snack syndrome misconception

Dr. Richard points out still another way people are likely to shortchange themselves nutritionally. A busy schedule combined with living alone or with a roommate on a different schedule usually results in skipped meals. If we work late one night or have a drink after work with a friend, we're much more likely to grab a quick snack or just curl up in front of the TV and forget about eating entirely. Another night we might go out and eat an enormous meal at a restaurant. The combination of eating very little or nothing at all, then stuffing the body, is very hard on it. This kind of erratic eating pattern combined with the sweet roll/sandwich syndrome sends many women to their doctors complaining of gastrointestinal problems, bowel disorders, spastic colon and constipation. This type of eating pattern also contributes

to weight problems, both overweight and underweight, which in turn are among the most common causes of menstrual disorders.

4. VD misconceptions

We are living in the midst of a VD epidemic, according to the New York City Department of Health along with most other authorities. One reason for the epidemic proportions of venereal disease is the number of misconceptions we have about it—that treatment of VD is painful and complicated, for example, and if you go for treatment, the whole world will know your secret. Actually, venereal disease responds quickly to simple antibiotic treatment, either shots, penicillin or antibiotic pills. Most private doctors will almost always honor a patient's desire for privacy and not disclose the problem to parents. Major cities also have free or inexpensive VD clinics where a person can be treated with the guarantee of privacy.

Still another misconception that helps VD spread is the number of women who feel that if they have something as bad as gonorrhea, they'll surely know about it. From 50 to 80 percent of the women affected with gonorrhea don't have symptoms in the early stages. A male usually does and should tell any woman he's had relations with of the condition so she can go for treatment.

Another misconception that can keep women feeling uncomfortable and can also tug away at a sense of well-being is the fear that *all* gynecological infections are venereal and therefore shameful and threatening. Actually women can have all kinds of nonvenereal infections, the most common one being an infection called Candida albicans or monilia. It isn't serious, but the itching and burning symptoms and the discharge, which has the look and consistency of cottage cheese, are very annoying and uncomfortable. This infection is seen quite frequently now because birth control pills make many women more susceptible. Taking antibiotics for other unrelated illnesses also increases the chances of becoming infected with Candida because the antibiotics kill many of the body's bacteria, including the protective ones in the vagina, which usually keep the Candida from growing. This infection responds quickly to a painless treatment, so no one should hesitate to go to a doctor if she suspects she has it.

Another common vaginal infection is called trichomoniasis. It's an amoeba infection and it's transmitted through sexual intercourse, though it can also be caught from contaminated laundry or toilets. Symptoms usually are itching and a thin, yellowish discharge. The condition responds quickly to drugs, and usually both the woman and her sexual partner must be treated so they won't continue to pass the infection between them.

A Pap smear is a routine, painless gynecological office procedure in which cells are collected from the cervix and prepared on a slide for microscopic examination. Many young women are under the false impression that this smear is *only* for cancer detection and necessary just for "older" women. Although the main purpose of the smear is for early cancer detection, it can provide the doctor with other valuable information, such as whether a woman is ovulating—very important if she is having trouble becoming pregnant—or whether any infection like trichomoniasis is present. Also, cancer of the cervix can occur in young women and most gynecologists feel that a woman should have an annual Pap smear as soon as she begins seeing a gynecologist.

5. One of the most common youth diseases— mononucleosis

Probably one of the most common youth diseases is mononucleosis or the "kissing disease" as it is sometimes referred to. Classic symptoms are sore throat, headache, swollen glands and a feeling of constant fatigue. There are some prevalent misconceptions related to "mono." First, it isn't really a kissing disease. This idea got started because of a study done on West Point cadets. School doctors noticed that in January, following the Christmas vacation when the cadets went home and had contact with females after a rather celibate academic semester, many cases of mono were reported. Studies show, however, that mono, though it is an infectious disease, is not highly contagious.

Another mono misconception is the idea that anyone suffering from it has to go to bed for months of rest. Dr. Richard points out that often the reason for prolonged bed rest is not physical, but mental. For emotional reasons the patient may want to take to his or her bed. Some period of rest is necessary, but it's not usually so long that it throws one's life out of kilter.

6. The currently fashionable disease—hypoglycemia

A currently fashionable disease with an aura of misconception surrounding it is hypoglycemia, or low blood sugar. There is usually a strong emotional component to this disease, too, and it has replaced the vapors, fainting spells and low blood pressure as an explanation for what is frequently an emotionally caused problem. True hypoglycemia is rare and is often the forerunner of diabetes; therefore, it is seen usually in people with a family history of this disease. Real cases of the disease can be successfully treated by reducing the starch and sugar content of the individual's diet. Getting to the root of the emotional stress causing the hypoglycemic-like symptoms—anxiety, dizziness, palpitations, sweating—will most often cause the symptoms to disappear, indicating that the patient was not a true hypoglycemic, but simply suffering from a stress syndrome.

7. Smoking only causes problems late in life

"I'm young, it's okay if I smoke now," or "I can always quit smoking later if it bothers my health" are two misconceptions that play havoc with the respiratory system. Even at eighteen, heavy smoking can cause problems. A person who smokes, gets a cold, gets over it, then coughs for weeks afterward should stop smoking and he or she will stop coughing. Persistent coughing long after a cold's symptoms are gone is a pattern that frequently ends in chronic bronchitis, which could become chronic a lot sooner than we think with continued smoking. The more long-range aspects of heavy smoking are probably already familiar to everyone.

8. Getting wet and chilled causes colds

Sitting in a draft, wet feet or an air conditioner blowing on your neck can all give us a cold—right? Wrong. The only way we catch a cold is to get one directly from someone who has one. And colds are very contagious. A British medical group did a special cold-catching study demonstrating that wet feet, drafts and the like did not affect the severity or the duration of a cold nor did these things have anything to do with catching a cold in the first place. A cold is contagious for a day or so before symptoms develop and then for a couple of days afterward, so actually when a cold is at its runniest and sloppiest, and when everyone is avoiding its owner, it is probably not contagious.

9. Who does and doesn't need an annual check-up?

Not so much an area of misconception as one of differing opinions, the annual check-up is something much discussed among doctors and young women alike. Many women worry that their doctors will think they're hypochondriacs if they come for a check-up, and although some doctors say it really isn't necessary especially under thirty, no one will think a woman is being hypochondriacal if she feels better having a check done once a year. All doctors feel, however, that we should be aware of our heredity when we plan a check-up schedule. For example, diseases like diabetes, heart disease, breast cancer (if an immediate female member of the family has had it) all have high heredity quotient. If any of these ailments runs in the family, a woman should tell her doctor and have the appropriate tests when she is having her regular routine medical check.

10. The square's misconception

The final, most serious misconception we can have about our health is that as a young adult it's square to take it seriously. Getting into good health patterns will not only pay off now, it will pay off throughout life, even lengthening it.

An update of current medical opinion

By Ellen Switzer

Before nineteen-year-old Judy S. left home for her sophomore year in college, she asked her family doctor for birth control advice. She was surprised when he suggested the method her mother and grandmother had used: a diaphragm with contraceptive jelly. Was he just old-fashioned? Should she seek the opinion of a specialist who might be more familiar with the newer forms of birth control?

Susan J. is married, twenty-four years old, and would like to work for at least two more years before starting a family. The birth control pills she has been using, besides providing contraception, have evidently controlled the heavy bleeding and the menstrual cramps she used to have during her periods. But a rise in her blood pressure has caused her physician to suggest discontinuing the pills. An IUD (intra-uterine device) would present too much likelihood of a return of the bleeding and cramps. Her doctor has suggested a diaphragm with contraceptive jelly or cream for her and/or condoms for her husband. Susan has always thought that those methods were little better than nothing at all. Her doctor assured her that new statistics show that the older methods, if properly used, are almost as effective as the IUD. If she were to use a diaphragm, and at the same time, her husband used a condom, the protection against conception would rival the pill's. Is he right?

Cases such as Judy's and Susan's were discussed recently in Miami Beach by more than 350 family-planning specialists at seminars sponsored by the American Association of Planned Parenthood Physicians.

One of the strongest and most surprising impressions that emerged from the meeting was the renewed emphasis being placed on the barrier methods of contraception—diaphragms with contraceptive jelly or cream, condoms, and foams. Judy's doctor was definitely not old-fashioned—he was right in the mainstream of current thinking about birth control.

"Two years ago, students in a master's semi-

nar at a well-known school of public health asked me to show them a diaphragm. They had never seen one," a director of a college health service told a colleague. "This year I have been prescribing diaphragms almost as frequently as pills." The reasons for this apparent return to old methods are logical. They have no serious side effects and are more reliable when used consistently than earlier statistics indicated.

Dr. Louise Tyrer, vice president for medical affairs of the Planned Parenthood Federation of America, said that diaphragms, foams and condoms—with a method failure rate of 2 to 4 percent per woman per year—may, with consistent use, be as effective as the mini-pill (the least frequently prescribed oral contraceptive) and IUD's. The fact that has given the barrier methods a bad name is what experts refer to as "user failures." One physician called it "the bureau-drawer syndrome." "It's sometimes easy to forget to use an intercourse-connected device," he said, "and when it's in the bureau drawer, it's obviously not going to prevent pregnancy."

A recently concluded two-year study published by the medical journal *Family Planning Perspectives,* found only 2 percent of the diaphragm users in the study to have had unwanted pregnancies. Of the thirty-seven users who became pregnant, twenty-two reported that they had "used the diaphragm inconsistently, or not at all."

The experts at the Miami Beach seminar pointed out another advantage of barrier methods. They emphasized repeatedly that a patient taking oral contraceptives must be examined regularly and must have medical help available should undesirable side effects occur. The same is true for IUD users. And the IUD is more likely to be expelled or cause problems in a woman who has never borne a child.

Dr. Tyrer had several suggestions to insure the problem-free use of the diaphragm. Even if your device comes with an inserter, learn to put it in by hand; by so doing you can make sure the device is correctly in place, covering the cervix. If you have either gained or lost a lot of weight or had a baby, have your doctor refit you. Your size may have changed.

Oral contraceptives

The amount of estrogen in the pill (the ingredient that causes almost all the undesirable side effects) has been lowered steadily and has now reached the lowest level at which the medication can still be considered effective.

The so-called "sequential" pill (estrogen throughout the cycle with progestin added for the last few days) has been removed from the market by the Food and Drug Administration, because it seemed to produce more problems than the combined estrogen-progestin pill.

A very rare pill-connected complication, not previously noted, is the appearance of benign liver tumors. Therefore, no woman who has any liver disease should take birth control pills. A woman who has contracted hepatitis should discontinue pill use until after she has recovered, and liver function tests have determined that the liver is not permanently damaged. Women with enlarged or tender livers, or mononucleosis, should also stop using the pill until their physicians give them a clean bill of health. (Very recent research has shown that pill takers over thirty who are also heavy smokers have a greater risk of coronary problems than nonsmoking or very light smoking pill takers. Pill users over forty who are also heavy smokers have a *substantially* greater risk of coronary problems, so much so, that researchers concluded it was unadvisable for such women to take the pill.)

IUD's

A new copper IUD, the Copper-T, was approved for general use in November, 1976, but is not yet available. In clinical trials, the device has proved to be safe and effective, and, according to Dr. Tyrer, its shape is not so easily expelled as other shapes. The device is small and is considered especially useful for women who have never had a child or for those who have suffered from cramps and heavy bleeding with other IUD's but still want to use this form of contraception. The Copper-7 IUD and the Progestasert, which are available, have similar advantages. [The Progestasert contains a time-released supply of the hormone progesterone, which gives it added contraception effectiveness. Progesterone has not been connected with side effects in birth control pills.]

Sterilization

Sterilization procedures for women are becoming simpler. The so-called mini-laparotomy (which involves a tiny incision in the lower abdomen) is being used by more and more physicians.

The number of vasectomies is increasing. Complications that were feared several years ago (arthritis was one) have not occurred. The physicians who reported these difficulties eventually reported that there was no correlation between the problem and the operation.

Reversible sterilization operations for women who have had tubal ligations, as well as for men who have undergone vasectomies, were

also discussed. Such reversal operations have occasionally been performed successfully, and new techniques of microscopic surgery make the outlook brighter. But good results are still rare, according to Dr. Joseph E. Davis, chairman of the Department of Urology at New York Medical College. "My advice to the patient who is not completely sure that he or she will never, under any circumstances, want another child, is to not have surgery," Dr. Davis says.

Abortion

The number of abortions in the United States is increasing. In New York City last year, there were almost as many legal abortions as live births. The vast majority of women seeking abortions come for this procedure very early in their pregnancies, often before they have missed a second menstrual period. Almost all such procedures are done by the suction method, in outpatient settings and with local anesthesia. Serious physical problems are very rare.

Second-trimester (over twelve and through twenty-four weeks) abortions are relatively rare and present more risk. Such abortions are done in hospitals, usually using the so-called salting-out method. This is done by introducing a saline solution through the abdomen into the uterus, which starts contractions that expel the fetus. A few medical school-affiliated hospitals and clinics have done second-trimester abortions using a form of suction, a method that, performed by experts, seems to result in few complications and is preferred by many patients.

What does it all add up to? There are still no perfectly safe, failure-proof, side-effect-free contraceptive methods. The pill is not for everyone, and all other methods, including even sterilization, fail occasionally. Abortion is obviously not a contraceptive method of choice, but for those who do not object to it on ethical grounds, it can be a safe, effective backup to the barrier methods.

If there is no revolutionary birth control method in the scientific pipeline yet, the available options continue to be effective, safe and acceptable.

Editor's Note: Ellen Switzer is a freelance author who writes frequently on law and medicine. Her latest book is The Law for a Woman.* *She is also the author of* There Ought to Be a Law.†

* Ellen Switzer, and Wendy W. Susco, *The Law for a Woman,* Charles Scribner's Sons, New York, 1975.
† Ellen Switzer, *There Ought to Be a Law: How Laws Are Made and Work,* Atheneum Publishers, New York, 1972.

WHICH WAY DO WANT TO HAVE

You have choices you didn't have before

By Wenda Wardell Morrone

My husband and I panted and puffed and blew our way through labor; we chanted and pushed, and then suddenly our son was there, a tiny slippery, raw mirror of his father. John was the second person to hold him. It was to both of us a tough, incomparable moment.

That was in 1970—a year, says Mrs. Ruth Watson Lubic, general director of the Maternity Center Association in New York City, that marked a shift in the attitude of couples toward their childbirth experience. Before that her agency received only a few letters each year asking wistfully, in effect, wouldn't it be nice if one could deliver at home, if various disadvantages of hospital births could be avoided.

Beginning in 1970 the letters increased and the tone changed; there was now a growing antipathy to hospitals. A labor like ours, directed and controlled by hospital and doctor, ceased to be regarded as a technological, human miracle; couples had become aware that leaving so much control in the hands of others meant having little real choice about the use of drugs or in-hospital procedures such as episiotomies. They began actively to seek other choices.

In the intervening eight years, every part of the so-called normal hospital childbirth has been questioned, from routines such as induced labor and separating infant and mother after birth, to the treatment of babies at birth, to the fundamental questioning of the role of both hospital and doctor. There have been many changes. Instead of the basic choices my husband and I faced of knocked-out/conscious, alone/together, couples can now pick from several kinds of deliver-ers, delivery settings and methods of controlling labor.

The change most closely tied in to the normal hospital routine is probably that of the midwifery service in Roosevelt Hospital in New York City. A group of five midwives conducts a private practice under the sheltering wing of the obstetrical service there. (Lay midwives are illegal in many states; formally trained midwives are R.N.'s with one to three years' additional specialized training. There are sixteen schools with nurse-midwivery programs and 1200 nurse–midwives coast to coast. They have become legal in almost all states, largely within the past five years.)

Nurse-midwives have been part of hospital clinics for some time, sharing examinations and deliveries with interns and established obstetricians. Now, at Roosevelt, the midwives as a group have their own patients, whom they follow similarly to an obstetrician, from initial visit through delivery, if pregnancy and delivery are normal. (Caesareans, for example, require a backup obstetrician, never more than a corridor away.)

The women choosing the service are, by and large, middle-class. "They are well educated, well informed. They have read the current literature and they know what they want," says Barbara Brennan, the nurse-midwife who heads the service. "You cannot tell them what to do. But if you explain what might happen, and what you might have to do if it does, then I find that they will trust you to do it." Patients have included doctors' wives, doctors, nurses; for most, it is the first pregnancy.

This is also a fair description of the women who have come to the Childbearing Center in New York City. Like Roosevelt, the Center has a staff of midwives, backed up by obstetricians, but there is one very big difference: the setting. The Childbearing Center is in a large, former private home that also houses the Maternity Center Association, sponsor of the Center. It is eleven minutes by ambulance from its main backup hospital.

Labor can be spent walking in a room or garden; one can time contractions in a neighborhood coffee shop (no food is allowed) or while making instant coffee in the Center's kitchenette. The father is, of course, present, and siblings are welcome to visit. Delivery is in a regular bed with a wide mattress in a gaily painted room. After a normal birth, the baby is examined by a pediatrician, and *twelve hours* later the family goes home. Because of this part of the program, women are not accepted for it un-

YOU (AND HE) YOUR BABY?

less the Center is assured that some support person (e.g., husband/mother) will be with the new mother and baby for at least a week after birth; the support person is encouraged to attend the classes that the Center gives throughout pregnancy.

A major aim of the program is to provide an alternative not to people who would ordinarily seek hospitals, but to those who would otherwise give birth at home. The home setting is possible because, while a hospital must accept all patients, the Childbearing Center can—and does—set rigorous criteria for "normalcy" and can at any point in pregnancy or labor transfer a patient who has become too high a risk to a hospital. (The responsibility for a hospital to accept all patients is also the reason that almost any alternative to regular hospital procedure will have better childbirth statistics: the problem cases ended up in hospitals.)

Dr. Thomas Dillon, head of obstetrics at Roosevelt, feels that midwifery programs may continue to be confined to large urban areas where there are enough potential patients, and where doctors are more open to new approaches. And yet in a small town in Pennsylvania, Dr. William Hazlett has for over fifteen years combined many of the features of these two programs and carried them a step further: Dr. Hazlett encourages fathers to deliver their own babies, and couples come to him from all over the Northeast for this reason.

Studies have shown that this participation by the fathers allows a special bonding process similar to that theorized between mother and newborn. Mrs. Eleanor Mullen, Dr. Hazlett's assistant, says that parents feel there is a special tie created from infancy on between a father and the baby he has delivered. What are causes célèbres elsewhere have been business as usual here for over a decade. And unlike Roosevelt Hospital or the Childbearing Center, Dr. Hazlett does not see his policies as examples to be emulated by others, nor himself as a missionary: "Until all the recent publicity, I thought this would all die with me."

Even within traditional hospitals there are changes in childbirth procedures. Enemas and episiotomies and pubic shaving are no longer routine in many hospitals. There is now an alternative to the Lamaze breathing techniques. Developed by a Denver obstetrician, Dr. Robert Bradley, it is based instead on recognizing and relaxing muscle tension to combat pain.

Beyond the hospital changes, there has also been a surge in home births, and with them a growth in the number of lay midwives. (Formally trained nurse-midwives do not, as a rule, deliver babies at home.) Lay midwives are largely self-taught. Sometimes they operate in loosely formed groups, thus adding to one another's knowledge. A midwife's reputation is by word of mouth; a woman seeking home birth has no concrete way of evaluating a midwife's skill or experience, except for the trust that may or may not be built up during the pregnancy.

Giving birth at home is a hard phenomenon to track, since it goes on outside the medical establishment. Doctors and clinics may refuse prenatal care to a woman who wants to deliver at home; it may even be difficult to register the birth of her child. And since lay midwives are illegal in many states, their patients tend to be very protective. But some facts have surfaced. California is generally believed to lead the trend. In a 1974 study of three hundred home births in California, we get a picture of the couples involved. While home births may have begun among the flower children, they haven't stayed there; only 10 percent of the study families could be considered "counterculture." The other 90 percent were statistically no different from the couples enrolled in any prepared childbirth course; they had college educations, cars, televisions, often their own homes. The medical establishment, dubious about such carefully planned nonhospitals as the Childbearing Center, violently rejects the concept of home births. Comments on those who seek home births range from "the category of the absolutely dumb" to "placing both mother and infant in abject jeopardy."

Several things are consistent throughout all the alternative approaches to childbirth. The least complicated, perhaps, is the cost. A normal pregnancy and delivery costs between $1000 and $2000, of which only a few hundred dollars is paid by medical insurance. (Childbirth is an "elective" procedure.) In contrast, the Roosevelt Hospital midwifery program costs $459, and the Childbearing Center, $575. A home birth costs even less; and many lay midwives are paid in groceries, or charge nothing. The lower price is tied to the concept of "normal." The Childbearing Center is in a building separate from a hospital, in part, says Mrs. Lubic, to see just how much a normal childbirth costs, a figure impossible to determine within a hospital, where each patient pays her share of the equipment overhead even if she does not have to use any of it.

The second consistency throughout these alternatives is the move away from doctors, toward almost anybody else. The most obvious example of this is in the supervision of a patient's labor. John and I were supervised largely by a revolving door of nurses who were strangers to us; our babies were delivered by doctors who sprinted into the delivery room and who had little time after the births to stay and share our high. It was what we expected; perhaps, in some ways, it made our experience very much our own. But when I contrast it to spending the same hours with one's husband, and also with women that one had come to know and trust over months of supervision and advice and care, I allow myself to remember, for the first time, some of the fear I felt behind my exhilaration.

Setting aside the labor, the management of pregnancy is different in a midwife's care. "I think women find it easier to ask questions of a midwife and to say what they want," says Barbara Brennan. "I think it helps them to think of pregnancy as a normal procedure."

Dr. Dillon of Roosevelt and Mrs. Lubic see their programs as prototypes of new kinds of medical service, where people can have only the care that they need; they don't claim—and don't want—to be able to handle problems that require advanced hospital procedures; they are only interested in helping women who have had normal pregnancies to give birth normally to normal babies. The major question appears to be What is a normal childbirth?

Proponents of each method define normal by different criteria. Obviously, those obstetrical services predicting a 50 percent Caesarean rate by the year 2000, think that normal is not, in fact, all that normal. Dr. Dillon, on the basis of two years of statistics, says that the midwives have found that normal can turn into abnormal too quickly; the facilities of a hospital are essential. Mrs. Lubic feels that by careful screening throughout pregnancy and labor, the abnormal rarely takes one by surprise and the short distance to the hospital is no threat. According to some lay midwives, "normal" does not include a guarantee of the baby's survival.

Normal/abnormal, acceptable/unacceptable risk: Where do you draw the line? A problem with defining "acceptable risk" is that normal birth has not been studied extensively. The forces that trigger labor, for example, are not fully understood, nor are the effects of maternal emotions on the fetus. In one study, pregnant monkeys were given blood tests at irregular intervals throughout their pregnancies. Nothing else was done to them, yet the rate of stillbirths was a full 15 percent greater than that of a control group. It's tempting to theorize that the labor heavily monitored and surrounded by technology may itself contribute to the fetal distress it is designed to treat. Homelike settings and midwives may contribute to normal labors. We don't know. The programs such as those at Roosevelt or the Childbearing Center are providing research as well as warm experiences.

One of the most important aspects of changes in approach to childbirth is surely that of the attitude of the parents. When I was newly pregnant, I was primarily thinking about not having a miscarriage; we took lessons in childbirth because my doctor asked, midpregnancy, if we were interested. Now many couples know what they want before they are even seen by a doctor or midwife; all the programs encourage—and sometimes receive—calls from couples as much as a year before they are pregnant. Such pregnancies are planned in every sense of the word.

This change in attitude has both good aspects and disturbing ones. On the plus side, being informed and planning ahead automatically means that a couple is taking more responsibility for the mother's and baby's care. To enroll in one of these programs, many couples, for example, have had to argue down protests of their families. These couples ask questions, the doctors and midwives involved with them agree; they don't accept routine answers. "They don't accept *any* routine," says midwife Brennan. "They will accept an enema, for example, if you explain why it is necessary in their case and what the effect will be, but they won't accept it as routine."

This increased responsibility is an essential part of the program at the Childbearing Center, planned and built into it. "If somebody were to ask me for the one goal we have," says Mrs. Lubic, "it is to provide families with the confidence that they can bring forth and rear a child."

The whole issue of responsibility/dependence/trust is central to the debate about childbirth, and it is a complicated issue. Some doctors are delighted when a patient takes responsibility. Dr. Hazlett will often take a chance on avoiding an episiotomy if the patient will share that responsibility. "Sometimes it turns out that she is right, sometimes there's a big tear. But that we decide it together—I like that," he says. But not all doctors do. "Dependency is a problem for a lot of providers," says Mrs. Lubic. And the bottom line is trust. The old doctor-as-God approach had as its base the well-meaning intent that it would be easier for a woman to "trust" her physician if she left everything up to him. The new feeling is that the more a couple knows and is allowed on what Mrs. Lubic calls "the decision-making team," the more the couple will trust that the care given is precisely the care needed.

But this changing attitude on the part of couples has its dark side, too. Pubic shaving, enemas, episiotomies, birth positions, circumcisions—all these are challenged. This pressure makes sense up to the point of getting individual and appropriate care. But frequently the concern goes beyond this and becomes what one doctor described as political: a couple wants or refuses a procedure regardless of what anyone says about the needs of their own case.

Perhaps the most important thing offered to us in all these alternative approaches to birth is the restoration of pregnancy as something normal, and I mean "normal" differently from what the professionals mean. It has seemed to me for a long time that the "normal" American woman spent a sensuous singlehood lighting somebody's pipe and then, upon marriage, went into a closet until she was old and unthreatening enough to come out and scrub the yellow wax out of the corners of her kitchen floor. Now pregnancy and childbirth are coming out of the closet. There may be many disagreements about how childbirth should be handled, but there is a fundamental agreement too: babies don't make first appearances wrapped tidily in blankets anymore. We bear them, with great effort and awe and a strength that we might have hesitated, only a few years ago, to call womanly.

ENERGY

Is gray winter weather really responsible for that absolutely yukky, low-energy depression so many of us get about this time of year? Is there some mysterious energizing force in sunlight that's missing in winter? Or is it purely physical; does the cold really take so much out of us that energy resources are depleted? Here are some answers.

New York psychiatrist Dr. Wilbert Sykes says winter blues and that low-energy feeling are primarily psychological. The explanation is different for different people. In childhood some people were probably responsive to their parents' winter depression and "learned" to be depressed too. It's a question of being conditioned by your environment. You expect to be depressed and full of ennui in winter, and every time the calendar registers "winter," you start to feel blah. It's true enough that winter limits your physical activities and shuts out many of the ways you might normally relieve your boredom and frustration—a walk outdoors, a game of tennis, a swim, even the pleasure of a green landscape. But there are many winter substitutes—winter sports, the invigoration of a walk in the snow or even a snowy landscape! Winter doesn't have to be low-energy time unless you make it that way.

Energy and boredom

The feeling of lethargy is so closely linked to boredom that psychologically it can be hard to separate the two. When you're bored, you feel as though you have no energy. There are two well-accepted explanations for boredom, according to Dr. Sykes. The first goes like this: You're consciously or unconsciously in conflict about something, with your energies equally split in two different directions. As a result, you feel bored and exhausted. The second explanation goes this way: You have only so much emotional energy for any task or tasks, and when that's gone you have no more and you feel physically as well as emotionally tired and bored. Both explanations are valid, one sometimes more than the other depending on the situation.

How to get more energy

Most of us have a lot more energy than we use. If we can find a way to release some of our unused energy, there'd be no problem with fatigue or boredom. According to Dr. Sykes, a lack of energy is often a hatrack for "I don't want to do it." You feel too tired to do something because you don't really want to do it.

• Face the fact that you don't want to do a particular thing and you'll frequently find that this

to keep it, especially in winter

admission releases enough energy to get you through the job. You realize you're really tired and that you're going to dislike doing whatever it is just as much later as now, so you may as well get it done now.

• Differentiate among your activities. Understand that the energy you expend cleaning the house isn't related to what you'll use sewing something terrific for yourself or making a meal you'll really enjoy eating. Changing the pace of your activities releases energy for new things.

• Don't keep thinking about conserving your energy. That orients you around fatigue. Think of energy as a muscle—the more you use it, the more you develop it and the better it works.

• Try to take the fears, self-deceptions and inhibitions out of your activities and you'll release the energy you spent in worrying and fussing for something more positive. For example: The young woman who's giving her first big dinner party. She spends hours worrying if the food will be right, the seating arrangements agreeable, whether the guests will enjoy one another. She could ease some of her doubts by convincing herself that she's doing the best job she knows how, then getting on with it. She'll have more positive energy to apply to the task.

Keep your energy level high

• Be in tune with yourself. Discover what makes you feel good or soothes you when you're tired and bored—a walk, a hobby, even pounding your fists in your pillow to release your anger. When you're feeling tired or blue, immediately move into some activity you like. In winter, this is especially important because weather subconsciously contributes to lethargy.

• Don't fall into energy-depleting habits. Eating too much or drinking too much can give you just the excuse you may be looking for. Then you can say, "I'm tired and sleepy because I ate—or drank—too much." Actually it may be just the other way around: you ate or drank too much because you were looking for something tangible to pin your fatigue on.

• Don't live out a "self-fulfilling prophecy." This may sound like psychological double-talk, but actually it just means that if you're feeling depressed and tired, and you give in to the feeling, letting it spill all over by reaching for a dreary dress and skipping a necessary shampoo, you'll find other people reacting to your mood. They'll leave you alone, feeling even more depressed than before. To keep your energy running high, make the extra effort to wear something you like, spend a little more time on your hair. Responses from others will be positive instead of negative and will help you get into a more positive, active mood.

• Remember the importance of a little vacation to renew energy. It doesn't mean you have to shoot your budget for a ticket to the Caribbean, even a weekend trip renews energies.

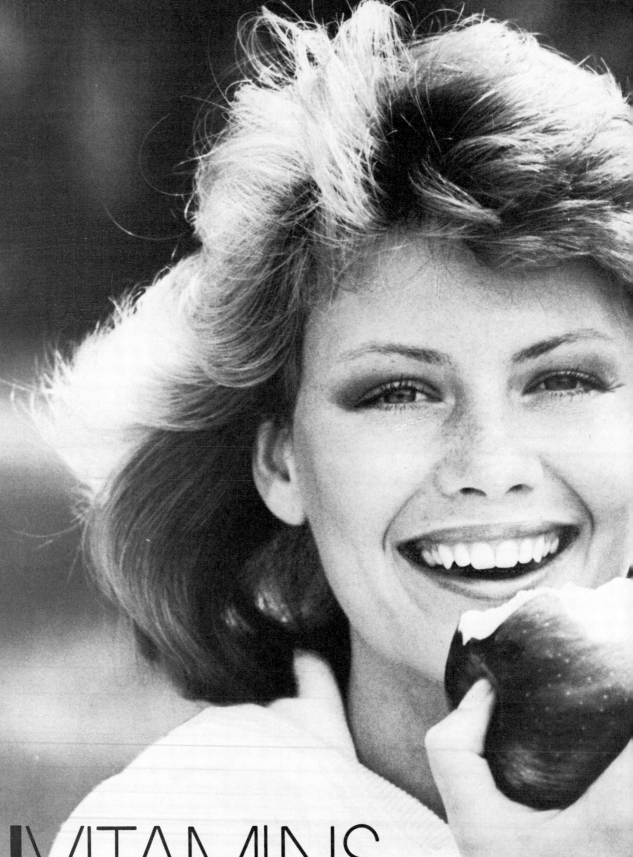

HEALTH

40

VITAMINS
How they affect your health and looks

The fascinating thing about vitamins is that everybody has an opinion about them. Given half a chance, almost everybody will expound a pet theory about how no one needs to swallow vitamin pills if he or she eats right or how vitamin such and such cured their hives, or gave them all kinds of energy and so on and so forth. Even the experts can't seem to agree on what vitamins do beyond certain limits. But there is agreement on the basics, and setting yourself straight on these can give you a much better perspective on what vitamins can and can't do for you.

VITAMIN A

Vitamin A is sometimes called the skin vitamin and though it is essential for the maintenance of healthy hair and skin, it is also important in helping to keep your eyes and the mucous membranes lining the respiratory system and digestive track healthy. Milk, liver, spinach, carrots, broccoli, lettuce, cabbage and tomatoes are all relatively inexpensive foods that supply vitamin A in large amounts. For example, roughly two ounces of beef liver supplies over six times the minimum daily allowance. You might be interested to know that a statistically significant number of North Americans lack appreciable reserves of vitamin A and 20 to 30 percent fail to consume the recommended daily allowance. Vitamin A is also one of the vitamins you can get too much of with resulting toxic effects, so don't prescribe pills for yourself. Eat wisely—it's virtually impossible to get too much through sensible eating.

VITAMIN B

Vitamin B is not a single vitamin but a complex of eight related vitamins frequently referred to as the nerve vitamins because of their effect on the body's nervous system. Actually the B vitamins affect everything from eyes to your thyroid, though their primary effect is usually considered to be on the nervous system. Good sources of most of the B complex vitamins are yeasts, inexpensive cuts of beef, whole grain cereals, liver, fresh leafy green vegetables. Women taking oral contraceptives sometimes are deficient in folacin, one of the B complex vitamins, and because of this, many doctors think this is one instance where supplementary vitamin pills are a good idea. Folacin deficiency is also seen in pregnant women.

VITAMIN C

Vitamin C is said to be the cellular vitamin because it assures the wholeness of the important body-building blocks, the cells and tissues. It is relatively nontoxic and the body usually gets rid of any excess vitamin C through excretion. Your body's need for vitamin C increases under periods of emotional stress, and when the stress is prolonged, supplementary vitamins in the form of pills are sometimes prescribed. Citrus fruits, liver, spinach, tomatoes, broccoli and most vegetables are good sources of vitamin C.

VITAMIN D

This is called the bone vitamin by many doctors and consequently it's extremely important for children to have an adequate supply. Excessive dosages of vitamin D can be toxic to both children and adults, so as with vitamin A, it's important to eat for health rather than dose yourself with pills. Your body makes vitamin D when exposed to sunlight. It's also found in fish liver oils and in foods enriched with it such as milk and some cereals.

VITAMIN E

Vitamin E is primarily an antioxidant, that is, it inhibits or reduces the oxidation of unsaturated fatty acids in the tissues. Contrary to what you may have heard, vitamin E has no proven effect on human fertility or virility. Beef liver, wheat germ, fruits and green leafy vegetables, nuts and mayonnaise are good sources.

YOUR VITAMIN QUESTIONS ANSWERED

These questions represent some of the most frequently asked about vitamins. The answers to some may surprise you because they explode some commonly held vitamin misconceptions.

I hear so much about vitamin A being good for skin. What does it really do?

Vitamin A does affect skin, but if you've been led to believe that swallowing large quantities of it will give you a radiant, glowing complexion, you're in for a disappointment. The most common link between vitamin A and skin is acne treatment. Oral vitamin A is prescribed for acne treatment, especially in cases consisting mostly of severe blackhead formation. But doctors do not agree about how effective this treatment is. It is always combined with other acne treatment and in no way considered to be a "Cure." Tretinoin, vitamin A acid, is frequently applied topically to acne patients giving considerable relief from symptoms, but Tretinoin is a special form of the vitamin, not the same thing you're swallowing in a vitamin pill.

Severe vitamin A deficiencies can manifest themselves in various kinds of skin lesions and rashes but the deficiency may be caused by a metabolic disorder that prevents the body from absorbing vitamin A efficiently. These kinds of problems are rare and a real vitamin deficiency is seldom found in people who have an adequate diet.

Would I be healthier and look better if I took a vitamin pill everyday?

The American Medical Association in its informative booklet "Vitamin Supplements and Their Correct Use," answers this question well: "Vitamins are essential to maintain life. The usual and most reasonable source of vitamins is food. A diet selected from the variety of foods available can supply all the vitamins a person needs. There might be times, however, when supplementation is necessary . . . when a person is unable or unwilling to consume an adequate diet, as during an illness, allergy, or emotional upsets. . . . The physician is trained to determine the most beneficial supplement and also to help the patient remove disturbing factors causing poor eating habits."

What's all the talk about vitamin E and fertility and sexual potency?

In the animal kingdom, vitamin E rightfully enjoys a well-earned reputation for helping to maintain fertility. But people are human. In many laboratory tests, animals deprived of vitamin E became sterile. When vitamin E was reintroduced into their diets, they became fertile again. No one has been able to prove that the same is true in humans. When deprived of vitamin E under laboratory conditions, humans do not become sterile. As for sexual potency, experiments have shown that vitamin E has no effect whatsoever on it.

I keep hearing so much about vitamin E and skin—that it promotes healing, lessens scarring from surgery and so forth. What's the story?

Vitamin E enjoyed a short-lived reputation as a wonder vitamin. But after a great deal of research, most medical authorities say that no need in human nutrition for vitamin E has been established. It does not promote healing nor does it lessen scars. Dr. Robert Auerbach, a New York dermatologist, says that many patients, after hearing about vitamin E's mythical "healing qualities," have treated surgical scars with it. When they return to the office six months later and the scar looks better, they say vitamin E did it. Actually, time did it. Scars tend to fade with time, lose redness and become flatter. If the patients hadn't used the vitamin E, their scars would have improved just the same. And in many cases, patients found that applying vitamin E directly to the skin has caused an irritating contact dermatitis instead of helping the healing.

Does anyone really know whether large doses of vitamin C will help fight off colds?

The only answer to this question is no. The controversy has raged on and off for years. Linus Pauling, the Nobel Prize-winning scientist who started the whole idea of fighting off colds with vitamin C, still believes it's effective. About all you as an individual can do is ask the advice of a doctor who is familiar with your general state of health. The doctor can then best determine the benefit of supplemental vitamin C for you.

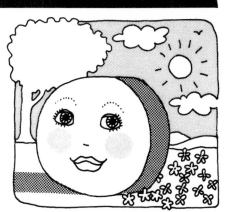

I have a case of severe acne. My doctor prescribed vitamin C as well as A. I understand the A, why the C?

Dermatologists frequently prescribe vitamin C for acne patients who are receiving vitamin A therapy. The vitamin C aids vitamin A absorption. In other words, the C helps make the A more effective. Vitamin C also is helpful in the healing process of some wounds, thus the possibility of it helping to heal acne.

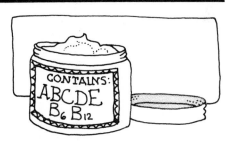

What's the story on the various skin preparations containing vitamins?

Medical authorities say they really don't know the long-term effects of using preparations containing vitamins. They do know that the addition of vitamins to skin creams will not produce any overnight miracles. Some vitamins like A, when applied directly to the skin of animals under laboratory conditions, cause local thickening, but whether this is true in humans and whether the thickening is good or bad is still unknown. Dermatologists definitely warn against "inventing" your own vitamin cosmetics—like opening vitamin capsules and rubbing the contents of vitamin E capsules on skin. Dr. Paul Lazar in Skin and Allergy News talks of the dangers of rubbing the contents of vitamin E capsules on skin. He reports treating at least twenty-five patients with a typical contact dermatitis that resulted from using vitamin E directly on the skin. Dr. Lazar says, "Just because a substance is relatively safe when ingested, doesn't mean it can be applied to the skin." If you want to use a vitamin cream, use one made by a reputable cosmetic manufacturer and wait until it's been on the market long enough for its effectiveness and safety to be known. You don't have to be the guinea pig.

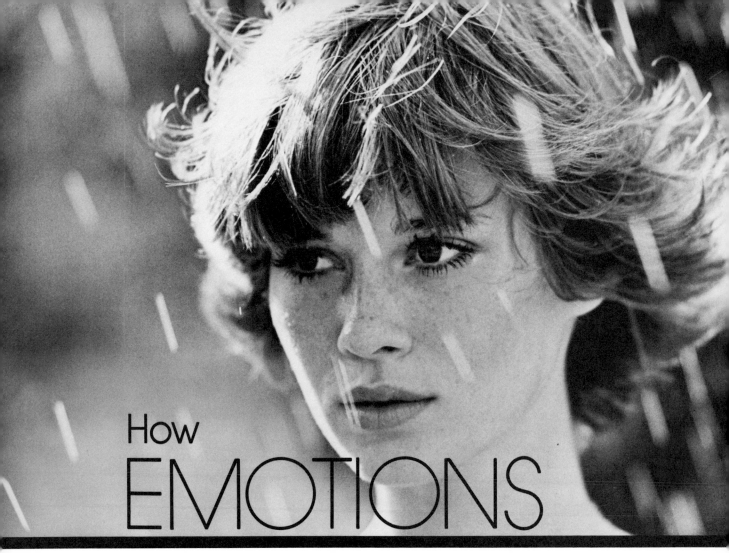

How EMOTIONS
play tricks with your looks

The role of stress and/or anxiety, the major culprit in emotionally caused beauty problems, is something doctors have a lot of suspicions about and very little scientific proof. It is difficult to get that proof because reaction to stress is a highly individual thing. Not everyone gets uptight to the same degree over exams, a sad love affair, a family crisis, death or whatever. And in order to get precise information on how stress affects us, specialists must be able to measure and control the amount of stress, something almost impossible to do in humans. In spite of the difficulties in evaluating the effects of stress, a lot of interesting things are known about how it affects your looks. Understanding how stress works on you can't stop its effects, but it certainly can help you to "roll with the punches" as the saying goes, so that you get back to your normal equilibrium as quickly as possible.

Emotions get expressed in your looks in ways that are familiar to all of us. If you're upset, you might opt to go to bed and escape your worries instead of washing your hair, for example. Next day the fact that your hair is oily just emphasizes the way you feel emotionally. Or, if you're

having a down day, you may not take as much time pulling yourself together in the morning as you usually do, so again, your looks reflect your emotions. The way you stand, sit and move all day can convey your down mood.

And conversely, if you're feeling great, you suddenly find everyone telling you how pretty you look today. These are subtle things that trace the sensitive pattern of your normal day-to-day emotional swings. But there are other less subtle and purely physical manifestations of your emotions. These are the kinds of things that are most likely to show up under high levels of stress and anxiety, maybe even anxieties you aren't aware of, and their effect on your skin and hair can be a problem, especially if the tension is spread out over a period of time.

Skin and lie detector test

Skin has been called "the mirror of your body," "the principal organ of communication between body and environment." Familiar expressions like a "thin-skinned person," "I'm ready to jump out of my skin," "saving your skin," "itching to do something," all point to the close connection between skin and emotions. An even more convincing demonstration of the skin's tie-up with emotions is the common lie detector test. It works in part by measuring the chemical output of the skin caused by the emotional factors of telling a lie.

Behind a blush—shame, anger

One of the most common physical displays of what's going on inside your head emotionally and one that almost everyone has experienced dozens of times is what doctors call an "emotional blush." It's that warm, burning or itching sensation that turns your cheeks a bright red. Some people experience the same thing on the neck and chest instead of the face. The emotions that cause it are usually shame, embarrassment or anger. The most frustrating thing about an emotional blush is that it puts your feelings right out there where everyone can see them. But unfortunately, this can't be helped. You can't control this kind of skin reddening. The parasympathetic and sympathetic nervous systems, not under direct control of the brain, are in charge of this kind of reaction, so all you can do is blush and forget it. The reaction only lasts a minute or so and then vanishes.

Stress and the adrenal gland

More lasting kinds of reactions occur when you are under a lot of tension, which causes your adrenal glands to produce more or less of certain hormones, thus changing the normal hormone balance in your body. This can cause physical changes that are extremely complex. In the skin area, stress seems to bring about an increase in oily secretions in the face and scalp. Stress also causes you to perspire more profusely and the perspiration combines with the oily secretions, emulsifying them. This emulsified oil flows more easily and coats your skin, giving it that familiar oily shine.

When skin breakouts flare up

If stress can cause an increase in oily secretions, it's not hard to take it one step farther and find an increase in breakouts too. Excessive oiliness and breakouts are always partners in crime. Most dermatologists find that when an acne patient reports a particularly bad flare-up, there's a good chance he or she has been under stress recently. It's so predictable, in fact, that dermatologists know there will be an influx of young patients around exam time.

When it comes to breakouts and acne, your own nervous habits frequently get into the picture and make things worse. Unconsciously, you may pick at your face, aggravating the situation further. There is probably little you can do about the situation that's providing the initial stress, but you can help prevent your picking from making matters worse. If your usual acne treatment doesn't seem to be working at this time, you can see a dermatologist too, and let him suggest something more effective. The important thing is not to let the condition build up

to such momentous proportions that this causes you even more anxiety.

Nervous habits complicate skin conditions

Many other skin conditions, like eczema, psoriasis, dermatitis of all kinds, can be made worse by stress. The stress *doesn't cause* the condition in the first place, but once you have it, long periods of tension can make it worse. Dermatologists point out that patients often complicate things by constantly scratching, which only further irritates an already irritated skin and a whole vicious cycle gets going. If you are under a lot of tension, it may be difficult for you to control the scratching. Some scratching, even if you have no skin problems, is a relatively common nervous habit. Asking your doctor to prescribe something to stop the itch and to soothe your skin is a good idea.

Your period and breakouts

One stress manifestation experienced by almost every woman is a change in the menstrual cycle. A missed or delayed period is frequently the result of stress altering your hormone balance. And although you're normally prepared to cope with the increased oiliness and the breakouts that often accompany your period, it may be the straw that breaks the camel's back if it arrives a week later than you thought. The best treatment is to do what you normally do for the oiliness and breakouts and not to worry about the change in your cycle. You'll probably be back to normal next month. If you're not, this is the time to get your doctor's advice.

Emotion and oily scalp

If your skin gets oilier as a result of stress, your scalp and hair will too. More frequent shampooing is the solution. If you suffer from eczema or other skin disorders, they can affect the scalp, too. This requires the help of a competent physician.

Stress and hair loss

The most controversial linkup of stress and hair is in the area of hair loss. Many dermatologists feel there is a direct connection between prolonged anxiety and moderate hair loss. Others are not so sure. Most agree, however, that the hair loss must be programmed into your genetic makeup in the first place. Just how much hair anyone loses in a lifetime is a matter of heredity. If it's in your genes to lose X amount of hair, stress may speed up the loss for a short time, but it probably doesn't cause you to lose any you wouldn't lose later.

Stress can and frequently does aggravate skin or hair conditions you already have or make a latent problem come to the surface. Fortunately, you usually return to normal quickly once the stress is removed. Knowing this can help you relax and you'll have fewer problems.

Millions of women under thirty-five are deeply, often needlessly, concerned about the appearance and health of their breasts. Which of these concerns are reasonable and which are needless are discussed here by a doctor.

Beauty and health guide to your
BREASTS

By Phillip Sarrel, M.D., and Ellen Switzer

- A nineteen-year-old woman whom we shall call Elizabeth is looking in a mirror, comparing her right breast to her left breast. That afternoon she had gone to a department store to buy a new bra. The saleslady had remarked, "You seem to be a size 34A on your right side and a 34B on your left. Of course, we can alter the bra . . . but isn't that a little peculiar?" Elizabeth had noted that her breasts were not the same size ever since she was about fifteen-years-old. She had always thought that her right side would catch up with her left. For several years she hadn't thought much about the problem. But the saleslady's remarks had brought back all her old worries. Was there something wrong with her? Was she just a freak? Was there anything she should do about the situation?

- Joan is also looking at her breasts. She is planning to get married next month and she has observed that her nipples are inverted. She remembers reading in a sex book that one of the ways a man can tell whether his partner has had an orgasm is that her nipples become erect. With inverted nipples, such an erection probably can't occur. Will this make her fiancé doubtful about his and her lovemaking abilities? If she has a baby, will she be able to nurse it? Do inverted nipples mean that there's something wrong with her breasts—for instance, might she have some disease?

- In the waiting room of a gynecologist's office, a twenty-three-year-old woman whom we shall call Pat sits trying to read a magazine. She's clearly terrified and gets more edgy by the minute. Four days ago, as she was examining her breasts, she found a small lump near her nipple. She reported this to her doctor who suggested that she come in for an examination. Pat is convinced that she has cancer.

For medical, psychological and cultural reasons, more young women are concerned about the health, shape and size of their breasts than about any other part of their anatomy. Research conducted by such organizations as the American Cancer Society indicates that women fear breast cancer more than any other disease.

Few women are entirely happy with the way their breasts look. There are some young women, who may look to others perfectly normal, who still worry about their breasts.

Elizabeth, for instance, is needlessly concerned. If she looked at her face, instead of her breasts, she would find that her left profile and her right profile are also not identical. Most human beings are asymmetrical: their right and left sides don't match exactly. This is particularly true of breasts. Elizabeth should either find a bra that stretches to accommodate her uneven cup size, or have the bra altered.

Joan's inverted nipples are a very common condition. There is no statistical evidence that cancer or any other serious breast disease is more common among woman whose nipples turn in instead of out. The information she received from her sex book is incorrect. Nipple erection is one of the *first* indications of sexual arousal, and does not prove that a woman has experienced orgasm.

There is also no reason why inverted nipples should keep Joan from breast-feeding a baby. She may have to put some effort into preparing her breasts during pregnancy, and, if she wishes to nurse, should tell her obstetrician about her plans, who will advise her on what techniques to use to bring up her retracted nipples so that the baby is able to suckle.

Pat, sitting in her doctor's office, shaking with fright, might have saved herself several sleepless nights had she been aware of the fact that breast lumps at her age are exceedingly common and that malignancy is so rare as to be statistically almost unrecordable. Other conditions that cause breast lumps are always quite harmless, and most don't need treatment.

1. Why are young women so much more concerned about the appearance of their breasts than other aspects of their figure?

The answer to this question is not simple; it involves cultural as well as psychological factors. Young girls learn at a very early age that American men regard breasts as the prime sexual symbol. They note that the young woman with prominent and well-shaped breasts is admired. A girl's own breast development occurs at a time in her life when she is most self-conscious—at the beginning of puberty. Puberty usually starts with a growth spurt, and most frequently the spurt is signaled by hands and feet that rapidly increase in size. This may make a young girl feel awkward and slightly embarrassed. Next, hair appears on her body. Breasts start to develop next, and shortly after she begins to round out, she may have her first menstrual period. All these drastic changes occur in a relatively short period of time, ranging from a few months to two years. The girl suddenly has to adjust her body image from that of a child to that of a woman. Of all the changes that occur, breast development is the most noticeable. She can watch herself change from month to month in the mirror. She can also observe in gym classes how her friends are developing. If she feels her breasts are different from those of her age-mates, she may become exceedingly concerned. Since she will rarely discuss her worries with anyone, her self-consciousness about her breasts may remain throughout her life.

2. Once breasts develop, do they look the same throughout the monthly cycle?

Breasts change during the cycle. They may appear larger and fuller just before menstruation. They may also be a little sore. This is owing to increased hormone production during that part of the cycle. Early in the cycle, the ovaries produce increasing amounts of estrogen. After the egg is released, about two weeks before the next period begins, another hormone, progesterone, is added. Both these hormones cause breast changes that result in enlargement, as well as increased sensitivity. This is normal.

3. What are the most common breast abnormalities in women under 35?

Two conditions may cause the breast lumps and irregularities that worry many women; both are nonmalignant, and rarely require treatment. They are cysts and fibroadenoma.

Cysts occur when the liquid that is secreted by glands in the breasts does not drain properly through the breast ducts. A cyst is usually fairly regular in shape (often about the size of a penny or a dime). It is easily movable when palpated. Cysts tend to occur just before menstruation begins and disappear by themselves after bleeding has started. Therefore, a young woman who in examining her breasts finds a small lump late in her cycle might just wait until her period is over and then examine herself again. If the lump is gone, nothing else needs to be done.

Fibroadenomas occur when the fibrous tissue that holds the breast together starts to grow in an abnormal way. They may occur in just one part of one breast, or appear in several spots on both breasts. A woman who has this condition should report it to her physician. Fibroadenomas are also not malignant.

According to Dr. George Crile, Jr., Consultant Emeritus in Surgery at the Cleveland Clinic and an internationally recognized authority on breast diseases, in women *under* thirty, a lump is most frequently diagnosed as a fibroadenoma. In women from thirty to thirty-five, it's apt to be a fluid-filled cyst. Dr. Crile recommends the removal of large cysts by draining them with a needle, under local anesthesia in the physician's office. He feels that entirely too many young women are subjected to needless physical and psychological trauma when cysts are removed through surgery in a hospital.

4. When should a woman start examining her own breasts?

The American Cancer Society recommends self-examination at age sixteen. This does *not* mean that a young woman should start worrying about cancer during adolescence. It simply helps her to become familiar with the feel of her normal breast, and to establish a habit of self-examination.

The best way to examine your breasts is to gently feel them with your fingertips. It sometimes helps to do this in the bathtub, when both breasts are slippery. It is, of course, easier to find lumps in small breasts than in large ones. Women with large breasts should lie down flat with one arm above their head, and examine their breast with the opposite hand. This way, it's easier to feel its outline to the chest wall.

In examining one's breasts, one is looking for any abnormality—anything that was not there the last time a self-examination was done. Breasts change during the menstrual cycle; it's a good idea to do a self-examination at the same time every month.

5. Who is most likely to get breast cancer?

Women over forty-five who come from families where breast cancer has been present in grandmothers, mothers and sisters run the highest risk. There are also some indications that women who are married have a slightly lower breast cancer rate than those who are single, that those who have breast-fed several children also have somewhat fewer breast malignancies than those who have not, and that Caucasian women have more breast cancer than Oriental ones.

6. Is there a way to find breast cancers before they become noticeable lumps in a self-examination?

Yes, there is an X-ray technique called mammography,* which can spot very small tumors before they can be felt. Perhaps the best available method of detecting very early breast cancer is a type of mammography known as xeroradiography. This technique will reveal tiny dots of calcium that are commonly present in breast cancer. When malignancies are this small, they are almost 100 percent curable.

7. What about the common myths about the causes of breast cancer?

Breast cancer is *not* caused by sexual intercourse, venereal disease, blows, bruises or bites, having babies or nursing babies, contact with someone who has cancer, or the use of contraceptive pills (though research is still being done on the latter, no conclusive evidence exists to link the pill with breast cancer).

8. When should a woman go to a physician for an examination?

Most physicians examine breasts as part of a routine annual checkup. If her doctor does not

---

* Editor's note: The American Cancer Society recommends breast X ray, either mammography or xeroradiography, for women fifty or older or for those who have any of a long list of predisposing breast cancer factors. They do not recommend it as a regular procedure for younger women. They do, however, point out that the publicity about the dangers of mammography have made many women forget about the primary benefit of a mammogram—that is, its ability to detect early and curable cancer. The Society urges women not to put off having a mammogram that her doctor feels is necessary for her just because she fears its negative side effects.

examine her breasts, the patient should ask her doctor to do so.

9. How do breasts change during pregnancy, and will they look the same later?

One of the first symptoms of pregnancy is often a slight swelling of the breasts, as well as occasional breast soreness. As the pregnancy progresses, breasts tend to get heavier and the color of the nipples turns from pink to brown. Women who would like to have larger breasts are often delighted with the change. Usually, breasts decrease in size after childbirth, and/or when the mother has stopped nursing. They probably will not have the same shape or size they had prior to the pregnancy.

10. Does breast-feeding improve or hurt the shape of the breasts?

If a mother breast-feeds several children, her breasts may become slightly larger and less firm, which tends to happen as a woman gets older in any case. Whether or not a baby is breast-fed is usually influenced by cultural factors more than by health standards. There is one organization called LaLeche League, that provides excellent information on how to breast-feed successfully, but which also tends to make women who don't wish to nurse feel as if there were something wrong with their maternal instincts. Many women and several physicians have expressed resentment about this attitude.

11. Is there any proof that birth control pills can cause breast cancer?

During Congressional hearings a few years ago, nonmedical witnesses cited studies that indicated that rats who had been fed huge amounts of estrogen over a long period of time developed breast malignancies. The amount given was twenty times larger than that in any oral contraceptive. What's more, animal experiments do not necessarily apply to humans. *There is no conclusive evidence that oral contraceptives have caused breast cancer in women.*

Formerly, physicians usually changed a woman who had a tendency to develop breast cysts or fibroid growths from oral contraceptives to some other forms of birth control. Now some feel on the basis of recent studies that this is not necessary. Actually, there is even more evidence that oral contraceptives may prevent the formation of the nonmalignant cysts, if these are caused by an uninterrupted flow of her own natural estrogen into her bloodstream. Women who have very irregular periods sometimes don't secrete any progesterone; as a result the secretion of estrogen without progesterone can lead to breast lumps.

Birth control pills may regulate menstruation, since most pills contain both estrogen and progesterone, so they tend to cure rather than exacerbate this problem.

12. Is not wearing a bra harmful?

Going braless is probably not a health hazard, unless a woman's breasts are very heavy. In that case she may develop a posture problem, or her shoulder muscles and tendons may become overstretched. However, any woman can probably preserve the shape of her breasts better if she uses some support, unless she is almost flat-chested. If one looks at pictures of women in primitive tribes who have never heard of a bra, one can't help noticing that the breasts of these women sag, often almost to their waist, by the time they reach early middle age. A member of a university medical faculty and his wife (who is over sixty) recently visited such a tribe. The women flocked around the wife to touch her firm, well-shaped breasts, apparently trying to convince themselves that what they were seeing was actually her natural endowment, and not some kind of artificial padding.

13. What are necessary and sensible precautions a young woman should take to insure the health and attractiveness of her breasts?

As we have emphasized throughout this article, breast cancer is exceedingly rare among young women under thirty. However, self-examination of the breasts once a month (preferably at the same time every month, usually after a menstrual period) is a good precaution. Lumps that don't disappear within a few days should be reported to a physician. Mammography may be recommended to women after a certain age who have a genetic history of breast disease.

Women concerned about breasts that are heavy or that tend to sag should keep their weight normal since heavy breasts sag earlier. A well-fitting bra will help maintain shape and comfort.

A young woman who finds that she is obsessed by concerns about her breasts, even though they have been found perfectly normal by her physician, may have an emotional problem and might consider professional psychological counseling.

Editor's note: Dr. Phillip Sarrel is an associate professor of gynecology and obstetrics at Yale University School of Medicine. Ellen Switzer, author of There Ought to Be a Law, *and* The Law for a Woman *is a free lance writer specializing in medical and legal subjects.*

HELP, I'M ALLERG

For at least thirty-one million Americans, summer is high season for allergies. Sneezes, wheezes, hives and a lot of other symptoms can make you anything from mildly uncomfortable to downright miserable. What can you do? If you have severe allergy problems, you'll want to see a doctor who specializes in treating allergies, but if your problems are less severe, here are some tips to help cut down your miseries this summer.

How does an allergen reach you?

Allergens or antigens are the medical names for the substances that cause allergic reactions. They can be divided into four categories: inhalants—pollens, grasses, plants and so forth; ingestants—foods; contactants—poison ivy, fabrics, cosmetics; injectants—bee and wasp stings and medicine injected into you. But these categories overlap and that gives people a lot of unexpected trouble. For example, a woman allergic to horses suddenly finds herself sneezing while picnicking in a field near horses on a windy day. The wind carries horse dander causing her to have an allergic reaction. Another example is a young woman allergic to a cat. She avoids petting an adorable kitten in a friend's home, but begins to wheeze anyway because the lively kitten

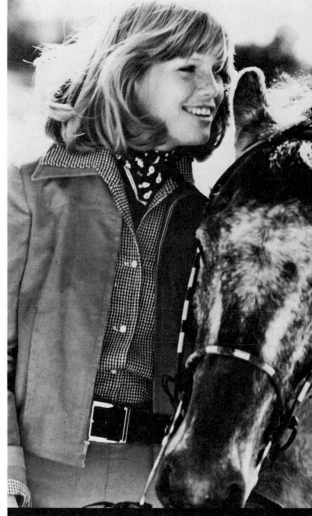

Wind can blow animal dander.

spreads its dander around by frisking and playing and even by napping on the sofa where the allergic woman sits.

Allergies have erratic patterns

Allergies are so frustrating because they aren't always predictable. A hay fever sufferer can have several good seasons, then a terrible one for no obvious reason. Or, even more bizarre, a woman allergic to strawberries can get a terrible case of hives from New Jersey berries, yet she can eat her fill of berries from California. The difference in soil probably accounts for a slightly different kind of berry. Some people allergic to eggs can eat hard-boiled eggs but not soft-boiled ones. Sometimes you get a severe

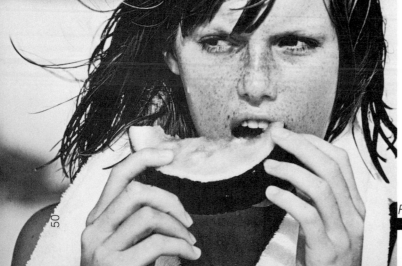

Foods sometimes cause allergies.

50

reaction to something you've eaten or inhaled for ages with no problems. This is because it takes considerable exposure to an allergen to cause symptoms in many people. Sometimes symptoms occur only under very specific circumstances. A food allergy may not be severe enough to cause trouble under normal circumstances, but a large quantity of the food eaten when there are other allergens present may cause trouble. The *combination* of allergens is what causes the reaction.

What can you do to protect yourself?

If you have pollen-induced allergies, check out the vegetation of any spot you're going to vacation in. For instance, east of the Rocky Mountains, trees usually pollinate in spring, grasses in summer and weeds like ragweed toward the end of summer. Thus you may think your allergy season is over, but if you travel to another part of the country it could be just the beginning or yet-to-come. Also, ragweed, probably the most troublesome pollen of all, pollinates about mid-August and continues until the first frost, but is not generally found west of the Rockies or in Europe. In mild climates, something is pollinating most of the year, so before you plan a trip, it's a good idea to see if there are any plants that you're terribly allergic to.

About one person in six is hypersensitive to insect stings such as bees or wasps. If you're

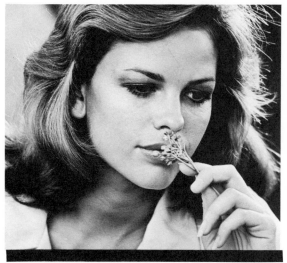

Inhaling pollen can cause trouble.

stung and symptoms seem severe, apply ice to lessen the absorption of venom, remove the insect's stinger as carefully as possible so that no more venom is pressed in. If symptoms seem to be getting worse, see a doctor immediately. To lessen your chances of being stung, don't walk barefoot on grass, don't eat outdoors without being aware of insects and don't use hairsprays, perfumes or lotions with sweet, insect-attracting scents. Don't volunteer to dump picnic refuse in insect-infested garbage cans. Also, wear light rather than dark colors—insects seem less attracted.

Molds are another common allergy producer. If damp, musty places seem to make you sneeze or wheeze, it's probably a mold allergy and you should avoid vacationing in very hot, humid climates. You might also be suspicious of foods like aged cheese, wines and beers, all of which have mold in them. Old houses, old bedding and furniture are possible offenders. If you're opening the vacation cottage at the beach, let someone else be first and spend a night there until things have been aired out.

Poison ivy is probably the most common summer allergy. About 75 percent of the population is susceptible to some degree. Besides watching where you're walking, remember that you can get poison ivy by touching your own or someone else's clothing that has touched poison ivy or by petting a dog or cat or other animal who has walked through it. Wind carrying the smoke of burning poison ivy can be lethal. Many people think they are doing the community a favor by burning the plant without realizing that the wind-borne smoke can infect people who can't see the fire and realize the danger. Kill it with chemicals; do not burn it.

Probably the most common protection against summer plant and grass allergies is the antihistamine pill. These pills help relieve runny noses and eyes, itching ad sneezing. There are many available by prescription and others that can be bought over-the-counter.

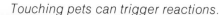

Touching pets can trigger reactions.

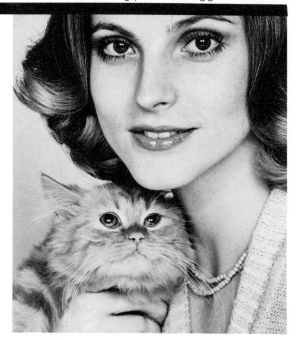

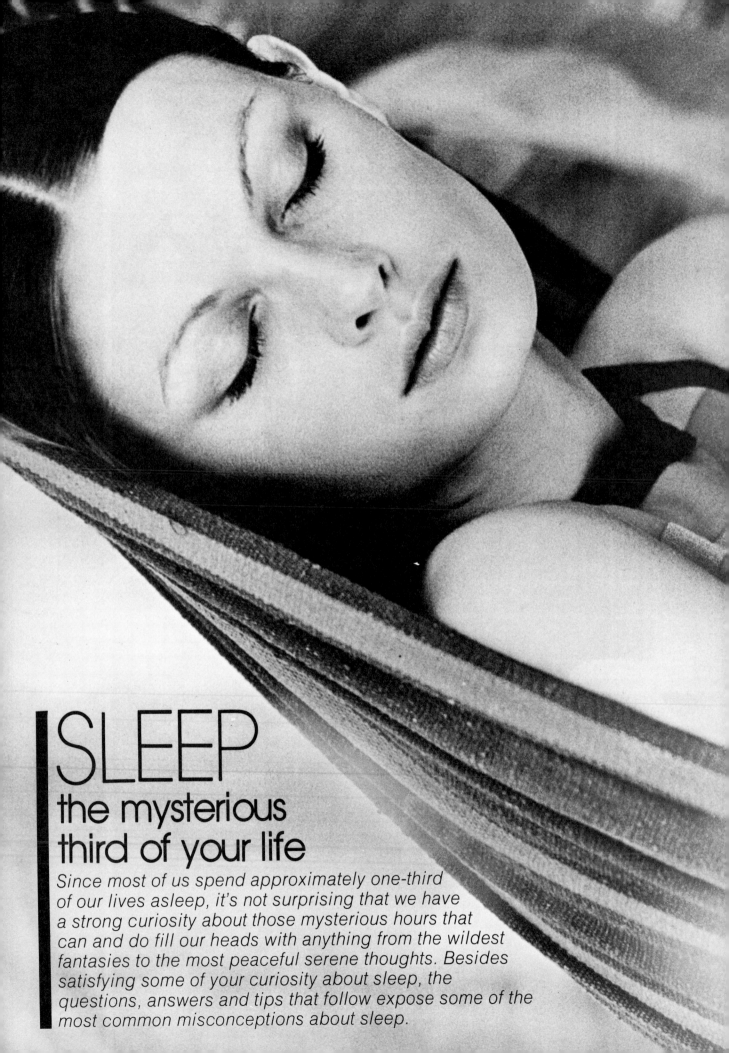

SLEEP
the mysterious third of your life

Since most of us spend approximately one-third of our lives asleep, it's not surprising that we have a strong curiosity about those mysterious hours that can and do fill our heads with anything from the wildest fantasies to the most peaceful serene thoughts. Besides satisfying some of your curiosity about sleep, the questions, answers and tips that follow expose some of the most common misconceptions about sleep.

Will lack of sleep cause bags or dark circles under eyes?

Lack of sleep for long periods may cause red-rimmed or dark-circled eyes. This usually happens after long periods of too-little sleep. Usually, the "dark circles" that people complain of are hereditary and are not affected by amount of sleep. Puffy eyes or bags under the eyes in the morning are frequently from normal nightly fluid accumulation in tissues under eyes.

Does everyone really need 8 hours' sleep a night?

Gay Luce and R. Julius Segal in *How to Avoid Insomnia* (original title *Insomnia*),* quote one statistical study that breaks it down this way: about 8 percent of the people surveyed slept five hours or less; 15 percent slept five or six hours; 62 percent slept between seven and eight hours. You have to let your body tell you what's right for you.

* Gay Luce, and R. Julius Segal: *How to Avoid Insomnia,* Paperback Library, New York, 1971.

If I occasionally can't get to sleep, is there any harm in taking a sleeping pill?

Authorities differ widely about usage of sleeping pills. Most pills are barbiturates with the potential for making their users dependent. Some people who take them find themselves slowly and subconsciously drifting into the habit of needing a pill to sleep. That's part of their danger. Besides the potential for dependence, most sleeping drugs interfere with the normal sleep cycle—usually the REM (or dreaming) part of the cycle. Studies have shown that disturbances of REM cycles have been known to cause emotional disturbances. If your sleeping problems are predictable—say occurring only after days of great stress—it's better to try to put yourself in a sleep-inducing mood (more about this, later) than to take sleeping pills. If you're the type who goes into a terrible tailspin when you occasionally just cannot go to sleep, you might talk to your doctor to see what he or she thinks about your taking a sleeping pill.

If I have trouble sleeping, will it affect my performance?

Your frame of mind is more likely to affect your performance, rather than the lack of sleep. If you allow yourself to get terribly uptight about the lost sleep, you may talk yourself into feeling a lot worse than you do—and that can certainly affect your performance. The effect of one night's poor sleep is usually not very devastating, especially on a young person, unless it is coupled with a lot of emotional tension. The best advice is to "cool it."

Sleep scientists also point out that many people sleep well, but just *think* they don't. Such thoughts as "I wish I'd go to sleep" or "Why can't I go to sleep?" run through your mind when you are actually asleep.

Why do I sometimes awake angry or depressed?

Sleep is not just a voyage into the unconscious. Even though you may remember nothing from that soft darkness of the previous night's sleep, your brain was active, you were having thoughts and dreams. There are many differing scientific views about exactly how and why we remember, or don't remember, what we dreamed or thought during sleep. But there is agreement that dreams or sleep thoughts can be deeply upsetting. Some behavioral scientists say most dreams are repressed—not remembered—because they are too disturbing to be consciously confronted. We sometimes use them as a means of thinking things we wouldn't dare think while awake. Whatever the actual process may be, the night's mental activities can leave residue feelings the next day that cause you unexplained anger or anxiety.

If I go to bed at 10:30 or 11 P.M. I fall asleep quickly. If I wait till 12:30 or 1, I have a terrible time falling asleep. Why?

Our bodies have a rising and falling rhythm that occurs in cycles. It accounts for the various sleep cycles we go through and it is present to a lesser degree during the day. If you feel drowsy at 10:30, your body is telling you it's in a downward cycle and this is a good time to go to bed. At 12:30 you may be moving into an upward cycle, and it will be difficult to go to sleep. By listening to your body clock you can fall asleep easily; by fighting it, you may have problems drifting off.

Can one get too much sleep?

Sometimes people who seem to sleep a great deal are using sleep as an escape. They escape whatever is bothering them or release themselves from boredom—going into the fantasies and intrigues of a dream world. If you feel you're using sleep as an escape, you might try to find out what you're escaping from so you can direct your sleeping time to something productive. It's sometimes necessary to get professional psychiatric help to get to the root of the problem, but it's usually worth it.

Can The Pill alter sleep patterns?

Good question, but there's no clear-cut answer. Animal studies show sex steroids (synthetic hormones in the pill are comparable) can alter animals' sleep patterns, so the same may be true in humans.

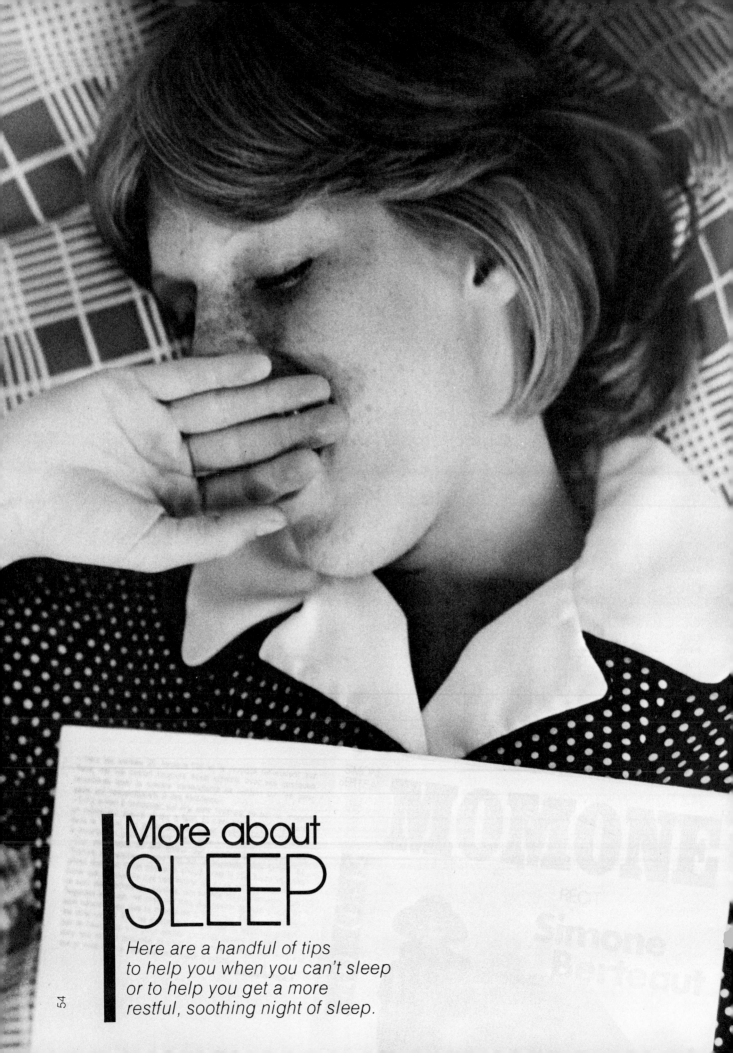

More about
SLEEP

Here are a handful of tips
to help you when you can't sleep
or to help you get a more
restful, soothing night of sleep.

Make yourself a pretty bed to sleep in

It may not make you sleep any better, but it certainly will make you feel better to fall asleep in the prettiest bed around. A few flowers in a vase on a bedside table is another luxury to allow yourself once in a while. You might scent a piece of cotton with your favorite perfume and tuck it under your pillow. It's always a good idea to place your bed in a way so that reading is easy and comfortable. A good reading light is another essential. If your bed has no headboard but "headed" by a wall, a pile of pillows resting against the wall or one of those little bedrests with arms would work.

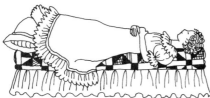

Rest those tired legs

When you've been on your feet all day, lie down with your legs up on some pillows—see sketch above. It's positively super. The fatigue goes; circulation is stimulated.

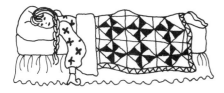

Caution for tummy sleepers

If you frequently wake up with a backache, one of the things you might consider as a possible cause is constant sleeping on your stomach. Many back doctors warn patients with low-back trouble that habitual stomach sleeping can contribute to their discomfort. If you occasionally have low-back discomfort or menstrual cramps, try this position: Lie on your side and slip a pillow between your knees. The pillow raises the top leg and takes the pressure off the lower-back area.

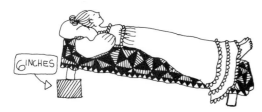

Get rid of early morning bags under your eyes

The sketch, above, shows you how to raise the head of your bed with two six-inch blocks of wood. Keeping your head elevated discourages fluid accumulation during the night—one of the main causes of the bags—and it's good for sinus and respiratory troubles, as well.

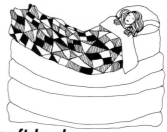

Hard versus soft bed: pillows or not

The kind of bed you sleep on is really mostly a matter of personal preference with a few exceptions. Anyone who suspects he or she is developing back problems—and thousands of Americans are—should try a firmer mattress. It gives the body more equalized support and doesn't allow your back to sag as the one in the sketch above does. Bedboards are fine if you happen to like the extra firm feel they give, but they really aren't necessary for most people. There are all sorts of myths that sleeping flat on your back without a pillow keeps you from aging so fast—but besides being terribly ascetic, it's doubtful if it has any beauty benefits. Sleeping with two pillows can be helpful to people who have respiratory or sinus trouble. It elevates the head and chest and discourages congestion from developing during the night.

Get into a presleep routine

Following a little routine before you go to bed can help you fall off to sleep more easily. It doesn't matter what you do—take a warm bath, read, have a glass of milk and a cookie. The idea is that by doing the same thing every night, you unconsciously begin to associate the routine with sleep and just by going through the motions of it, you begin to feel drowsy.

Bedtime relaxer to try

If you have a night or two when that soft drowsy feeling seems to evade you entirely, try this relaxing idea. Lie flat on your back. Try to relax, say, the calf muscles of one leg, then continue to relax each muscle of that leg separately as much as you can. You'll know you're succeeding when the leg feels so heavy you feel you can't lift it. Work all the way up your body until it feels limp and heavy. Your whole body will feel deeply relaxed—and if you're lucky, you'll be asleep before you get to your arms!

Don't overstimulate yourself just before bedtime

Almost anything that makes you feel sleepy is the right thing to do before bed. But many people find that strenuous exercising—which you might think would tire you out—actually stimulates the body and makes falling asleep difficult. A little mild exercise is fine, but save the heavy stuff for another time. Any frantic activity—cleaning house, sewing up a storm— can leave you with that wide-awake feeling and makes falling asleep a bit difficult.

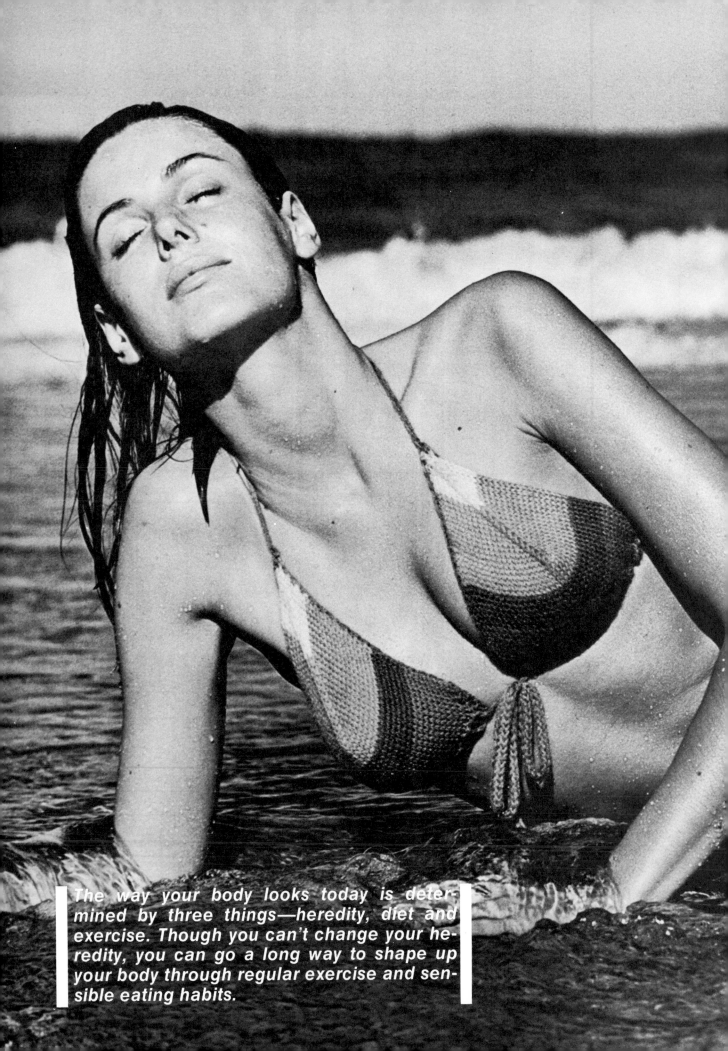

The way your body looks today is determined by three things—heredity, diet and exercise. Though you can't change your heredity, you can go a long way to shape up your body through regular exercise and sensible eating habits.

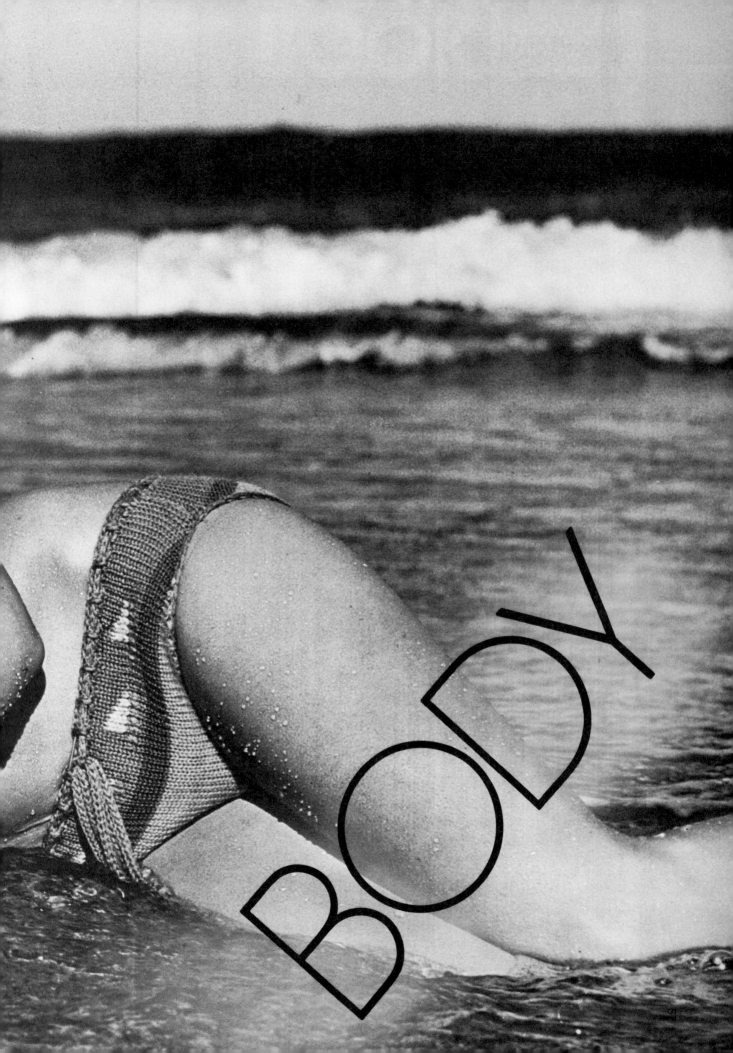

FIND YOUR BO

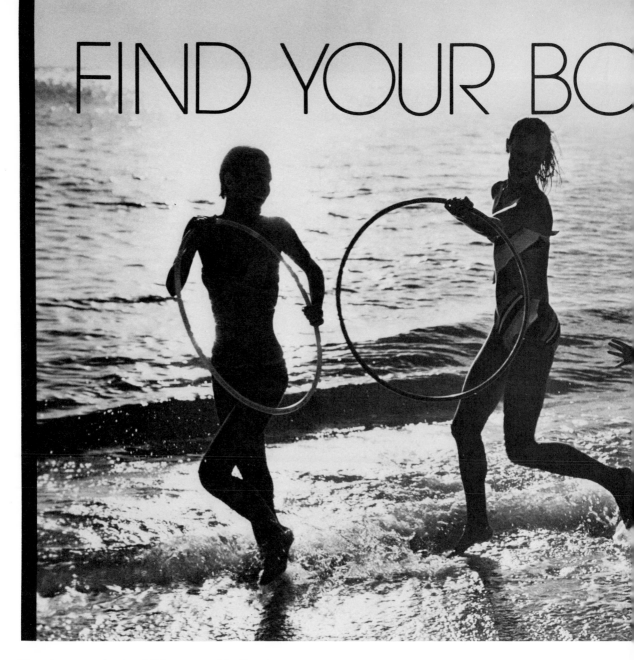

The shape you're in at this moment in time is no accident. It's the result of the body type you inherited from your parents and the product of years of good—or bad—eating habits plus exercise. If you're not happy with your body, there's a lot you can do about it. In fact, two out of the three things that determine its looks are under your control—diet and exercise. Even with the ability to control two-thirds of the factors that determine how your body looks, you may still be unhappy about how it shapes up. Usually this is because your expectations are out of synch with reality. You must work with a certain set of givens—i.e., your inherited body type. If you realize that you're an ecto- or endomorph or a mesomorph and that there are certain limitations to what you can and can't expect from this particular body type, you will be more realistic and thus happier with your body.

In the quiz here answer "yes" or "no" to *all* questions to determine your body type, then read on to pinpoint some of the givens for that particular body type so that you can bring your expectations more in line with what's realistic.

I

	YES	NO
Were you thin as an infant and toddler?	☐	☐
Do you tend to be slender now, with more angles than curves?	☐	☐
Do you find it difficult to put on weight?	☐	☐
Do you feel you have a lot of "nervous energy"?	☐	☐

II

Were you average weight and proportion as an infant and toddler?	☐	☐
Does your body seem dense and compact to you?	☐	☐
Is your muscle structure well formed and obvious to you?	☐	☐

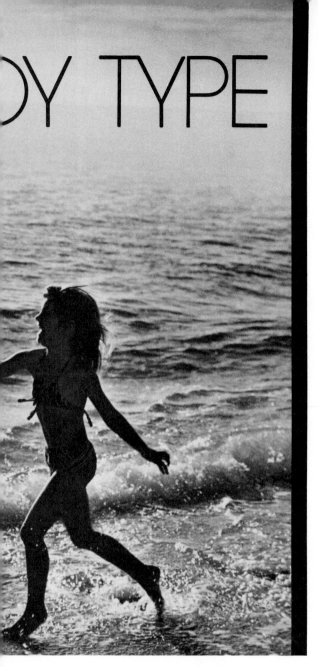

)Y TYPE

and know what to expect from it

How to interpret your answers

Rarely is one a perfect type, so you probably won't find yourself answering "Yes" to all the questions in any one group. But the group where you have the most "Yes" answers is probably the one that most closely represents your body type. If you're split evenly between two groups—which can happen—your body type probably falls half and half between the two. Then read the descriptions of both types below and base your body image expectations on the information that seems to best apply to you.

Body type characteristics

THE ECTOMORPH

Ectomorphs tend to be slender and to stay that way throughout their lives. These are the people who have trouble putting on rather than taking off weight. In many respects, you're fortunate because if you eat sensibly, overweight should not be a problem for you. If your ideal body image is Sophia Loren's you're never going to attain that ideal. You can, by eating well-balanced meals and getting proper exercise, have a very attractive well-proportioned body, but voluptuous you'll never be!

MESOMORPH

Mesomorphs have well-muscled, well-proportioned bodies that are often associated with success in sports. You can become overweight by overeating, but if you eat sensibly and exercise, you should have no trouble keeping trim. Weight, when you do put it on, tends to distribute itself evenly over your body.

ENDOMORPH

The endomorph has a round, soft, curvy body that's reminiscent of the women in Rubens' paintings. You have more of a tendency to put on weight than the other two body types and it generally settles through the stomach and hip area. This body type can be attractive and well-proportioned and it can have a very appealing sensual quality because of its curvaceousness. Endomorphs do need discipline and exercise if they are going to maintain their proper weight. The chief problem here arises when an endomorph wants to be an ectomorph. For her, this slender angular body is not realistic. (More about body types on page 102, ff.)

	YES	NO
Do you have a relatively easy time controlling your weight?	☐	☐
Do you rather enjoy competition, especially sports?	☐	☐

III

	YES	NO
Were you a plump baby and/or toddler?	☐	☐
Are you inclined to voluptuous curves today?	☐	☐
Does a lot of your weight tend to be put on below the waist?	☐	☐
Do you have a hard time controlling your weight?	☐	☐
Do you enjoy socializing, especially when it's focused around eating?	☐	☐

Making sense of the DIETS

There are probably almost as many different kinds of diets as there are dieters, and making sense of them all is enough to drive you to . . . food! Here is some common sense that will help, plus a little reassurance that anyone can lose weight and lose it for good by practicing sensible eating habits.

HIGH PROTEIN DIETS

High protein diets are those on which you eat protein almost exclusively. Very lean meats, chicken and fish, cottage and pot cheeses and eggs make up the bulk of such a diet. The most well known of these diets is probably the Stillman Diet, developed by the late Dr. Irwin Stillman. Some people refer to the Stillman diet as the "water diet" because you are required to drink at least eight glasses of water a day.

Pros: You do see rather spectacular results from this diet, often during the first week or ten days. It can be quite effective for people who want to lose just a few pounds quickly.

Cons: Even its originator, Dr. Stillman, cautioned that a dieter must supplement this diet with vitamins because this kind of limited eating doesn't provide you with all the nutrients you need. Also, an exclusively protein diet sets up certain chemical reactions in your body that can be dangerous, especially for people with such diseases as diabetes and others. In addition, the diet is boring and very difficult to stay on because the foods you can eat are so limited. In his later years, Dr. Stillman began to change his thinking on dieting and to come around to the low carbohydrate point of view, saying that most of us do need some carbohydrates, especially over a long period of dieting. Generally, a high protein diet that excludes almost all carbohydrates and concentrates only on proteins should not be tried unless your doctor recommends it and supervises you carefully while you're on it.

LOW CARBOHYDRATE DIETS

These diets are called low or minimal carbohydrate diets because they encourage the dieter to eat protein and fats (as contrasted with high protein diets that don't allow you to eat fat), but almost no carbohydrates. You are permitted fatty meats like steak, even bacon, fish, poultry, eggs and some dairy products. The Atkins Diet, originated by Dr. Robert Atkins, is probably the most well known of these. Putting yourself on one of these diets will automatically force you to eat fewer calories because carbohydrates are high calorie foods. They are also the foods most readily turned into fatty tissue.

Pros: This kind of diet does reduce calorie intake and cause weight loss. It provides you with plenty of body-building protein, plus some fats for energy.

Cons: Everyone needs some carbohydrates and it's very difficult for the dieter who needs to lose a lot of weight to know just where to draw the line on eliminating them. Some people can get by with very few. Others experience a sharp drop in blood sugar with accompanying feelings of mental inefficiency and irritability and fatigue. A doctor's advice on how to regulate your carbohydrate intake on this kind of diet is essential. There is also a psychological drawback with a minimal carbohydrate diet. Carbohydrates cause your body to hold water. When you cut down on them, especially when you cut down to practically nothing, your body dumps a lot of water quickly, resulting in a quick loss of pounds on the scale. You can only lose so much water, however, and after a few weeks the water loss isn't so dramatic and neither is your weight loss. It can be difficult to get by this plateau without being discouraged, but you will continue to lose weight—just more slowly.

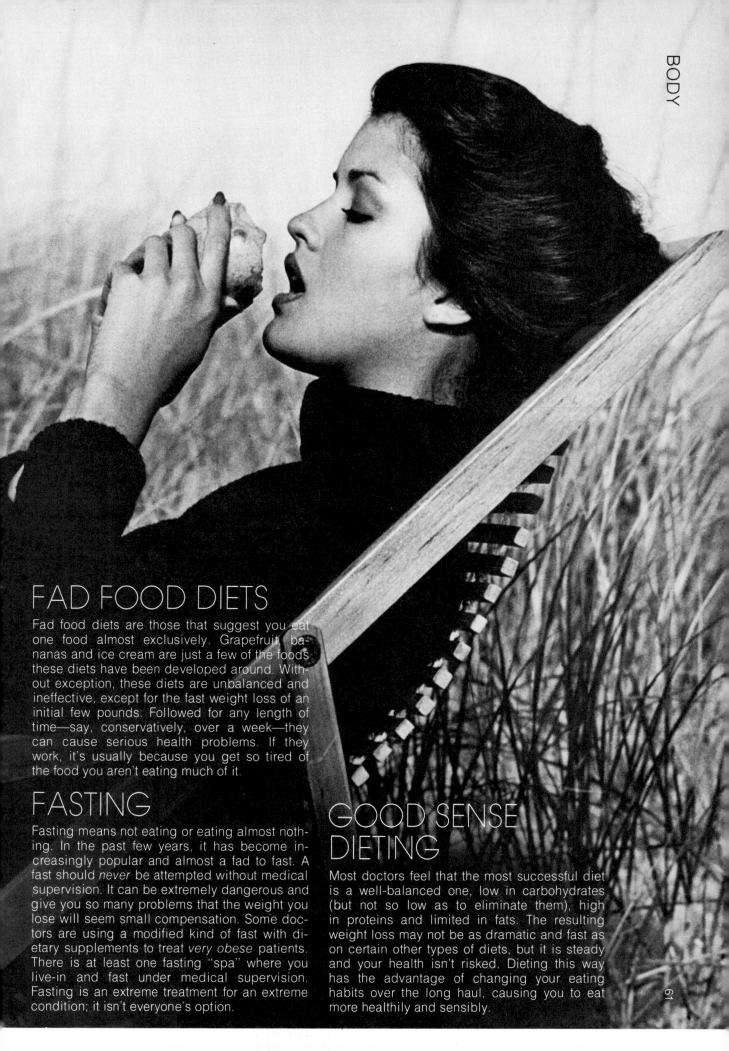

FAD FOOD DIETS

Fad food diets are those that suggest you eat one food almost exclusively. Grapefruit, bananas and ice cream are just a few of the foods these diets have been developed around. Without exception, these diets are unbalanced and ineffective, except for the fast weight loss of an initial few pounds. Followed for any length of time—say, conservatively, over a week—they can cause serious health problems. If they work, it's usually because you get so tired of the food you aren't eating much of it.

FASTING

Fasting means not eating or eating almost nothing. In the past few years, it has become increasingly popular and almost a fad to fast. A fast should *never* be attempted without medical supervision. It can be extremely dangerous and give you so many problems that the weight you lose will seem small compensation. Some doctors are using a modified kind of fast with dietary supplements to treat *very obese* patients. There is at least one fasting "spa" where you live-in and fast under medical supervision. Fasting is an extreme treatment for an extreme condition; it isn't everyone's option.

GOOD SENSE DIETING

Most doctors feel that the most successful diet is a well-balanced one, low in carbohydrates (but not so low as to eliminate them), high in proteins and limited in fats. The resulting weight loss may not be as dramatic and fast as on certain other types of diets, but it is steady and your health isn't risked. Dieting this way has the advantage of changing your eating habits over the long haul, causing you to eat more healthily and sensibly.

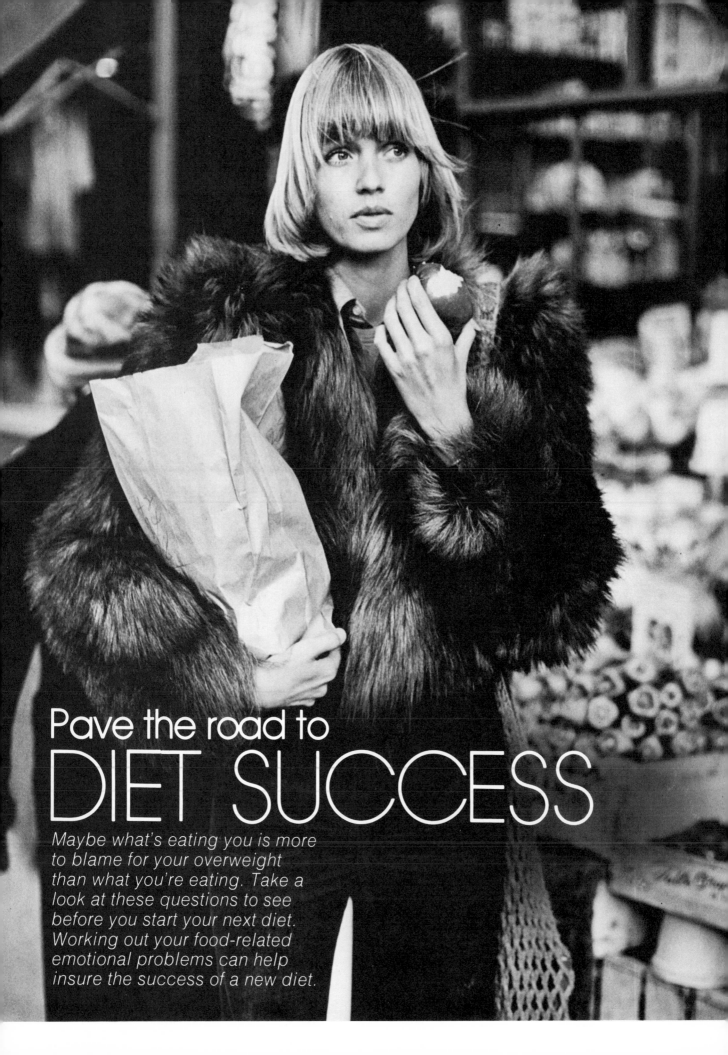

Pave the road to
DIET SUCCESS

*Maybe what's eating you is more
to blame for your overweight
than what you're eating. Take a
look at these questions to see
before you start your next diet.
Working out your food-related
emotional problems can help
insure the success of a new diet.*

If you can't seem to stick with any diet—and if it has ever occurred to you that sometimes you seem to be actually sabotaging yourself—then you probably need to work on underlying psychological problems: the hang-ups that cause you to cheat on your diets in the first place.

Perhaps you overeat because food is a great comfort, a way of "mothering" yourself. In that case, what you need to do is try to improve the quality of your life, to tackle the things that make you feel you *need* the solace of extra eating. In other cases, your fat itself may serve some secret, surprising purpose, and just recognizing what the purpose is can be a help. Identifying your own hang-ups is difficult, of course, but some of the very personal and probing questions that follow (based on the self-examination suggested by psychologist Dr. Frank J. Bruno in his book *Think Yourself Thin**) may strike a responsive chord. Try writing out your answers, where it's called for, because as Dr. Bruno says, "Just writing something out helps you think more clearly about it." Here are the questions:

* Frank J. Bruno, *Think Yourself Thin*, Nash Publishing Corporation, California, 1972.

1. When you're angry, do you usually hold it in or do you let people know what's bugging you? Does the fact that you're overweight upset anyone close to you—your mother, for example, or your husband? And if it does, are you secretly happy to see this person disturbed?

Overeating can be a way of expressing "forbidden" defiance and anger (even anger against yourself). As one teen-ager said to psychiatrist Dr. Haim Ginott, "My mother can take away my telephone and TV, but she cannot take away my fat."

2. Are you happy with your sex life? Are you tuned in to your sex needs or do you deny them or feel that "sex isn't really important"?

One woman may turn to food as a substitute not for sex but for the affection and reassurance she craves when her sex life is unsatisfactory; others turn to food when their sex lives are active—and generating (unacknowledged—and threatening) conflicts.

3. Make a list of things (and people) that frustrate you. Are you generally disappointed with

your life? And did you, as a child, form the habit of eating when you were tense, lonely or bored?

If so, you are probably vulnerable to occasional compulsive eating binges, which you've rationalized as celebration or solace. But there are better ways to pamper yourself: a hot fragrant bath, a movie, a new pair of fur-lined gloves.

4. How would you describe yourself to someone you'd never met? Do the faults outweigh the virtues?

If so, you may have such a poor opinion of yourself that you eat—once again—for comfort. Or you may feel that, as a fatty, you have the body you really deserve.

5. Make a list of situations you're afraid of or dislike because they make you nervous. Does overweight actually help you to avoid any of them (i.e., does it keep sexual approaches to a minimum . . . or does it prevent you from seeking a more desirable job)?

If so, you might try facing your fears and thinking of how you would handle the new problems that might come up if you were slim.

6. How do you feel about your body? Are you proud of it or ashamed? Have you thought you might become a different person if you lost weight, that in fact the "you" you are now might in some way die?

It could help if you remind yourself that weight loss is gradual, so there is time to adjust to a new body image . . . and the new way others may react to you.

If you're super-honest in your answers, you'll surely gain some insights into your own special diet blocks. The insights alone may suffice to get you back on your diet—for real. Or you may decide to seek professional help, as many young women do—from a doctor or therapist. If you decide on a doctor, find one who will take time to help you understand your problem, not just hand you a printed diet and give you a canned pep talk about self-discipline. To be a successful dieter, it's helpful to concentrate not only on what you're eating—but also on what's eating you!

FINDING THE DIET
That works for you

Not every diet works for everyone, even though it may be a sound, sensible diet. The reason for this is that we all have little psychological preferences that make some diets appealing and others dreary. Many diets rely on your having to count calories, others require you to measure food and still others group foods into allowed and disallowed groups. Any of these systems works, you just have to pick the one—or the combination—that's most agreeable to you. We give you one excellent diet, starting on the next page which works by categorizing foods and limiting quantities. Others follow.

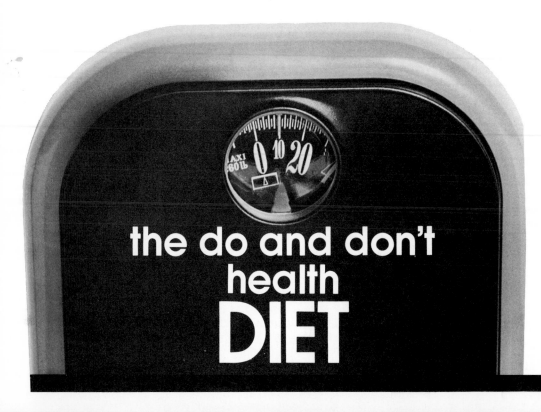

the do and don't health DIET

Devised by Phyllis Starr Wilson with Dr. Morton Glenn, assistant professor of clinical medicine, New York University School of Medicine, this is not a rigid menu-by-menu regimen; it lets you pick and choose what you like from a list of proteins and carbohydrates, thereby avoiding many fats and automatically cutting calories. Its big advantage is that it's a sensible eating plan that you can adopt as a lifetime eating pattern.

do	don't	do	don't

MEATS, 1st week:
chicken, veal, fish, shellfish—broiled, roasted or baked; 3 oz. portion for lunch 6 oz. portion for dinner (see following section for easy way to measure.)

MEATS, 1st week:
avoid beef, lamb, pork and anything that includes them, like bacon, sausages; never fry or saute anything when you are on this diet. Nothing smoked or canned in oil like smoked salmon or sardines in oil.

BREADS
Thin-sliced white, wheat, rye—1 slice or ½ hard roll at breakfast; 1 slice or ½ hard roll at lunch.

BREADS
No pumpernickel that has molasses or caramel in it; thus higher sugar content; no bagels, English muffins, no bread at all at dinner.

2nd week:
lean beef, lamb or pork— once a week for lunch, once for dinner. Chicken, veal, fish, shellfish for all other meals—3 oz. for lunch, 6 oz. for dinner.

2nd week:
Don't eat more than a 2 oz. portion of beef, lamb or pork for lunch; 4 oz. portion for dinner.

DESSERTS
Fruits. Special treat once a week, ice cream in Dixie cup size portion instead of a glass of skim milk or fruit.

DESSERTS
No cakes, pies, cookies, puddings, ice cream (except as listed in ''Do'' list).

3rd week, and following:
lean beef, lamb or pork— twice a week for lunch and twice for dinner. Chicken, veal, fish, shellfish for all other meals.

3rd week and following:
Don't have more than portions allowed above.

MISCELLANEOUS
Dressing—mustard, tomato cocktail sauce, commercial salad dressings with only 3 calories per teaspoon (Italian dietetic salad dressings are usually only 3, but check label); dressings you make from lemon juice and tomato juice.

MISCELLANEOUS
No oil or salad dressings that contain it; nuts, doughnuts, seeds, chocolate, jams, jellies, honey.

VEGETABLES
(Some items here are not vegetables, but they are usually eaten as such): asparagus, eggplant, green beans, peas, lettuce, spinach and all greens, squash, string beans, tomatoes, broccoli, cabbage, cauliflower, cucumbers, green peppers, radishes, turnips, carrots, celery—½ cup cooked portion of any of above for dinner; if still hungry, ½ cup of a second is allowed. Eat any quantity of raw vegetable from above list, any place, anytime (except tomatoes, 1-a-day limit).

VEGETABLES
Corn, lima beans, yams, spaghetti, macaroni, kidney beans, navy beans, avocado, olives. Never fry or saute vegetables.

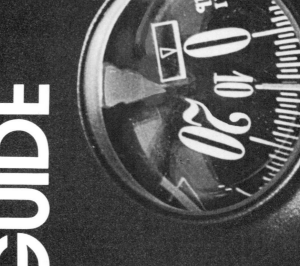

FRUITS
All fruits, except those listed in ''Don't'' fruit list. If canned, or frozen, must be in water, not syrup. Especially low-caloried fruits are berries (½ cup portion); cantaloupe (½ cup portion). Allow 3 fruit portions a day.

FRUITS
Don't eat grapes, cherries, watermelon. Don't eat any dried fruits—apricots, dates, prunes, etcetera. Stay away from syrup-packed fruits—even if you wash syrup off, some is absorbed. No large sizes in fruits; only choose the medium to small apple, orange, etcetera.

DAIRY FOODS
Cheese—hard cheeses: 1 slice for breakfast and 2 slices for lunch (as a substitute for meat, of course); cottage (4–6 oz.) or farmer (2–3 oz.) cheese. Eggs—1 or 2 a meal, can be used as main course instead of meat—boiled or cooked in nonstick pans. Pure skim milk—1–2 glasses a day.

DAIRY FOODS
Avoid all spreadables like Brie, cream cheese, Camembert, except cottage and farmer cheese. Never exceed 2 eggs a meal, 4–6 a week; never fry or scramble in butter or margarine. No whole butter or 99 percent fat-free milks, no cream, non-dairy or synthetic creamers. No butter or margarine.

FOOD GUIDE

What to expect from this diet

1ST WEEK

Do expect to lose at least 2 pounds, probably more in the first week. Some women lose 3 to 5 pounds depending on their capacity for retaining or expelling water.

Don't be fooled by any loss over 2 pounds—it's only a water loss, which will return in the third week once your body's metabolism stabilizes.

Don't stop dieting after the first week just because you've lost the 5 pounds you wanted to. It will take you 3 weeks to really lose the 5 pounds in fat.

2ND WEEK

Do expect to lose about 2 pounds per week. A 5-pound loss takes 3 weeks; a 10-pound loss about 8 weeks.

Do realize that you are still in the water-loss phase of your diet and this loss does not noticeably change your measurements unless it's drastic, whereas fat loss does. In the second week your clothes may still feel snug even though you've lost 4 pounds because 2 of them were water.

Do measure your body and write down the results so that you can compare them now with those at the end of the third week.

3RD WEEK

Don't be discouraged. You may not see a weight loss at the end of this week, but to cheer

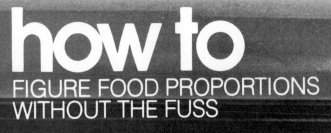

how to
FIGURE FOOD PROPORTIONS
WITHOUT THE FUSS

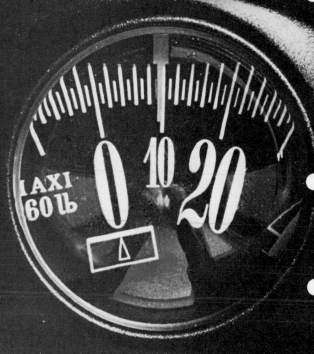

● HAMBURGER AS A MEAT MEASUREMENT

All over this country, the standard measurement of the average commercial hamburger (not the jumbo or super ones for which you pay extra) is the top of a medium-sized mayonnaise cap. They fit into these like a cookie into its cutter and weigh 3 oz. You can roughly judge many portions in comparison to this. For instance, if the piece of steak you eat is double the thickness of the hamburger, you can safely eat half a piece (only half the diameter). One medium lean lamb chop or pork chop is about the same size as the 3 oz. hamburger. One medium chicken thigh is about the same size, too.

● MEASURING SANDWICH MEATS

There are usually three kinds of sandwich measurements in the United States. Most coffee shops serve 3 oz. of meat in their sandwiches. Restaurants catering to women or light eaters serve 2 to 3 oz. The delicatessen or specialized sandwich shop usually serves super sandwiches—heroes, etcetera—these tend to contain 4 oz.

● OPEN-FACED SANDWICHES

These are great DO's for eating lunch out. In the standard coffee shop you can order a regular sandwich, eat only one piece of the bread and the 3 oz. of meat or chicken. Avoid salad mixes like egg, chicken or tuna salad—they are all loaded with calories because of the mayonnaise. Don't put mayonnaise on any sandwich; substitute mustard if you must; better still, have it plain.

● FIGURING VEGETABLES

If you're in doubt about the half-cupful portion, practice measuring cooked vegetables at home. It's roughly a scoop or Dixie cup portion, and your eye will soon get used to the right amount. If you're served any more when you're out, just leave the rest on the side of your plate.

yourself up, measure your body. You'll probably see a reduction here. What's happened is that an actual fat loss has replaced a water loss and it shows up in your measurements, though not on the scale.

4TH WEEK

DO expect to take roughly 4 more weeks to lose all 10 pounds, but be compensated by the fact that you're through the third week—the worst one, known as the quitter's week. The going should be easier and more routine now.

DON'T—now that you've learned about water loss and retention, try to restrict salt in your diet in hopes of keeping the water loss permanent. It doesn't work that way; the body eventually restores the balance.

DON'T

FALL FOR THESE DIET FADS AND FALLACIES

Can you really diet and still eat all you want of certain foods?

Diets that advocate eating all the steak, bananas or whatever you want bank on the fact that the dieter will soon tire of these foods and eat little of them. Dieters do—that's why we're allowing unlimited low-caloried raw vegetables. You'll see that after you've eaten as much as you want of them you'll automatically stop the stuffing. Diets that offer inordinate amounts of certain foods can work in terms of weight loss, not only because people get tired of the same food and cut down, but because they usually have been eating too much of everything, so that concentrating exclusively on limited food choices automatically cuts out others, thereby reducing calories. Such diets don't work in the long run—you can't continue to eat that way—so the dieter often gains the weight back. *Glamour's* Do and Don't Diet is a well-balanced way of eating that retains the appetite to good all-round nutritional habits. While you are on it, you are simply on a minimal version of a lifetime plan for healthful eating. Since it's so nutritionally full, you don't risk

harming your health, which brings us to vitamins and deficiencies.

Do you have to take vitamins when you diet?

Not on this diet. The only deficiency possibility that could come up is from settling too exclusively on a few favorite items and not getting enough Vitamin A. You can get the A from a simple all-round daily-maintenance type vitamin. Don't waste money on the single therapeutic ones. Be sure you include 1 citrus fruit in your choice of fruits to take care of C needs.

Are chemically pure foods more healthful than those with additives and preservatives?

Dr. Glenn suggests that if the package lists more chemicals than food, like some of the "convenience" items—such as dessert toppings, which are practically all chemicals, avoid them. But with some chemicals such as those that prevent spoilage, help in appearance and taste, there is the risk of eating unhealthful or unappetizing food.

Is organic food more healthful than other foods?

It is only more expensive, and for the dieter it can be a trap. Some of the new combination grain cereals are so high in calories, Dr. Glenn says they should actually be considered unhealthful.

DO

FOLLOW THIS DAILY GUIDE

Breakfast: egg or slice of cheese; slice of bread; fruit; black coffee or tea.

Lunch: open-faced sandwich; glass of skimmed milk; fruit. Dinner: veal, chicken or fish; one or two vegetables; fruit; glass of skimmed milk, black coffee or tea.

This is a typical selection for the first week of your diet. Don't hesitate to make substitutions within the general lines of the Food Guide Do's and Don'ts.

FOLLOW THESE TIPS FOR EATING OUT

Appetizers: tomato (not cream of) soup, clear consommés, broths.

Main course: fish, chicken, veal, shellfish, baked or broiled, no rich sauces; leave potatoes on plate. Remember, 2 shrimp cocktails can be a main course.

Dessert: cantaloupe and berries—without cream; black coffee or tea. Dr. Glenn says it takes only 3 weeks to establish the black coffee habit.

Sandwiches: they're great for diet lunches if you eat only 1 slice of bread, ½ the roll. Dr. Glenn suggests not ordering the hamburger without the roll. It isn't satisfying and you'll probably want something later. In this case, ½ a roll is better than none.

	sun	mon
morning	½ CUP BLUEBERRIES 1 OZ. READY-TO-EAT CEREAL ½ CUP SKIM MILK 1 SLICE TOAST 1 TSP. MARGARINE BEVERAGE	1 CUP STRAWBERRIES ⅓ CUP COTTAGE CHEESE WITH CINNAMON ON 1 SLICE RAISIN TOAST ½ CUP SKIM MILK BEVERAGE
noon	SPINACH OMELET (2 EGGS, ½ C. SPINACH) ½ MEDIUM TOMATO LETTUCE 1 SLICE BREAD 1 TSP. MARGARINE ½ CUP SKIM MILK 1 SMALL ORANGE BEVERAGE	4 OZ. BAKED SCROD 1 TSP. MARGARINE BROCCOLI CASSEROLE* ½ CUP SLICED PEACHES ½ CUP SKIM MILK BEVERAGE
evening	ROAST CORNISH HEN* ½ CUP WAX BEANS ½ CUP CHOPPED BROCCOLI 1 TSP. MARGARINE 4 OZ. BAKED RUTABAGA PRUNE YOGURT WHIP* BEVERAGE	CURRIED CHICKEN WITH RICE* ½ CUP CUT GREEN BEANS TOSSED GREEN SALAD 2 TSP. VEGETABLE OIL AND VINEGAR 2 APRICOT HALVES WITH 1 T. CAN JUICE ½ CUP SKIM MILK BEVERAGE

GLAMOUR'S
low-cost, low-calorie
DIET

With the cost of food where it is today, the dieter has a double problem—not only trimming down her food intake but her financial output. That's why we asked Weight Watchers International, Inc.®, to work out for *Glamour* readers this special 1-week budget diet based on their well-known and successful program, which changes, or reeducates, the dieter's eating habits so that she chooses nutritious, slimming food and eats it at the right time of day, instead of fattening unnutritious food anytime she feels compelled to. Here you will find a week's worth of delicious but inexpensive menus with recipes (even a few special dinner party ones). There are also alternate lunch suggestions for women who either eat lunch out or take it along to the office. And all without having to count a single calorie—it's already been done for you.

tues	wed	thurs	fri	sat
1 LARGE TANGERINE 1 OZ. READY-TO-EAT CEREAL ½ CUP SKIM MILK BEVERAGE	½ CUP GRAPEFRUIT JUICE 1 OZ. HARD CHEESE 1 SLICE TOAST ¾ CUP SKIM MILK BEVERAGE	1 SMALL ORANGE 1 POACHED EGG 1 SLICE TOAST 1 TEASPOON MARGARINE ½ CUP SKIM MILK BEVERAGE	½ MEDIUM GRAPEFRUIT 1 OZ. HARD CHEESE 1 SLICE TOAST 1½ TEASPOONS MARGARINE ½ CUP SKIM MILK BEVERAGE	½ CUP ORANGE JUICE 1 SCRAMBLED EGG 1 SLICE TOAST 1 TEASPOON MARGARINE ½ CUP SKIM MILK BEVERAGE
ACOS WITH PIMIENTO DRESSING* ¼ MEDIUM CUCUMBER CELERY RADISH ROSES 1 MEDIUM APPLE ½ CUP SKIM MILK BEVERAGE	ZINGY BEEF PATTIES* ½ MEDIUM TOMATO, SLICED ½ MEDIUM PICKLE LETTUCE 1¼ TEASPOONS MAYONNAISE 1 CUP SKIM MILK ¼ MEDIUM PINEAPPLE BEVERAGE	½ CUP MIXED VEGETABLE JUICE 4 OZ. TUNA FISH 2 OZ. SLICED ONION 1 MEDIUM RED PEPPER, SLICED 1 SLICE BREAD ½ CUP BLUEBERRIES 1 CUP SKIM MILK BEVERAGE	LIVER AND ONIONS AU FENNEL* 1 CUP KALE 1 SLICE BREAD ½ CUP SKIM MILK 1 SMALL PEAR BEVERAGE	4 OZ. BROILED LEMON SOLE ½ CUP SAUERKRAUT WITH ⅛ TEASPOON CARAWAY SEEDS 2 OZ. SLICED BEETS ½ CUP PINEAPPLE CHUNKS 1 CUP SKIM MILK BEVERAGE
SOYBEAN LOAF WITH MUSHROOM SAUCE* ½ CUP ZUCCHINI 1 TSP. MARGARINE LETTUCE WEDGE WITH 2 TSP. MAYONNAISE RUSSIAN DRESSING* ½ CUP ORANGE AND GRAPEFRUIT SECTIONS 1 CUP SKIM MILK BEVERAGE	½ CUP TOMATO JUICE CRÈME FISH PIE* 4 OZ. BAKED WINTER SQUASH ½ CUP SPINACH WITH NUTMEG BAKED BANANAS* 1 TABLESPOON YOGURT BEVERAGE	LENTIL SOUP WITH HAM* TOSSED GREEN SALAD WITH 1 MEDIUM TOMATO 2 TSP. VEGETABLE OIL AND VINEGAR 1 MEDIUM APPLE ½ CUP SKIM MILK BEVERAGE	1 CUP ONION BOUILLON BAKED FISH WITH CIOPPINO SAUCE* 1 CUP CAULIFLOWER WITH PIMIENTO STRIPS ½ CUP PLAIN YOGURT OVEN STEWED PRUNES* BEVERAGE	AMERICAN CHOP SUEY* ¾ CUP SUMMER SQUASH LETTUCE WEDGE WITH RUSSIAN DRESSING* ½ MEDIUM GRAPEFRUIT, BROILED ½ CUP SKIM MILK BEVERAGE

dieter's tip sheet

FOR EATING LUNCH OUT OR
TAKING IT ALONG TO THE OFFICE
Make a selection or selections in each category.

- APPETIZERS

Tomato or mixed vegetable juice
Plus beef or chicken or onion bouillon

- ENTRÉES

Choice of open-faced sandwich (i.e., 1 slice enriched or whole grain bread): broiled steak; grilled cheese and tomato; sliced chicken, turkey, roast beef or 3 oz. ham.

or

Choice of an individual can of tuna or salmon; boiled shrimp with 1 teaspoon mayonnaise; cottage cheese with fruit or vegetable; 2 medium eggs, poached or soft or hard-cooked or scrambled without fat; 3 oz. frankfurter; all-beef hamburger patty; 3 oz. smoked fish. (With any nonsandwich entrée, you may have 1 slice of enriched or whole grain bread.)

- ACCOMPANIMENTS

Green pepper rings, sliced cucumbers, dill pickle, tossed salad with 1 teaspoon vegetable oil and vinegar or 1 teaspoon mayonnaise, sliced tomato.
Plus choice of baked potato, enriched rice or noodles instead of bread.
Plus cooked vegetable.

- BEVERAGE

Choice of hot or iced tea or coffee, or skim milk.

- DESSERT

Choice of melon, grapefruit or orange sections, pineapple or other fresh fruit.

menu notes

- Take your choice of beverage: tea or coffee.
- You might want to turn a ½ cup of skim milk into a between-meals or before-bed snack.
- The fruit allowed at lunch might also be taken as a snack or added to your milk shake.
- All dishes with asterisks have recipes that follow.
- Wherever menu calls for skim milk, you might want to substitute instant nonfat dry milk reconstituted —it's less expensive. (Equivalents are on nonfat dry milk package.)

sun

roast cornish hen

1¼ lb. oven-ready cornish hen
1 c. chicken bouillon, divided
2 T. chopped celery
salt and pepper to taste

Place hen in small baking pan. Add ½ cup bouillon, celery and seasoning. Bake at 350° F about 40 minutes or until tender, basting 2 or 3 times with remaining bouillon. Remove skin and discard liquid before serving. Divide evenly. Makes 2 servings.

PRUNE YOGURT WHIP

1 c. plain yogurt
8 medium dried prunes, pitted and quartered
½ tsp. lemon juice

Combine all of the ingredients in blender container or food processor container with double-bladed steel knife. Process until smooth. Divide evenly into two dessert dishes. Chill. Makes 2 servings.

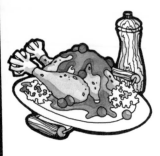

mon

broccoli casserole

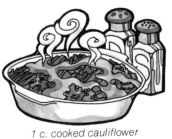

1 c. cooked cauliflower
½ c. evaporated skim milk
¼ c. water
1 packet instant chicken broth and seasoning mix
¼ tsp. basil
salt and pepper to taste
2 c. cooked chopped broccoli

Place cauliflower, milk, water, broth mix and basil in blender container; process until smooth. Season to taste. Place broccoli in 1 quart ovenproof casserole and cover with sauce. Bake at 375° F for 20 minutes. Divide evenly. Makes 2 servings.

curried chicken with rice

8 oz. boneless, skinned chicken, coarsely diced
2 oz. chopped onion
1 tsp. curry powder
¾ c. chicken bouillon
2 T. chopped celery
½ c. tomato puree
½ medium apple, diced
½ c. diced carrots
½ tsp. lemon juice
salt to taste
½ c. cooked enriched rice

Place chicken and onion in nonstick skillet. Cook over low heat until lightly brown. Sprinkle curry powder over chicken and stir to blend. Add bouillon and celery. Simmer 10 minutes, stirring occasionally. Add tomato puree, apple, carrots and lemon juice. Simmer 20 minutes or until carrots are tender and sauce is thickened. Season to taste. Serve over rice. Makes 1 serving.

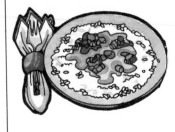

tues

tacos with pimiento dressing

4 oz. cooked ground veal
1 tsp. chili powder
¼ tsp. paprika
1 tsp. dehydrated onion flakes
¼ tsp. salt   ¼ tsp. onion powder
dash hot sauce
1 c. lettuce shreds
2 T. Pimiento Dressing
2 taco shells

Cook seasoned veal in nonstick pan for 5 min. Add ½ to taco shells; top with mixed lettuce and Pimiento Dressing. Serves 1.

PIMIENTO DRESSING

1 jar (7 oz.) pimientos, drained
2 T. cider vinegar
2 T. prepared mustard

Mix in blender till smooth: 1 cup.

soybean loaf & mushroom sauce

2 lbs. cooked, dried soybeans
2 c. tomato juice
1 T. plus 1 teaspoon Worcestershire sauce
4 packets instant chicken broth and seasoning mix
2 tsp. onion flakes   1 tsp. sage
garlic powder to taste
2 medium green peppers, diced and blanched
2 c. each cooked diced celery and carrots
salt and pepper to taste
2 medium tomatoes, sliced
Mushroom Sauce, below

Mix first 7 ingredients. Put 2 cups in blender till smooth. Put aside. Repeat with *remaining* soybean mix. Fold in vegetables. Season. Fill large nonstick loaf-pan. Top with tomatos. Bake 400° F 45 min. till firm. Serve with Mushroom Sauce. Serves 4.

MUSHROOM SAUCE

½ c. canned drained mushroom stems and pieces
2 tsp. ketchup
1 packet instant beef broth and seasoning mix
¼ bay leaf   ⅛ tsp. thyme
⅛ tsp. browning sauce
dash garlic powder
1¼ c. water
2 tsp. cornstarch, dissolved in 2 tsp. water

Cook first 7 ingredients 2–3 min. Add water. Bring to boil. Cook low heat 5 min. Add cornstarch. Cook till thickens. Serves 4.

RUSSIAN DRESSING

2 T. plus 2 tsp. imitation mayonnaise
2 tsp. ketchup
2 tsp. chili sauce
Worcestershire sauce to taste

Combine in small bowl. Divide. Serves 2.

wed

zingy beef patties

12 oz. ground beef
2 T. dehydrated bell pepper flakes, reconstituted
1 T. dehydrated onion flakes
2 tsp. prepared mustard
2 tsp. prepared horseradish
2 tsp. Worcestershire sauce
½ tsp. chili powder
salt and pepper to taste

Combine ingredients; mix we shape in two equal patties. Br on rack 3 to 4 inches from he source for 5 minutes. Turn, br 4 minutes or more till dor Makes 2 servings, 1 patty eac

crème fish pie

¾ c. water   1 pkg. instant chicken broth and seasoning m
1 T. cornstarch, dissolved in 1 T. water
½ medium green pepper, diced and blanched
½ c. canned drained mushroom stems and pieces
¼ c. diced pimientos
1 T. parsley
2 T. evaporated skim milk
¼ tsp. Worcestershire sauce
dash nutmeg, salt, white pepp
12 oz. cooked fish, flaked
6 oz. cooked potatoes, whippe
1 T. imitation (or diet) margarin
paprika

In a large saucepan comb water and broth mix; bring to boil. Stir in cornstarch; cook u sauce is clear. Add green p per; simmer 3 to 4 minutes, s ring occasionally. Add mu rooms, pimiento, milk, parsl Worcestershire sauce, nutm salt and pepper. Stir to comb Fold in fish. Pour into a 1-q shallow ovenproof casser Combine potatoes, margar salt and pepper. Spread o fish mixture. Sprinkle with prika. Bake at 400° F for 20 r utes or until throughly hea and potatoes are golden bro Divide evenly. Makes 2 servir

baked banana

½ c. orange juice
½ tsp. lemon juice
1 tsp. cornstarch
1 T. margarine
1 medium banana, peeled and sliced
dash nutmeg

Combine juices in sauce Dissolve cornstarch in jui Cook, stir constantly till th Stop cooking. Add marga Put banana in small shallow ing dish. Pour sauce. Spri nutmeg. Bake at 375° F fo minutes or till bananas tender. Divide evenly. Serve

thurs

lentil soup with ham

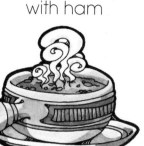

3 c. water
4 oz. cooked, dried lentils
oz. cooked ham, finely diced
1 oz. onion, finely diced
¼ c. finely diced carrot
¼ c. finely diced celery
1 lettuce leaf, finely chopped
packets instant chicken broth
and seasoning mix
½ bay leaf
pinch thyme
salt and pepper to taste

Combine all ingredients, except
lt and pepper, in a saucepan.
mmer 30 minutes, or until veg-
bles are tender and soup has
ckened. Season to taste.
kes 1 serving.

fri

liver and onions au fennel

4 oz. onion, thinly sliced
½ c. water
1 packet instant chicken broth
and seasoning mix
½ tsp. paprika
½ tsp. Worcestershire sauce
salt and freshly ground pepper
to taste
6 oz. liver
fennel seeds to taste
garlic powder to taste
1 T. imitation (or diet) margarine

Combine onions, water and broth
mix in a medium saucepan.
Bring to a boil, cook until onions
are tender. Drain. Add paprika,
Worcestershire sauce and pepper. Set aside. Sprinkle both
sides of liver with salt, pepper,
fennel seeds and garlic powder.
Lightly brown each side in a
large hot nonstick skillet. Place
onions over liver, continue cooking, covered, 3 to 5 minutes
more or until liver is done to
taste. Remove from heat. Dot
with margarine. Makes 1 serving.

baked fish with cioppino sauce

1½ c. tomato juice
1½ T. wine vinegar
1 T. dehydrated onion flakes
1½ tsp. chopped fresh parsley
1½ tsp. vinegar-packed capers
1 tsp. basil
1 tsp. lemon juice
½ tsp. rosemary
⅛ tsp. garlic powder
1 lb. fish fillets (grouper, cod or
halibut)

Combine all ingredients except
fish in medium saucepan. Simmer about 20 minutes. Place fish
in an ovenproof casserole, pour
sauce over fish. Bake at 350° F
for 20 minutes or until fish flakes.
Divide evenly. Makes 2 servings.

oven-stewed prunes

16 medium dried prunes
1 c. water
½ lemon, thinly sliced
small piece cinnamon stick

Place all ingredients in 2-cup
ovenproof dish; cover. Bake at
350° F for 1 hour or until prunes
are very tender. Discard lemon
slices and cinnamon stick. Divide prunes and syrup evenly.
Makes 4 servings.

sat

american chop suey

1 medium green pepper, diced
4 oz. onion, diced
¼ c. celery, diced
2 packets instant beef broth and
seasoning mix
2 garlic cloves, minced
1½ to 2 tsp. basil
2 c. tomato juice
12 oz. cooked ground beef patty,
cut into ½-inch pieces
1⅓ c. cooked enriched elbow
macaroni
salt and pepper to taste

In a large saucepan, combine
first 6 ingredients. Cook over
medium heat for 2 to 3 minutes,
stirring occasionally. Add tomato
juice, cook for 15 to 20 minutes
or until slightly thickened. Stir in
beef, macaroni, salt and pepper.
Heat throughly. Divide evenly.
Makes 2 servings.

bonus banana milk shake

(You must omit ½ cup skim milk
from one meal if you drink this
bonus shake.)

½ c. skim milk
1 ripe medium banana,
peeled and sliced
1 tsp. lemon juice
¼ tsp. vanilla extract
2 to 3 ice cubes

Combine all ingredients except
ice cubes in blender container;
process until smooth. Add ice
cubes, 1 at a time, process-
ing after each addition, until
crushed. Divide evenly. Makes 2
servings.

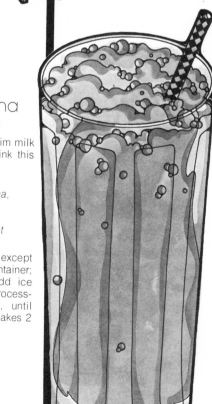

20

GREAT IDEAS WE BET YOU NEVER HAD ABOUT DIETING

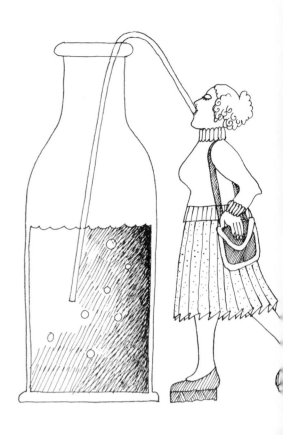

Sound and solid as the internist and psychologist who put them together, these great dieting ideas come from the book The Psychology of Successful Weight Control.* *It was written by Mary Catherine Tyson, M.D., an internist, and her late husband, Robert Tyson, Ph.D., a psychologist and writer.*

1. Identification with a trim body is quite different from identification with one that's too heavy.

What image do you have of yourself? Your answer will depend on your sex, age, education, occupation, family and general background, and particularly on the sort of body you have and what you think of it. The key word in the concept of body image is identification. . . .

You may have noticed that when you dress for a formal occasion you actually feel more formal because of your clothes. When you dress in sports clothes, you feel casual and relaxed. Children are resentful when they must wear clothes they consider inappropriate. The problem is they are not identifying with the clothes.

*Mary Catherine Tyson and Robert Tyson, *The Psychology of Successful Weight Control,* Nelson-Hall Company, Chicago, Illinois, 1974.

2. Identifying with your body is more important than identifying with clothes.

Your body as the very real physical part of you, greatly affects how you feel. Is it strong, so that you feel strong? Is it attractive, permitting you to feel attractive?

When a person identifies with an overweight body, she is in an unhappy situation. She enters a room with the unspoken, perhaps even unrealized, thought, "I am a fat person entering this room. Everyone sees it. That's the sort of person I am." A person's body image, favorable or unfavorable, has a strong impact on how she acts. Poise and self-confidence depend on it.

When you lose weight, you can look forward to the reward of improved body image and its accompaniments.

3. Eating equals love.

A baby has three main interests in life: sleeping, elimination, and eating. No one knows exactly how the world looks to an infant, but it seems probable that eating, in addition to satisfying hunger, is rewarding because it brings warm contact with the mother. Eating is associated with early experiences of affection. Animal experiments suggest that the physical contact may be more important than the eating itself in establishing the mother–child bond. . . . We could express this relationship as eating equals love.

A mother is pleased if her baby eats, and she is anxious if the infant refuses to eat. So, in addition to eating as a response to hunger, a baby soon eats to please its mother. She probably becomes increasingly aware that she can also control her mother by not eating. She learns to manipulate this most important person in her life by eating to please her and not to annoy her.

A mother gives, and her child receives and takes in. This is a picture of complete protection. How tempting it is to prolong this blissful state—and some people do in fact cling to it.

How food may serve as a symbol of love is illustrated by the girl who began to gain weight when she went to an out-of-town college. Her physician found out that almost every detail of her existence prior to her leaving home had been taken care of by her mother. Neither of these women realized how much the daughter's dependence had been built up. Suddenly there were all the details of clothes, cleaning up a room, etcetera, to attend to. It was no accident that the young girl ate excessively. Eating was a symbolic effort to make up for the absence of her mother's care.

This situation illustrates the close relationship between food and affection. When love is not received from the outside world, the dependent person often tries to compensate by feeding herself. But being good to oneself with food obviously cannot replace the missing care of a mother or a father. And since the behavior is never completely successful, the effort to compensate symbolically continues. Of course, food is also a reward in its own right, and a reward for which a person pays an exorbitant price. When the girl in our story gained insight into her behavior, she was able gradually to seek affection in more adult ways.

4. Biting and eating can express anger

There is a theory that when a mother denies her baby her breast or a bottle, the infant interprets the denial as rejection. She may respond with one of the few weapons in her possession, her mouth. Thus, biting is thought to be the expression of her anger at mother's "rejection."

Biting and eating as expressions of anger were demonstrated by a young man who ate large amounts of food whenever he was angry. This man had learned as an infant to be aggressive with his mouth. He had to learn to find less damaging ways of expressing anger than overeating.

5. Watch out for those times when you are tired, bored, worried, angry or feeling sorry for yourself

These are the moods that easily trip you up and make you turn to eating for comfort. Awareness will help you control yourself. See if you can do something direct and practical about what is really bothering you.

6. Study the attitudes of family members and of friends

People who know you become accustomed to you as you are—overweight. If you reduce, they can become sincerely concerned because you "don't look like yourself" and they may fear that you are overdoing it. They may be heard saying to each other, "I don't think she looked at all well. She's much too thin!"

Occasionally a relative of a dieter becomes so worried that he telephones the dieter's doctor to report his misgivings and to suggest that the diet be interrupted. Or he may offer the same suggestion to the husband or wife of the dieter. Some husbands and wives, without being aware of it, feel safer with a spouse who is overweight and therefore less attractive to the opposite sex, so they may urge the poor dieter to give up her attempts. The real danger in this is that the dieter may wish to believe what she hears and return to the comfort of overeating.

7. Open your mind to change as you lose weight

For example, as you reduce, gradually spend more time at some sport you enjoy. Habitual views can limit your horizon. Let the pleasures of reduced weight lead you to a richer life.

8. Respect your opponent— your appetite

Overeating is accurately described as an addiction. It is a very, very tenacious habit. It may not sound as formidable as other sorts of addiction, but do not underestimate it. Know your enemy and you will have a better chance of defeating it.

9. The liquid diet is not less fattening

Some people accept the belief that a liquid diet is less fattening than a solid one. The form of the food has nothing at all to do with its caloric value. Otherwise, babies, who are naturally on an all-fluid diet, would not triple and quadruple their weight in so short a time.

The Depressed Eater

10. How your body uses alcohol

If a large amount of food is eaten in one sitting, it is gradually digested and used by the body, either converted to energy or stored as fat. If a large quantity of alcohol is consumed at one time, most of it is immediately converted into body heat or soon excreted. The same amount of alcohol taken slowly over a period of many hours is likely to be converted to fat. So, if you plan to have a drink or two, remember that alcohol is less fattening if consumed quickly and at one time than if it is divided between two separate mealtimes. This of course does not apply to the fruit, sugar, and other additives in the drinks.

11. Alcohol can play a trick

When the dieter who has a few drinks one eve-

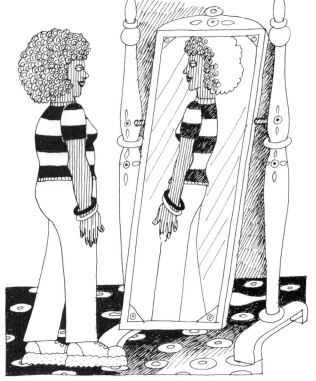

ning steps on a scale the next morning, she may be elated because she has lost weight. It appears that in spite of the extra food and drink, she is doing well!

Depending on what she consumed, the lower weight might actually be genuine loss of fat. The dehydrating effect of alcohol, however, could be the cause. Alcohol combines with body fluid and is excreted with it. The lowered weight may be due to a loss of water that had combined with alcohol, not of fat. Thirst leads to an intake of water to make up for the loss, and that lost weight is soon restored.

12. Habits put on weight

Habit has you put butter on bread when you make a sandwich. Can you eat a sandwich without butter? Sure you can. True, it doesn't taste as good, but you can easily endure it. Mustard, ketchup, and low-calorie dressings may compensate in part.

Butter and other rich spreads add flavor and texture, but they do very little to fill you up. One of the dieter's main needs is to achieve the sensation of fullness without too much cost in calories. Study your habits as you shop and as you cook. See how many fattening additives you can eliminate.

Putting butter on toast, for example, is a common custom that you can change. Another is putting butter on a baked potato. How can you prepare that dish without butter is a question heard repeatedly. The answer is that you can do it easily. An omelet can be made with much less butter than usual without creating cooking problems and with little noticeable difference in taste. Serve vegetables with only a touch of seasoning and herbs, and no butter. There is no sacrifice of bulk.

13. Recipes may be right for some people but not for you

Recipes in cookbooks, newspapers and magazines are generous in their recommended quantities of sugar and shortening. The flour content is usually needlessly large. Salt added to dishes will not add to your permanent weight, but it makes you thirsty. Salt, as butter and other fats, combines with the water you drink and causes a temporary but discouraging increase in your weight.

These ingredients can almost always be reduced or sometimes eliminated entirely with little change in flavor. Make it a habit to question the ingredients in your cooking.

14. How to cut out fat

All meat has some fat, but the proportion varies enormously in different kinds of meat and in different cuts from the same animal. Pork and lamb are particularly fatty and should be selected carefully. Choose lean meat no matter what type it is. Cut off as much fat as you can before cooking. The fatty borders of chops, for instance, can be cut off. Layers of fat on a roast can be trimmed off. Prick the skin of a chicken, turkey, and duck before and during cooking so that the fat can drain away. . . .

15. Life is possible with little or no frying

Skillful deep-fat frying can leave comparatively little absorbed fat in food, but even this small amount adds up to a large number of calories. Avoid frying in deep fat. Use utensils with non-stick surfaces, and apply as little fat or oil as possible to eliminate burning or sticking.

Avoid packaged fried foods. Whether fish, fowl, or meat, they usually have thick layers of rich batter that are a menace to your total calorie allowance.

Broil meats whenever possible. Broiling drains off fat just as roasting does. Boiling is another method that eliminates the need for fat as an aid in the cooking process. Some manufactured meats, such as frankfurters, contain a considerable percentage of fat, and this can be reduced by slicing and boiling them for a short time. Some spices are lost in boiling, but the sacrifice in flavor is not great and is a small price to pay for elimination of the fat.

Basting a roast or a fowl with butter or fat adds flavor, but don't do it. And gravy prepared from meat drippings is not for you. Dehydrated gravy mixes and tomato sauce should be used instead. Stuffing for turkey or chicken needs no more fat than that that comes from the fowl. If you crave stuffing, limit yourself to a very small portion, for it absorbs a lot of fat.

Potatoes baked with a lamb or beef roast are positively delicious, but they are blotters for released fat. Potatoes, boiled or baked, may be enjoyed by a dieter if she realizes that it is not the potato itself but the butter or gravy that is forbidden. Heavy sour cream, too, should be avoided.

Bologna, salami, liverwurst, meatloaf and other ready-to-eat meats may have as much as 30 percent fat added to them, and should be eaten in limited amounts. Another high-fat product is breakfast sausage. A pan in which sausages have been fried is flooded with dislodged fat. If sausages are on your diet list, press them firmly on paper towels after frying to remove as much of the fat as possible.

16. Keep your mind open and you will be surprised at the ingenious ways you will discover or devise to economize on calories

Concoct a tasty Russian dressing using ketchup and low-calorie mayonnaise. A combination of lemon juice, salt and pepper, tomato juice and herbs makes a delicious dressing for lettuce, watercress, and other leafy vegetables.

Dehydrated soups are relatively free of fat and satisfy your hunger because of their large but harmless water content. Cereals, both hot and cold, share with potatoes the fact that it is what you put on them that is largely to blame for their being fattening. Low-fat milk and artificial sweeteners together with some fresh fruit make cereals appealing and fairly low in calories.

Foods especially prepared for dieters are not essential to a successful diet. Such foods typically offer a reduced proportion of fat, sugar or carbohydrate, and are often stacked on store shelves marked "Diet Foods." Some doctors do not recommend these foods for they believe reducing should be accomplished by forming new eating habits and by limiting intake of ordinary foods and avoiding others altogether. They point out that diet foods are not ordinarily on hand at restaurants or at friends' homes and that reliance on these foods may cause a problem. Other doctors believe that the dieting person has a lot of difficulties to cope with already, and she should make use of every aid that is safe, including diet foods.

Read the list of ingredients on bread wrappers carefully. Some breads are low in salt and others in fat, and certain kinds are made with a large proportion of whole grain flour with added hulls. The latter are less fattening than bread made with ordinary refined flour because hulls are almost entirely nonnutritive. They add bulk but are for the most part passed through the digestive tract without being absorbed. Crackers vary enormously in shortening and salt content. Read the labels!

17. Everything weighs something

When you weigh yourself and find that your weight is up a few ounces, and you have been careful to stay with your diet, remember that even drinking an extra glass of water or wearing slippers changes your weight. Don't become gloomy for no reason.

18. Buy something that's too small

If you weigh thirty pounds too much now, figure out what size clothing you would need if you lost six or seven pounds. Make a liberal guess. Buy something that size—a dress or a jacket—even if you have to argue with the salesperson. When you're tempted to break your diet, think about that outfit. Imagine yourself wearing it. When you actually do lose the weight and can wear your new clothes you will feel triumphant!

19. Eat your meals in the same place each day

Whenever possible, use the same chair and sit at the same place at the same table in the same room when you eat your meals. This helps because you learn to associate your diet with those particular surroundings. This reinforces the new eating behavior you are teaching yourself.

20. How you can take a second helping

Take half of the total amount of food you're allowed on your plate. Then take the rest as a second helping. You know you are fooling yourself, but it will help you.

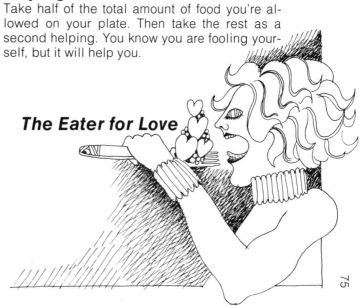

The Eater for Love

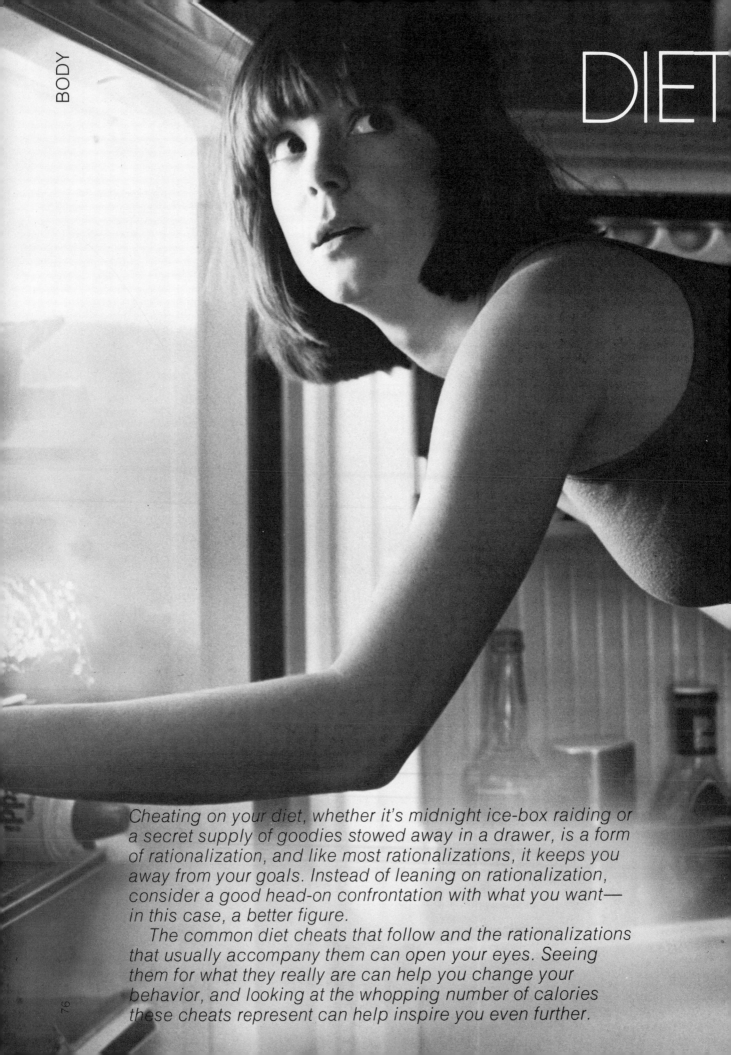

DIET

Cheating on your diet, whether it's midnight ice-box raiding or a secret supply of goodies stowed away in a drawer, is a form of rationalization, and like most rationalizations, it keeps you away from your goals. Instead of leaning on rationalization, consider a good head-on confrontation with what you want— in this case, a better figure.

The common diet cheats that follow and the rationalizations that usually accompany them can open your eyes. Seeing them for what they really are can help you change your behavior, and looking at the whopping number of calories these cheats represent can help inspire you even further.

CHEATERS Are you one? How to stop

THE STASHER

The stasher loves chocolates or cookies or candy bars or who knows what. She rationalizes that if she stashes them out of sight, no one will know her guilty secret. If you're a stasher, remember:
● Be honest enough to put your "hoard" out in the open so you'll have visual confrontation with your habit.
● Keep a written record of how much you eat from the cache and figure the calories on a weekly basis. You'll be shocked.
● Try to train yourself to buy low-caloried substitutes for your forbidden nibbling, then break yourself of nibbling altogether.

CALORIES
1 CHOCOLATE BAR 152*
1 PIECE BOXED CHOCOLATE CREAM CANDY . . 49
1 CHOCOLATE CHIP COOKIE 70
1 OATMEAL COOKIE 80

THE MIDNIGHT RAIDER

The midnight raider does her work when everyone else is asleep. She wakes, checks the clock (and her appetite), rationalizes that it's been a long time since she's eaten last and that no one will catch her anyway, and she heads for the fridge. In the words of one veteran raider, "I just pull up a chair next to the refrigerator and go to work." Next morning there's a stomach full of guilt to live with. To counter these rationalizations, remember:
● Late-night eating gives you no chance to work off the extra calories.
● Your metabolism slows down when you sleep so you don't really need anything more.
● If you absolutely must snack, keep a supply of fresh vegetables and fruit to nibble. A glass of skim milk and a graham cracker or plain sugar wafer cookie won't add too many calories, either.

CALORIES
BOLOGNA SANDWICH 370
COLA TO WASH IT DOWN (8 oz.) 96
1 CUP CHOCOLATE ICE CREAM 272
1 GRAHAM CRACKER 17
1 SUGAR WAFER 18
1 CUP SKIM MILK 95
1 FILLED COOKIE 91

*ALL CALORIES ARE APPROXIMATE.

THE DESSERT INSTEAD OF DINNER EATER

"I'll just have this piece of cake and skip dinner" is the philosophy here. To bypass a meal in favor of a goodie is not so bad occasionally. But, if you're of this mind-set, it probably doesn't happen occasionally, it happens a lot, depriving you indefinitely of good nutrition and the kind of eating habits that could solve a weight problem. Instead of being a meal skipper:

● Try collecting low-caloried dessert recipes that let you eat dinner including a dessert.
● Remember all the times you ate the dessert—and the dinner, three hours later.
● Think ahead. If you know a big dessert is coming, eat smaller portions of everything else. If you're planning the meal yourself, make the main course low-caloried, say chicken or a very lean cut of meat.

CALORIES
SMALL PIECE OF GERMAN CHOCOLATE CAKE 200
CINNAMON STREUSEL CAKE 350
AVERAGE PIECE APPLE PIE 250
AVERAGE PIECE PECAN PIE 300

THE TASTER

Many cooks have eaten the equivalent of a full meal long before anything gets to the table—a taste of this, a mouthful of that. Granted you do have to do a little tasting, but don't make a career of it. Remember:

● Taste only when necessary.
● Taste the smallest amount possible.
● Keep your recipes as accurate as possible to eliminate most tasting.
● Ask friends or whoever is eating with you to taste instead of doing it all yourself.

CALORIES
TABLESPOON WHIPPED CREAM 50
TABLESPOON GRAVY 45
TABLESPOON HARD SAUCE 64

THE ABSENTMINDED EATER

If you've been putting on pounds and you're sure you don't overeat at meals, you may be a victim of the "absentminded eater" cheat. This cheater consumes mounds of popcorn, potato chips, and so on while watching a movie or TV. How much you've eaten may never occur to you until your hand hits the bottom of the empty bowl. If you're this kind of cheater:

● Remember this is real diet trouble because you are unaware of your habit.
● Consciously try to avoid buying snacks at home or out.
● Don't eat your date's snack. If you find you do, ask him to help you discipline yourself or maybe make a pact to break the habit together.

CALORIES
1 CUP PLAIN POPCORN 40
POPCORN WITH 1 T. BUTTER 140
10 POTATO CHIPS 75
1 oz. CORN CHIPS 164
1 oz. CHEESE SNACKS 133
1 oz. PRETZELS 110

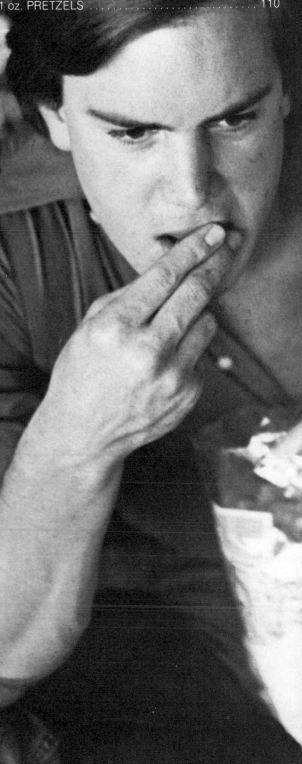

THE OCCASION EATER

"I have to eat the candy if it's a birthday present." The cheater here rationalizes that because it's a special occasion, the calories don't count. The scale will indicate otherwise.

● If you can't trust yourself with a food gift, give it away.

● If the "special occasion" is a party, head for the low-caloried hors d'oeuvre like fresh vegetables without the accompanying dip.

● Have a "whiskey and water" drink, or wine instead of high-caloried mixed drinks.

● Add ice to your old drink instead of having a second.

● If it's a birthday party, a dinner party or holiday eating feast, admit you're dieting and ask for small portions.

CALORIES

DAIQUIRI 190
1 CHEESE PUFF 59
1 PIZZA ROLL APPETIZER 40

HOW MANY CALORIES DO YOU PERSONALLY HAVE TO CUT TO LOSE WEIGHT?

If you have decided you need to trim off a few pounds or more, or if you really just want to be sure you stay at your present weight without letting extra pounds creep up on you, how do you figure the calories it will take? A few simple mathematical steps will tell you. Suppose your present weight is 130. Multiply it by 15 (the number of calories a moderately active person needs to replace per day for every pound of body weight) to get the total calories you are presently eating per day. For example: 130 × 15 = 1950. If you're happy with your weight, don't exceed 1950 calories. To lose, decide on how many pounds you want off in what period of time. Let's decide on losing 5 pounds as an example. Since it isn't medically sound to try for more than two pounds per week unless you're doing it under a doctor's care, you would decide to lose the five pounds over a three-week period. To find out how many calories you have to cut from your present intake per day, multiply the number of calories to a pound, 3500, by the number of pounds you want to lose, five. For example: 3500 × 5 = 17,500. Now divide the number of weeks they are to be lost in, here it's three weeks. For example: 17,500 ÷ 3 = 5833. Next divide that number of calories, 5833, by seven, the number of days in a week. Example: 5833 ÷ 7 = 833. Now subtract the number of calories you need to cut daily, 833, from your present intake. Example: 1950 − 833 = 1117. You will have to limit your daily calories to 1117 for three weeks in order to lose the five pounds. After three weeks, when you've happily lost your five pounds, you'll want to figure the daily caloric maintenance you'll have to keep to hold the five pounds off. To find that, multiply your present weight, 125, again by 15. Example: 125 × 15 = 1875. That's how many calories you'll have to consume daily to hold your new weight.

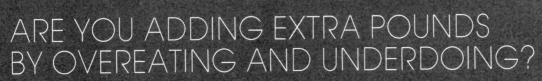

ARE YOU ADDING EXTRA POUNDS BY OVEREATING AND UNDERDOING?

One out of every two Americans is a winter weight gainer, and the usual gain is seven or more pounds. Part of the gain is due to decreased activity—winter laziness. In fact, Charles T. Kuntzleman, national program director of the Y.M.C.A. Fitness Finders Program, believes that most weight gain, summer or winter, is more a matter of underdoing than overeating. Another point of consideration is that muscle tissue burns calories, while fat tissue burns none; therefore, the better your muscle tone, the more calories you'll dispense with. If that doesn't convince you to do something about lazy winter slump—or any season slump—perhaps the approximate calories expended in an hour of these activities will.

TYPICAL WINTER ACTIVITIES	CALORIES for an hour of activity
CROSS COUNTRY SKIING	1200
DOWNHILL SKIING	594
ICE SKATING (LEISURELY)	350
BOWLING (CONTINUOUSLY)	270
RAKING LEAVES	480

TYPICAL SUMMER ACTIVITIES	CALORIES for an hour of activity
BACKPACKING (20 lb. PACK)	450
TENNIS	426
BIKING (5½ m.p.h.)	240
JOGGING	660
SWIMMING	430

Are you obsessed with being THIN?

By Barbara Coffey

Not every diet turns out to be a good one. As you'll see in the case of the young woman in this article, a diet can sometimes turn into a tragedy. No one knows exactly why some young women become obsessed with thinness and turn dieting into a compulsion, but it's a fact that they do and their number seems to be increasing. It wouldn't be fair to discuss diet and body image without paying serious attention to what happens when dieting goes haywire.

Anorexia is a medical term that means loss of appetite, but anorexia nervosa—the thinness disease—is not a normal, end-of-the-meal loss of interest in eating; it is loss of all appetite, so extreme that it can mean voluntary starvation.

Once thought to be a rare and bizarre disorder, anorexia has become so common that most of us can recite its symptoms as easily as those of the flu. They are frightening symptoms—total loss of appetite, drastic weight loss, erratic eating binges followed by guilt and desperate induced vomiting, laxatives or fits of activity to burn up the calories.

One young woman, whom we will call Cynthia, is typical both of the causes of the syndrome and of all its symptoms. Nineteen now, and a sophomore in college, Cynthia was sixteen when she first developed anorexia, thus falling well within the norm—90 percent of all anorexics are women, and most of them are between the ages of fourteen and twenty-two.

"I was and still am very quiet," says Cynthia. "I'm not the type to yell or fight or be boisterous. Food was my way of expressing myself, I guess." Not eating, she explains with some insight, was a kind of passive resistance to a father who tried to control every aspect of her life from the grades she earned to the way she rode a horse. The constant pressure was very hard on Cynthia, who, like many anorexics, is a driver–achiever; she was and still is a straight-A student.

"There was also a feeling of competition with my mother," she goes on. "My mother is very slim and works at it. She and my father divorced; she remarried when I was six and maybe I felt I had to compete with her on a thin-ness level or I'd lose the affection of my step-father, and he'd leave just as my father had.

"I didn't think people liked me," Cynthia continues, "and I thought if I were thinner, they would like me more." At sixteen, Cynthia weighed 105 pounds and stood five-foot-three. But many anorexics do start out overweight; once they begin dieting, however, they continue to the point of starvation.

The crisis in Cynthia's life came at the end of a summer spent at her father's beach house. She dieted the entire summer. "I guess it got so bad because there were just the two of us and I felt so controlled. Some days, all I'd eat was an apple." When her mother and stepfather came to pick her up, they were shocked at Cynthia's weight—seventy-six pounds—and at her lack of energy and total loss of enthusiasm for anything. They took her immediately to a doctor, who hospitalized her to prevent her from literally starving herself to death.

In the hospital, behavior modification therapy was begun. Behavior modification is one of the two most common methods used to make anorexics gain weight. The other, gastric tube feeding, is limited in duration. Eventually, the anorexic must begin to eat on her own.

Cynthia's treatment was standard. "They put me in a hospital room and took away all my privileges. I had no phone, no books, no TV, nothing. They'd just bring me my meals, and when I gained a quarter of a pound, I got a privilege returned. I felt desperate and isolated, yet I wouldn't cooperate. I'd make friends with one of the interns and get him on my side and he'd sneak in a book or some other diversion. I became a real pro at manipulating people—something I'd never felt I could do before. What made me maddest about the hospital was that when I did cooperate and eat and gain, it was natural that sometimes my weight would fluctuate and I'd lose a bit, even though I was eating. If I lost just one quarter of a pound, I'd go back to ground zero, no privileges again. I thought that was terribly unfair, but now I realize how urgent it was that I gain some weight.

"All during that time, I felt that everyone was trying to control my life," Cynthia recalls, "and I didn't want to give up the one thing that I could control—my weight."

Several months later, when she had gained enough weight to be out of physical danger, Cynthia came home. But she still would not eat normally. "I'd try not to eat without causing a commotion. Sometimes I'd eat like crazy, then make myself throw it all up." The pattern continued for almost one more year. "Finally," Cynthia says, "I just got tired of feeling crummy all the time, so I started to get better. I love riding, and my family had really sacrificed to buy me a super horse. I wanted to ride that horse in competition, but I knew at eighty-six pounds, I couldn't possibly control her. I gained the weight," she says with resignation in her voice.

Cynthia at first, and later her mother, father, stepfather and two brothers as well, underwent psychiatric treatment to try to discover what caused her anorexia.

I asked Cynthia whether she felt, three years later, that she was over her anorexia. Her weight is normal now, even a few pounds over. "I think it's done with now," she says. "I think I know the difference between an anorexic body and a normal one. [Many anorexics develop a distorted body image. They become unable to recognize that they look cadaverous; the image that stares back at them from the mirror is never thin enough, and often appears overweight to them, even at a starvation level. Many anorexics are unable to pick their own body from a group of pictures.] I don't want to look and feel that way again. I have too many things to do with my life now; I'm committed to becoming a doctor. I do think I want to diet off a few pounds, but I think I can control it now."

Can Cynthia control it? According to Dr. Richard Green, associate director of the Department of Psychiatry at Long Island Jewish—Hillside Medical Center, many anorexic women become "cured" in the sense that the threat of starvation is dismissed. But the anorexic tendency stays with them for life; the anorexic is obsessed with thinness. Dr. Green, an authority on anorexia nervosa, explains the difference between the anorexic's view of thinness and a normal person's: "An anorexic pursues thinness not because she wants to look prettier or more fashionable, but because she is *obsessed* with thinness."

Interestingly, a preoccupation with food is common to the anorexic. Roughly 25 percent of all anorexics have compulsive eating binges followed by depression and attempts to undo the calories. They are also often likely to be closely involved with the cooking and preparation of foods for others.

Dr. Green feels that the causes of anorexia nervosa are complex and vary from patient to patient. Some themes, however, predominate, among them: a feeling of not belonging to a family unit or peer group and a sense of lack of control over one's own life, a feeling that something or someone is running you and supplying the goals. In searching desperately for something that's truly their own to control, anorexics seize on their bodies. As Dr. Green points out, "Anorexia can be an attempt to control the victim's whole world through her eating habits."

A common pattern among adolescent anorexics is a fear of an inability to deal with the complexities of impending womanhood, and/or a reluctance to accept society's standard definition of femininity. Indeed, many anorexics reverse their femininity: not eating causes menstrual periods to stop and breasts to shrivel, so that anorexic young women look more like young boys than ripening women.

Not all cases of anorexia nervosa are so dramatic as Cynthia's. Many anorexics don't abuse their body badly enough to require medical treatment. But emotional damage is still a danger. Dr. Green points to five signs of anorexia or of the tendency to anorexia:

1. A constant preoccupation with food, either with eating it or not eating it.
2. A strong involvement with preparation of food for others without any interest in eating it oneself.
3. An overly enthusiastic pursuit of thinness, even when family, friends and standard weight tables regard one as far too thin.
4. Weight loss severe enough to cause periods to stop.
5. Weight loss of 25 percent or more of normal body weight, with no apparent physical cause. (This condition in itself justifies a clinical diagnosis of anorexia nervosa.)

Most anorexics can be helped through psychiatric treatment and by the sympathetic attention of friends and family. The difficulty lies in getting the anorexic to allow herself to be helped. Since anorexics usually do not see themselves as too thin, they ignore the major symptom of their disease. Ordinarily, anorexics seek help, or are willing to be moved in that direction, only when they begin to suffer severe physical discomfort—extreme fatigue, dizzy spells, loss of interest in their surroundings. For that reason, it may be useful, when dealing with an anorexic, to bide your time and urge her to accept help when real physical difficulties have surfaced. Dr. Green emphasizes, however, that it's imperative to get immediate medical treatment for an anorexic who has lost 25 percent of her normal body weight.

To a degree, anorexics may be yet another casualty of our increasingly pressured society. The sense of aloneness and isolation that many young adults feel is reflected in the enormous popularity of groups like Hare Krishna and the Sun Myung Moon movement, and the widespread interest in Eastern philosophy and religion. These groups offer a sense of belonging; the Eastern philosophies offer a retreat, if brief, from the pressure to achieve and compete. They are reflective, slowed-down systems of belief that encourage the individual to turn inward in order to escape from the frantic, hectic pace of life.

Sooner or later most of us learn that it's necessary to slow down and experience ourselves and our own private universe. I asked Cynthia at the end of our conversation what she thought would happen if she did not, as she plans to, accelerate her college courses and enter medical school early. I suggested that it might be rewarding for her to take a little time out to find out who she is. "I think it would be great," she exclaimed with enthusiasm, "but I don't have the time."

There's nothing simple about the causes of anorexia, but maybe something so simple as expanding our values can help to make everyone feel it's all right to take things easy now and then, to feel our ways slowly and to mature with the sure knowledge that we do belong. Most importantly, we belong to ourselves, and ultimately, control a major part of our lives.

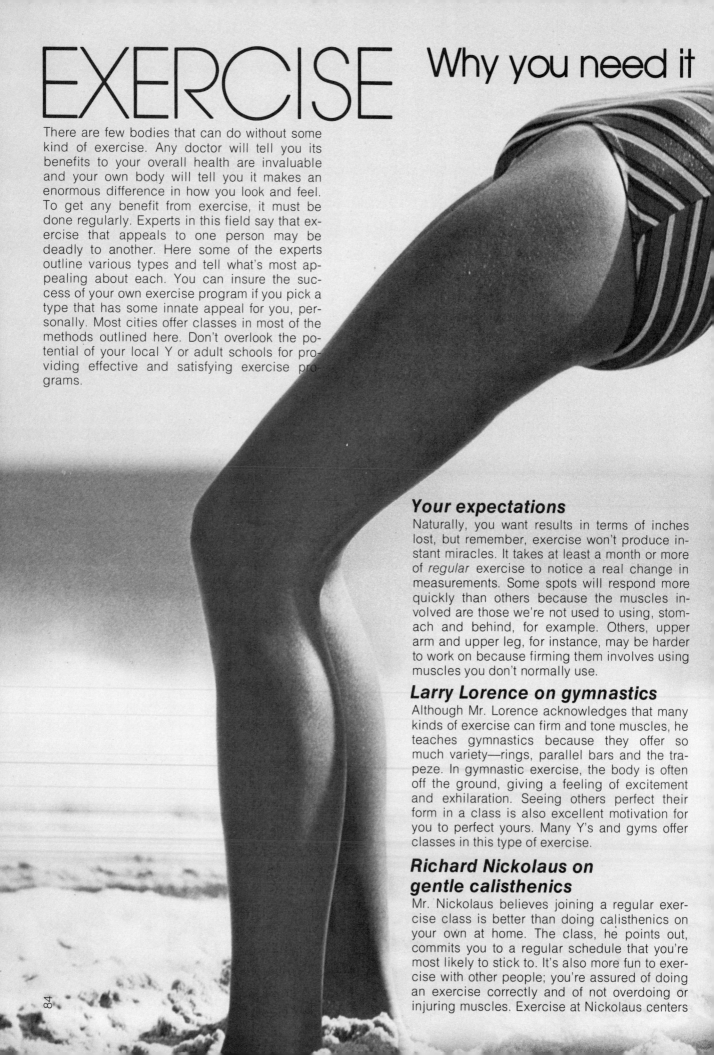

EXERCISE

Why you need it

There are few bodies that can do without some kind of exercise. Any doctor will tell you its benefits to your overall health are invaluable and your own body will tell you it makes an enormous difference in how you look and feel. To get any benefit from exercise, it must be done regularly. Experts in this field say that exercise that appeals to one person may be deadly to another. Here some of the experts outline various types and tell what's most appealing about each. You can insure the success of your own exercise program if you pick a type that has some innate appeal for you, personally. Most cities offer classes in most of the methods outlined here. Don't overlook the potential of your local Y or adult schools for providing effective and satisfying exercise programs.

Your expectations

Naturally, you want results in terms of inches lost, but remember, exercise won't produce instant miracles. It takes at least a month or more of *regular* exercise to notice a real change in measurements. Some spots will respond more quickly than others because the muscles involved are those we're not used to using, stomach and behind, for example. Others, upper arm and upper leg, for instance, may be harder to work on because firming them involves using muscles you don't normally use.

Larry Lorence on gymnastics

Although Mr. Lorence acknowledges that many kinds of exercise can firm and tone muscles, he teaches gymnastics because they offer so much variety—rings, parallel bars and the trapeze. In gymnastic exercise, the body is often off the ground, giving a feeling of excitement and exhilaration. Seeing others perfect their form in a class is also excellent motivation for you to perfect yours. Many Y's and gyms offer classes in this type of exercise.

Richard Nickolaus on gentle calisthenics

Mr. Nickolaus believes joining a regular exercise class is better than doing calisthenics on your own at home. The class, he points out, commits you to a regular schedule that you're most likely to stick to. It's also more fun to exercise with other people; you're assured of doing an exercise correctly and of not overdoing or injuring muscles. Exercise at Nickolaus centers

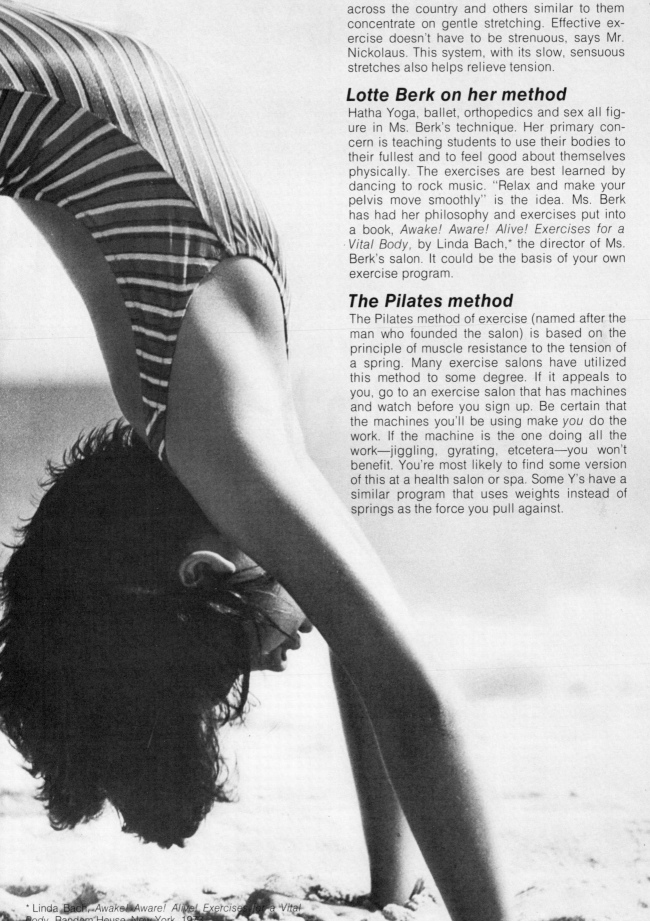

what kind works best for you

across the country and others similar to them concentrate on gentle stretching. Effective exercise doesn't have to be strenuous, says Mr. Nickolaus. This system, with its slow, sensuous stretches also helps relieve tension.

Lotte Berk on her method

Hatha Yoga, ballet, orthopedics and sex all figure in Ms. Berk's technique. Her primary concern is teaching students to use their bodies to their fullest and to feel good about themselves physically. The exercises are best learned by dancing to rock music. "Relax and make your pelvis move smoothly" is the idea. Ms. Berk has had her philosophy and exercises put into a book, Awake! Aware! Alive! Exercises for a Vital Body, by Linda Bach,* the director of Ms. Berk's salon. It could be the basis of your own exercise program.

The Pilates method

The Pilates method of exercise (named after the man who founded the salon) is based on the principle of muscle resistance to the tension of a spring. Many exercise salons have utilized this method to some degree. If it appeals to you, go to an exercise salon that has machines and watch before you sign up. Be certain that the machines you'll be using make you do the work. If the machine is the one doing all the work—jiggling, gyrating, etcetera—you won't benefit. You're most likely to find some version of this at a health salon or spa. Some Y's have a similar program that uses weights instead of springs as the force you pull against.

* Linda Bach, Awake! Aware! Alive! Exercises for a Vital Body, Random House, New York, 1973.

Creating new
BODY IMAGES

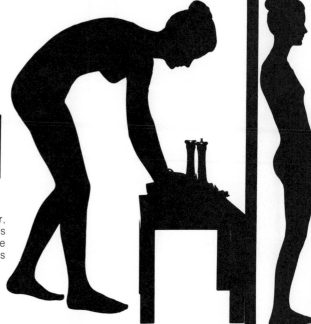

Most of us are aware of being over- or underweight, of having good or bad legs, a thick or thin waist, but few of us are aware of our own body attitudes. The way you habitually sit, stand or walk is probably much more obvious and familiar to others than it is to you. Although exercise, over the long haul, has vast potential for changing your body, creating a new body image by becoming aware of how you do small, everyday things can make an instant positive change in your body image. It can make you *appear* five pounds slimmer, it can make you look vital and fresh instead of tired and draggy. The only trick to changing body attitudes is to become *aware* of them—to think about sitting, standing and walking correctly until it becomes part of you. Here are some tips that will help, worked out by *Glamour* with Jennifer Yoels, who coauthored the fascinating book *Re-shape Your Body, Re-vitalize Your Life,** which you might enjoy.

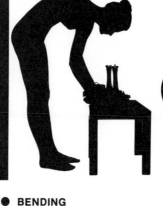

● WALKING
Left: Girl is stepping forward with heel, neither leg in position to bear body's weight. *Right:* body aligned, tummy in, buttocks contracted, weight on forward leg. Back leg is in position for next step.

● BENDING
Above: With feet together, heels bear most of the body's weight. *Right:* weight is borne by forward leg, body is aligned correctly.

● TYPING
Far left: Slumped shoulders, chair is too close, inhibits movement, neck will tire. *Near left:* Looking slimmer, less tiring position.

● LIFTING
Right: Makes your back do the work. *Below:* All muscles used. When stooping for something heavy, center yourself in front of it, walk to it, stoop.

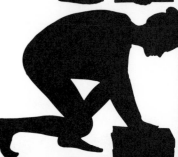

* Yoels, Jennifer, and Dr. L. Larry Leonard, *Re-shape Your Body, Re-vitalize Your Life*, Prentice-Hall, New Jersey, 1972.

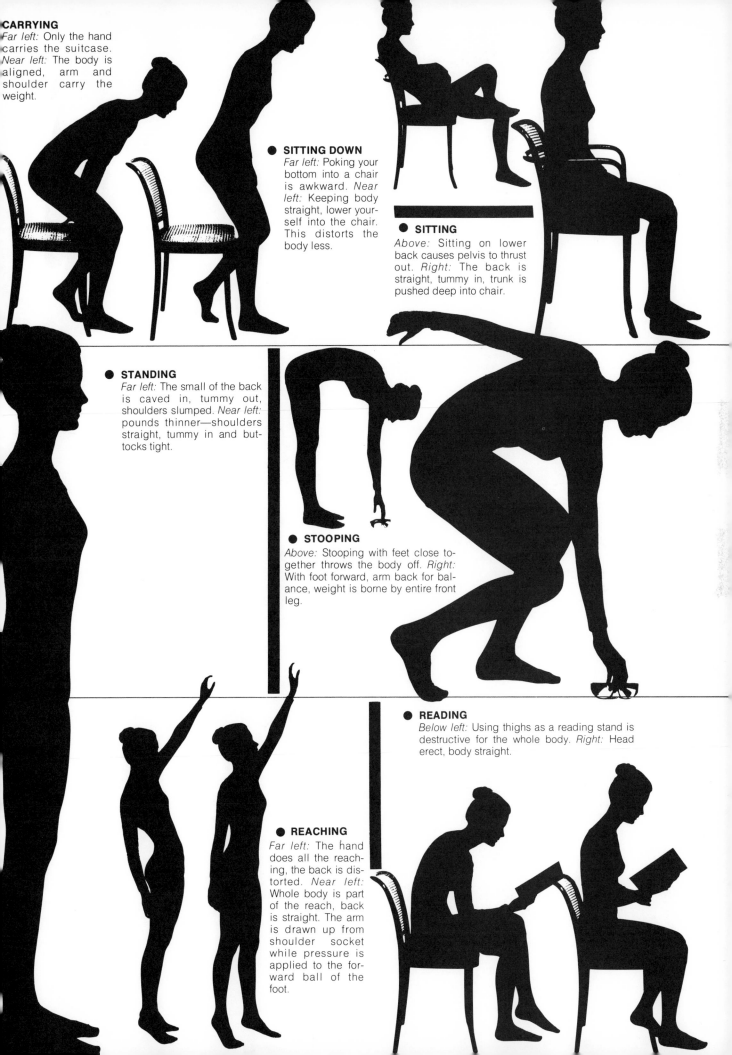

CARRYING
Far left: Only the hand carries the suitcase. *Near left:* The body is aligned, arm and shoulder carry the weight.

● **SITTING DOWN**
Far left: Poking your bottom into a chair is awkward. *Near left:* Keeping body straight, lower yourself into the chair. This distorts the body less.

● **SITTING**
Above: Sitting on lower back causes pelvis to thrust out. *Right:* The back is straight, tummy in, trunk is pushed deep into chair.

● **STANDING**
Far left: The small of the back is caved in, tummy out, shoulders slumped. *Near left:* pounds thinner—shoulders straight, tummy in and buttocks tight.

● **STOOPING**
Above: Stooping with feet close together throws the body off. *Right:* With foot forward, arm back for balance, weight is borne by entire front leg.

● **READING**
Below left: Using thighs as a reading stand is destructive for the whole body. *Right:* Head erect, body straight.

● **REACHING**
Far left: The hand does all the reaching, the back is distorted. *Near left:* Whole body is part of the reach, back is straight. The arm is drawn up from shoulder socket while pressure is applied to the forward ball of the foot.

TEST what shape you are in

If you could talk to the ninety-six million adult Americans who exercise regularly—forty-four million walk, eighteen million ride bikes, fourteen million swim, fourteen million do calisthenics and six-and-a-half million jog—you'd find out that most of them still don't feel they get enough exercise to keep them fit. Do you? Or do you belong to the category of nonregular exercisers, most of whom, according to the President's Council on Physical Fitness and Sports, paradoxically believe they do get enough? In order to find out for sure what kind of physical shape you're in and what kind of endurance you have, take these tests.

Walking test

The object of this test is to determine how many minutes (up to 10) you can walk on a level surface at a brisk pace without undue difficulty or discomfort. Time yourself; don't stroll, don't run, but walk briskly. Note after how many minutes you begin to feel tired and if and when your pace has to slow down in order to continue walking. If you couldn't walk for 5 minutes, you're not in first-rate shape and need some sort of exercise program. If you walked more than 5 minutes, you're in fair shape but still need an exercise program. Breezing through the full 10-minute walk means you're in good shape and probably already are an exerciser. If you would like a booklet of suggested exercises especially geared to results on the tests here, write to: The President's Council on Physical Fitness and Sports, Donohoe Building, Rm. 3030, 400 6th St. S.W. Washington, D.C. 20201.

Walk-jog Test

In this test alternate walking 50 steps (left foot strikes ground 25 times) and jogging 50 steps for a total of 10 minutes. When you jog, try to land gently on the heel of your foot, rocking forward to the ball. If you can't do this, try a more flat-footed style; jogging on the balls of your feet will make your legs very sore. Timing: Walking at the rate of 120 steps a minute (left foot strikes the ground at one-second intervals), jog at the rate of 144 steps per minute (left foot strikes ground 18 times every 15 seconds). If you can't complete the 10-minute test, you need regular exercise, perhaps some form of sports activity. Those who complete the test but get tired and winded are pretty good, but could be even better with more regular exercise. Breezers-through are in good shape and already exercisers.

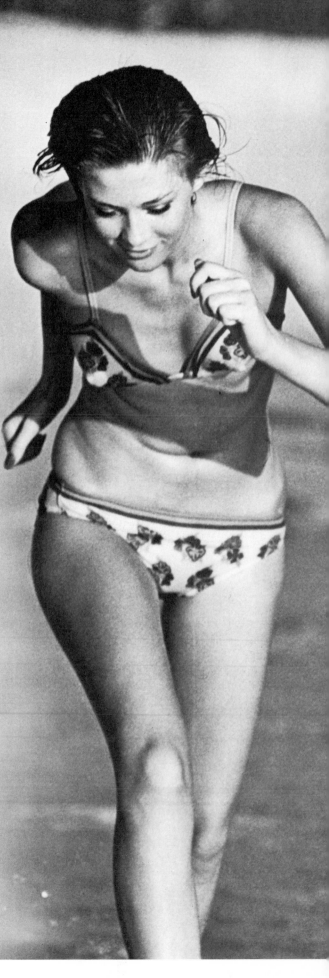

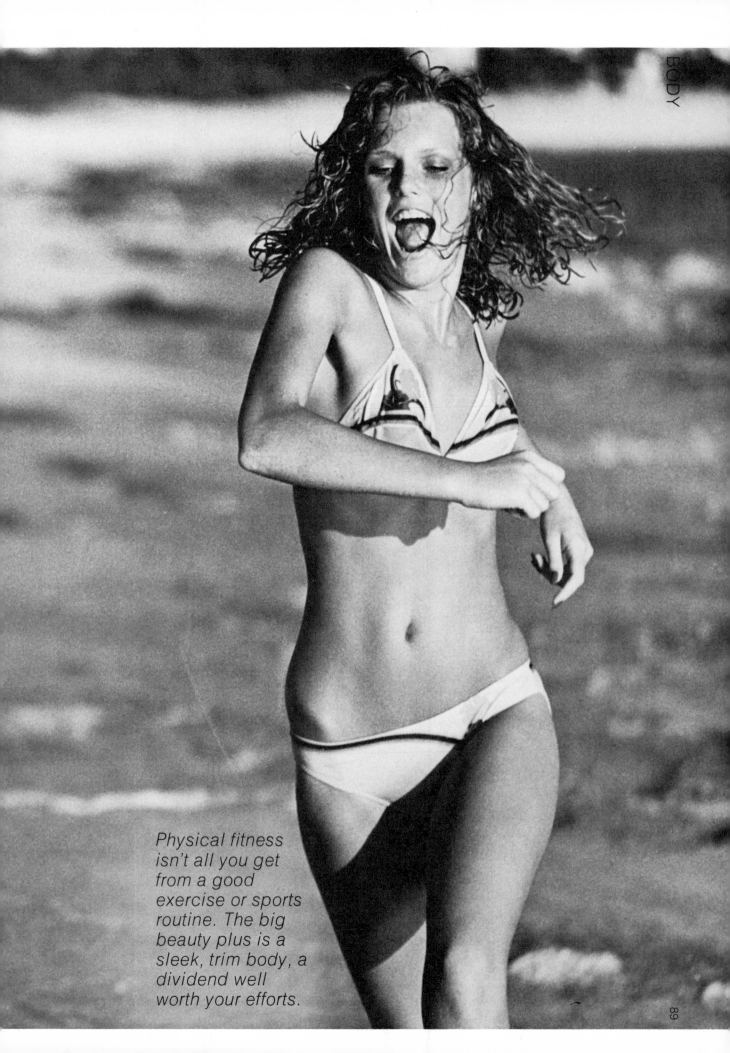

Physical fitness isn't all you get from a good exercise or sports routine. The big beauty plus is a sleek, trim body, a dividend well worth your efforts.

EXERCISE
Do you get the most out of it?

You'll get the most from exercise if you do the kind that increases your heart rate, thus stimulating your entire metabolism. And that doesn't have to mean dull old push-ups. It is likely that your favorite sport fits into this category of stimulating exercise, but you must follow a few rules to get all the figure-sleeking benefits as well as the long-term healthy ones.

Exercise to stimulate

Metabolism-stimulating exercise is often called aerobics and defined by doctors as any activity that pushes your heart rate up to 130 or 150 beats per minute, depending on your age and duration of activity. This activity should be done regularly, 4 to 5 times a week. Regular aerobic exercise gives you a sleek body, but most of all, it stimulates your body processes so they work more efficiently and leave you with more energy. One other plus according to doctors is that sports like swimming, cycling, tennis and skiing are excellent aerobic exercises and exciting to do, so you won't get bored and quit after a few weeks as you might with calisthenics. Dr. Samuel Fox, chief of the Cardiology Exercise Laboratory at Georgetown University, points out that young adults who establish a life pattern of aerobic exercise have a much better chance of avoiding serious heart, respiratory, circulatory and metabolic diseases than nonexercisers. Another interesting fact about aerobic exercise is that its benefits continue after you stop exercising. For example, if you cycle 3 times a week, this amount of exercise will have a carry-over benefit toward your total body functions for several days following the exercise. It's not necessary to cycle everyday to make progress.

Swimming

Swimming is a first-rate aerobic exercise and it uses most of the body's major muscle groups. But Dr. Fox points out: "Swimming" too often means hopping in a pool or the sea, meeting a friend there and standing around talking. That's not exercise. You should swim with a steady, even pace until you're really tired; rest, then swim again. Work up to 20 minutes and see if you can cut your rest periods down to 2 or 3. Before doing any strenuous exercise, check with your doctor to see that you're physically able to do it. If you like swimming and want to center an exercise program around it, consider joining the Y or a health club so that you can swim all year long.

Tennis

Tennis, especially singles, gives your body a real workout. Play for the fun and exercise and don't get worked up when you lose. Anxiety or anger defeat the purpose of aerobic exercise. Again, if you find it impractical or too expensive to play tennis regularly, alternate tennis with something else you enjoy.

Cycling

Bicycling is another good aerobic exercise. Dr. Fox says 15 to 20 minutes of cycling at approximately 13 miles an hour 3 to 4 times a week appears to be an adequate program. Don't cheat by picking downhill riding all the way. Ride where it's not too hilly but you still have to do some pumping. Ride to work or school everyday and you'll have your exercise for the week done. Buy a speedometer to see how fast and how far you go.

Skiing

Skiing is more than fun, it's one of the best exercises there is. The workout combined with lots of fresh air compound the health benefits and make skiing just about unbeatable. If you don't ski or don't live close to a ski area, try cross-country skiing. You can do it most anywhere there's snow and the exercise is just as valuable as downhill skiing. If you really want to keep skiing a serious exercise, you have to do it regularly, like any exercise, or combine with something else you can substitute when skiing isn't practical.

Running and Jogging

Doctors agree that running and/or jogging is first-rate exercise for your body, lungs, and heart. The trouble is, most people get bored with it before long. It doesn't offer the appeal and stimulation of a real sport. It is, however, excellent to fill in with when you can't play tennis, swim or whatever. Some tips about running or jogging. Do it at an even pace, don't rush, and don't pound your heels down on the ground—this can cause tendon damage. Work your way up to at least 15 minutes of running 3 times a week if you plan to make it your main form of exercise.

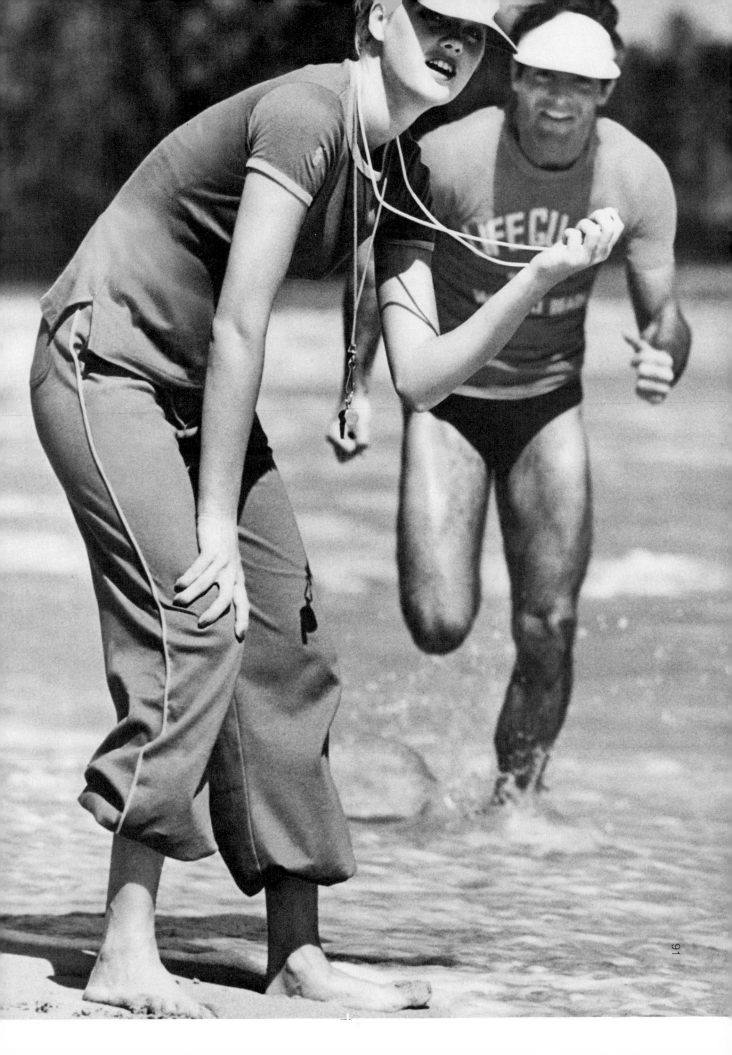

YOUR BODY— WHAT SAGS FIRST

Nothing really sags first, or last, if you make the effort to keep your body in shape through regular exercise, explains Dr. Fritz Fuchs, chief of the obstetric and gynecology staff of one of New York's largest teaching hospitals. But depending on your particular heredity and what stresses your lifestyle puts on your body, he says, different women have to concentrate on different areas. We've numbered the most common trouble areas in the order most people think of them declining: 1. breasts 2. stomach 3. lower hips and backside 4. upper arms 5. underchin and neck 6. legs. It's obvious where the idea that a woman's breasts and stomach sag first comes from—and logical although not consistently true. Since the number one stress on most women's bodies from eighteen to thirty-five is childbirth, it's the breasts and stomach that are usually singled out. And it is a fact that not just having children affects your figure, but also how many you have, how they are spaced and whether or not you breast-feed them. Regardless of the stresses, according to Dr. Fuchs, if you're a faithful exerciser you'll be rewarded with a trim, healthy body. Forget the misconceptions about what goes first and think of exercise as a way—the only way—to give your body the kind of firm muscular substructure it needs to see you through life.

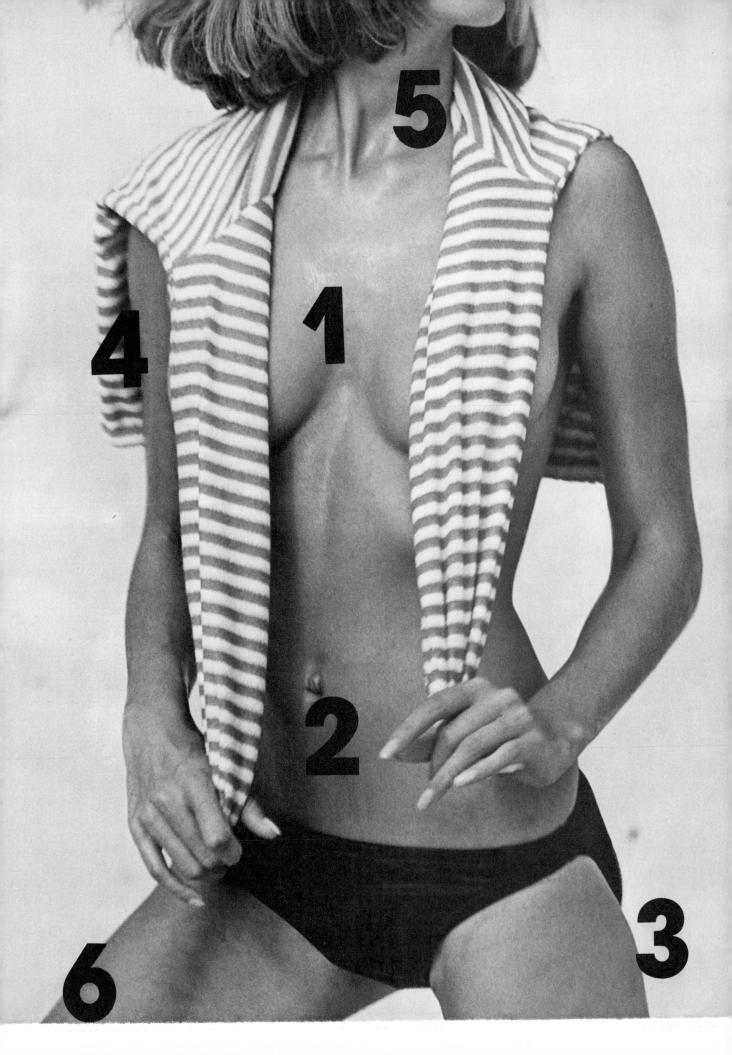

buttocks and thigh firmer

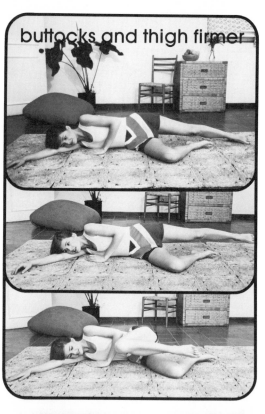

EXERCISE

For the active life

These exercises won't just help you smooth out an accumulation of bumps and bulges, they're also a great way to keep healthy and to stay in shape for your favorite sport.

Exercise left: Lie on side, head resting on outstretched arm, other arm on floor for support. Bend underneath leg. Raise top leg to hip level. Bend and straighten leg 15 times. Repeat on opposite side. All exercises by Marjorie Craig.

● Tip: Exercise is most effective if you don't let working leg touch floor.

Exercise below: Lie on back. Raise body from floor. Raise one leg, bending at knee, and touch fingers to toes. Lie back and repeat with other leg. Do 10 times.

● Tip: *Roll* spine gently as you raise body. Don't jerk; it's bad for your back.

stomach firmer

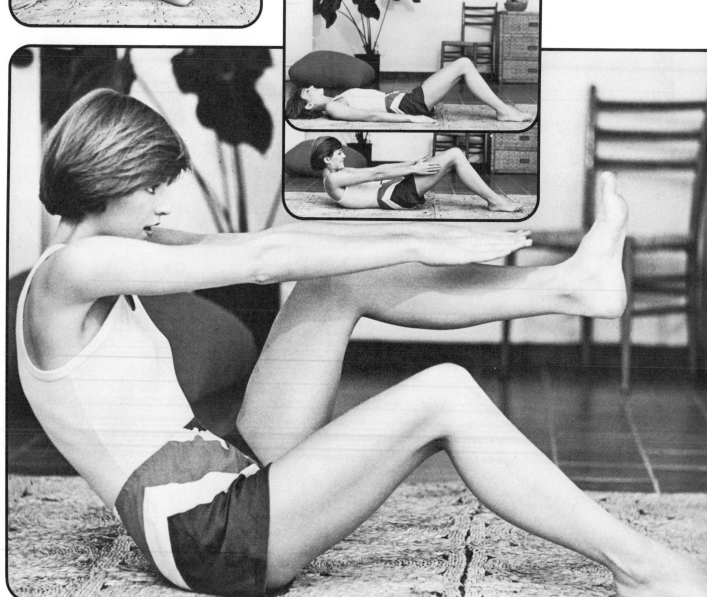

buttocks and thigh firmer

Follow pictures below. Clasp hands, face palms toward ceiling. Lower body, bend knees, hands to floor on left. Straighten up, arms high, bend knees again and place hands on floor in front. Straighten, arms high, hands on floor on right. Do 5 or more, each side.

● Tip: It's a good spine stretcher, works best when you stretch *up* as you raise your arms.

Stand as in top picture, right, feet apart. Tuck in pelvis and bend at waist, keeping back straight, arms hanging down. Bring elbows up, press in at sides. Bring arms behind you and slowly back to bent position pressing in hard. Repeat 10 times.

● Tip: Keep knees flexed and back as straight as possible to get the most benefit from this exercise.

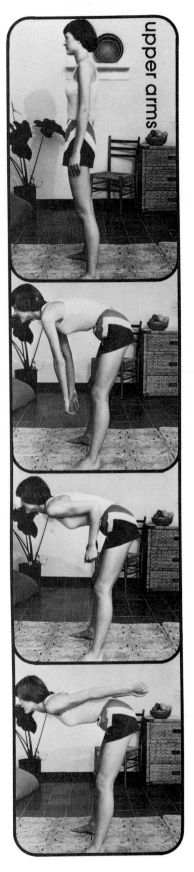

upper arms

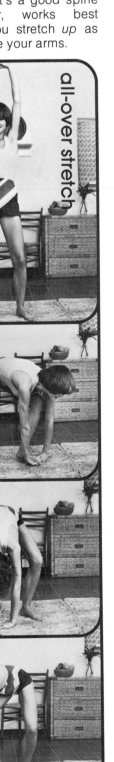

all-over stretch

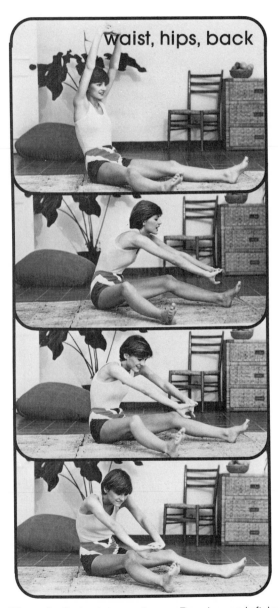

waist, hips, back

Sit as in first picture *above*. Bend over left leg, as far as you can without straining. Come up and bend between legs. Come up and bend over right leg. Do 10 times each leg.

● Tip: To avoid strain, keep knees relaxed. Bend slowly and smoothly.

hip, buttocks firmer

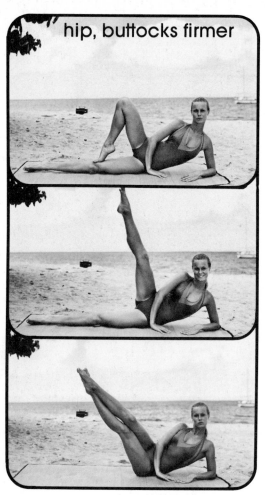

stomach tightener

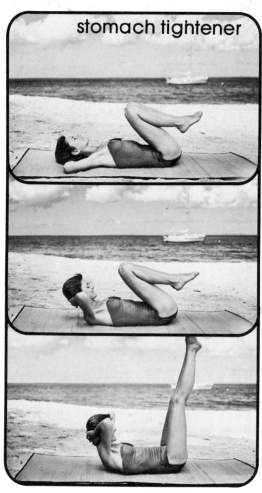

Left: This is really a dancer's stomach exercise. 1. Lie on back, hands behind head, bending knees on chest. 2. Lift head and shoulders, while you breath deeply. 3. Extend legs so that body weight is centered on waist. Return to position 2, then 1.
● Tip: Do not arch spine when extending legs.

Below: This is a belly-dancing exercise. 1. Tilt pelvis forward. 2. Lift right hip. 3. Tilt pelvis back. 4. Lift left hip.
● Tip: Do this in a gentle, undulating motion, very rhythmically, until you're tired.

Above: A jazz beat inspired this. 1. Lie in this position. 2. Extend top leg high into the air, keeping leg turned out. 3. Lift leg on floor to touch extending leg. Return to position 2, then 1. Repeat, opposite side.
● Tip: Keep spine off floor as you reach with lower leg.

Below: This is a ballet exercise. Stand as in picture 1. 2. Begin lifting and stretching ribs on left side as you bend right leg. 3. Lean forward and fold body over right leg. Slide hips to center, leaning body between legs (not shown). 4. Slide hips over left leg. 5. Stretch ribs on right side as high as possible while keeping left leg bent.
● Tip: Bend with back straight.

waist trimmer

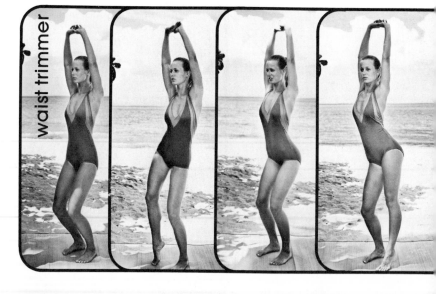

whole body stretch

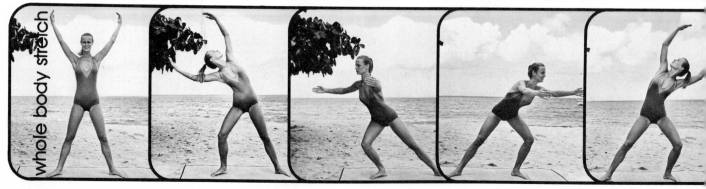

MORE EXERCISE

These "dancercises" are as much fun to do as they are for you. Do them indoors or out, wherever the mood strikes you.

Anything from tap dancing to jazz inspired these exercises. To get some fun from them, use your whole body and do them with a sense of rhythm. The amount of times you do each will vary depending on you. Work up only to the point of strain, don't push yourself beyond this.

leg firmer

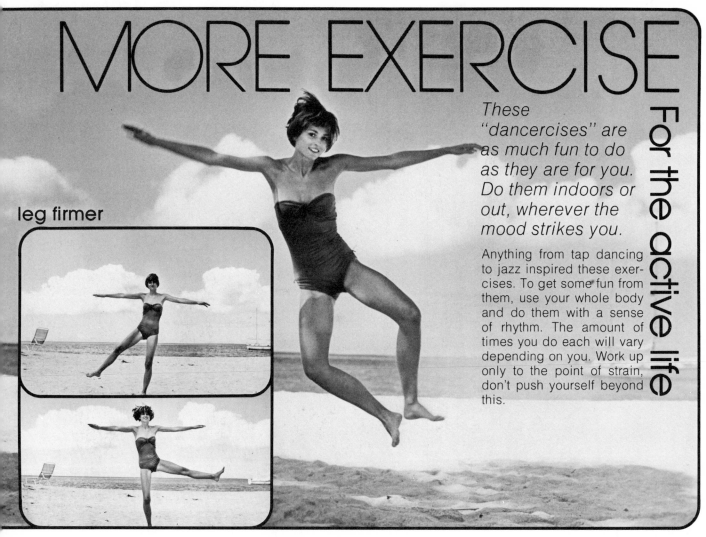

Top: The "Bell Kick," a tap dancing step you might have seen Gene Kelly do, inspired this leg firmer. 1. Jump twice on left leg. 2. Jump twice on right leg. 3. Step 1 and jump up, clicking heels together on count 2. Repeat on opposite leg.
● Tip: You'll get a nice sense of rhythm from this if you count as you do it. Count 1, 2, as you jump on each leg, 3 and 4 as you actually jump up and click heels together.

thigh firmer

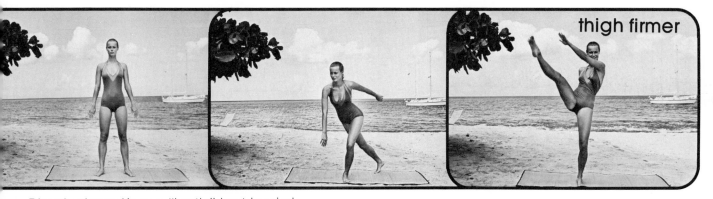

Directly above: Keep a "hustle" beat in mind—or exercise to hustle music—as you do this kick. 1. Stand with feet apart. 2. Bend left knee while extending right leg behind you. 3. Kick right leg high and try to straighten left leg. Return to position 2, then 1. Repeat on other side.
● Tip: Keep your movements smooth and stretch your spine long; it will look more graceful and you'll get more out of the exercise.

How long before those bulges start to budge?

No two bodies are alike—either in shape or metabolism. That's part of what makes keeping in shape such a challenge. But diet and exercise are a combination that work for everyone and the chart below will give you an idea of how long it takes before you see results in pounds. Conscientious exercise can start paying off in as little as 2 weeks in terms of firmer muscles. The pound loss is based on a diet of about 1200 calories a day. The less you weigh or the shorter you are, the less fuel your body needs, so bear this in mind and stay close to the 1200 figure. Also, the closer you get to your ideal weight, the longer it takes to lose pounds.

Present Weight	Amount You Want to Lose	Time It Takes
115–125	5	4 weeks
	10	8 weeks
126–135	5	3 weeks
	10	6 weeks
136–145	5	2½ weeks
	10	5 weeks
	15	8 weeks

No one should be fooled into thinking exercise alone will shape up a really overweight body. It won't. That's why the pound-loss figures are based on a low-calorie diet. But exercise can make even an overweight body appear trimmer and help smooth out the bulges. The sooner you begin exercising, the sooner those bulges go, so start shaping up now. Stomach and waist respond first, hips and thighs take a little longer.

The right proportions make the difference

Any body, even if it's a few pounds heavier than it should be, will look better if everything is in proportion. Check yourself out against the guidelines here, remembering that they are ideal and few women fit them perfectly.

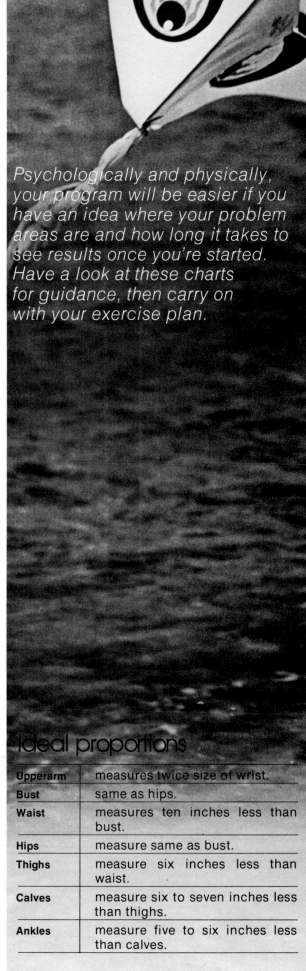

Psychologically and physically, your program will be easier if you have an idea where your problem areas are and how long it takes to see results once you're started. Have a look at these charts for guidance, then carry on with your exercise plan.

Ideal proportions

Upperarm	measures twice size of wrist.
Bust	same as hips.
Waist	measures ten inches less than bust.
Hips	measure same as bust.
Thighs	measure six inches less than waist.
Calves	measure six to seven inches less than thighs.
Ankles	measure five to six inches less than calves.

BODY SLIMMING

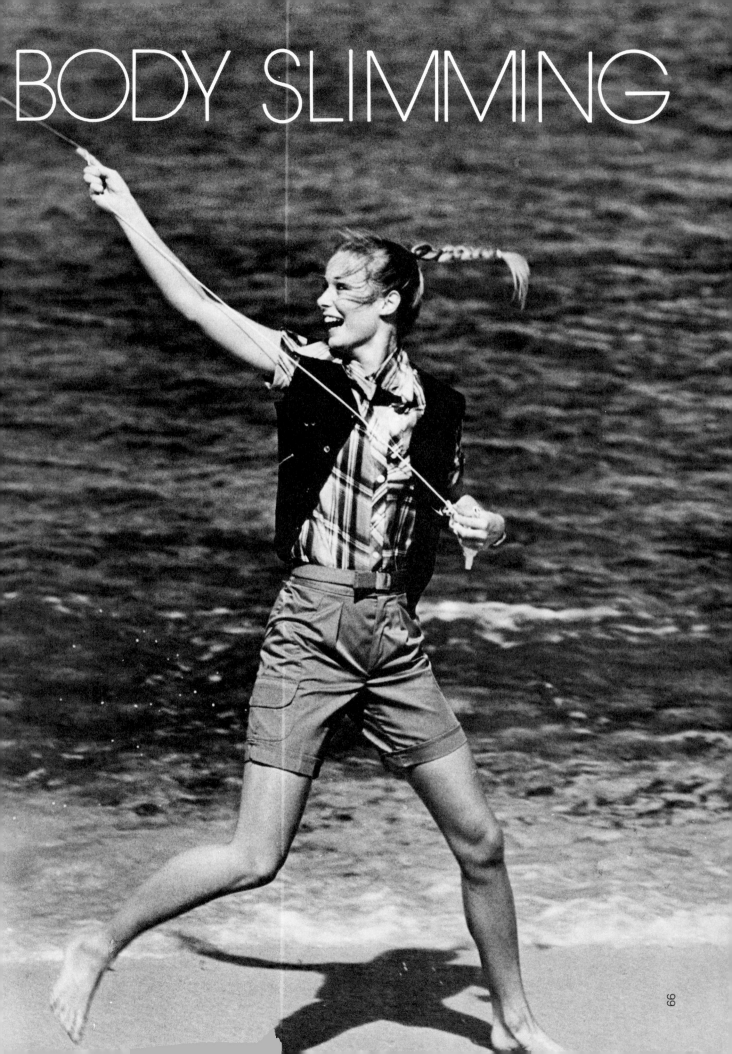

BODY SHAPING

You won't find it hard to spare time to do these body-shaping exercises because they can be part of a day's fun at the beach, by the pool or even in your backyard or bathroom. All you need to get started is a big bath towel, which acts as a force to pull against, making the exercises doubly effective. For best results, do exercises at least five times a week, everyday is better yet. Before you start any exercise routine, check with your doctor to be sure you're in good shape physically to do them.

for abdomen, hips, buttocks

Right: Place towel behind heels on ground. With back straight, reach between legs with right hand to pick it up. Stand, as center, towel in left hand. Drop towel behind you, bending knees, back straight. Repeat 6 to 10 times.

for entire torso

Stand as in photo, right. Bend at waist to the left, keeping arms and knees straight. Touch right hand to left foot. Return to standing position; alternate, touching left hand to right foot. Repeat 15 times.

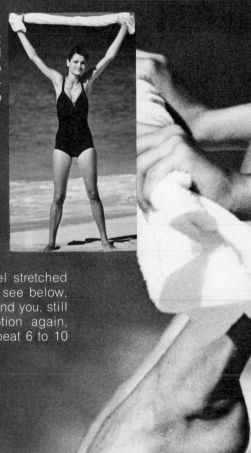

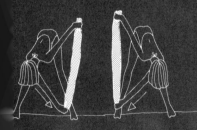

Stand as in picture, left, with towel stretched taut. Slowly raise arms over head, see below, keeping towel taut. Bring towel behind you, still taut, then reverse this whole motion again, crossing and uncrossing arms. Repeat 6 to 10 times.

for arms, back

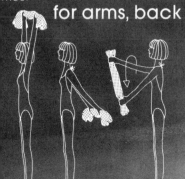

Exercises to do with a towel

for entire leg

Sit with legs extended, towel held with 2 hands out in front of you. Without changing towel position, bring knees to chest: see large photo left. Then extend knees over towel and stretch legs, illustration above right. Hold. Return to original position and repeat 4 to 8 times.

for inner leg

Place towel on floor or any smooth surface. Stand on towel, feet apart, see below. Slowly slide feet together, pushing towel up between ankles as you slide. Repeat 10 times.

How to find the
SPORT THAT'S RI
and be really good at it!

By Barbara Coffey

More and more men and women are becoming interested in taking up a sport because they realize that exercise is essential to good health, and one of the most enjoyable ways to get it is through sports. What still holds some people back is a sense of inferiority about their ability to excel in and enjoy a sport. They say they aren't the "athletic type"—usually meaning subliminally that they are worried about their body type—and shy away from exposing themselves on the courts or from competing with others. If you are one of these people, the chances are that whatever your physical or temperamental drawbacks are in terms of body build, you can overcome them with some motivation and awareness of what goes into being good at a particular sport.

Your body type does affect your game, but probably not in the way you think. Some researchers feel that unless you're a professional athlete where endurance and body build are crucial, the fact that you're tall and thin, muscular and average height or short and plumpish aren't so important to your performance in a particular sport as they may be to your *enjoyment* of it.

Dr. William Sheldon, who developed in the early 1940s what has become a classic concept for classifying body types, holds that certain characteristics of temperament also seem to go with each body type. His three basic body types are the ENDOMORPH, who is round and soft with a tendency to gain weight easily; the MESOMORPH, who is muscular, densely built, and often considered the classic "athletic type"; the ECTOMORPH, who is the tall stringbean type. Rarely is anyone a perfect type, most of us are a mixture of all three with one type predominating, although some individuals are pretty well split between two types.

According to Dr. Sheldon's theory of correlation between body type and temperament:

Endomorphs tend to be relaxed, outgoing, affectionate, interested in food and of an even, harmonious disposition. Mesomorphs tend to be aggressive, competitive, extroverted, and

like to take risks. Ectomorphs tend to be tight, restrained and shy, and to love privacy. These are generalizations, of course, and Dr. Sheldon's methods of research have been questioned, but since several different groups of researchers working at different times and places with people of various ages came to pretty much the same conclusion, it's difficult to dismiss the idea.

This concept has been taken further by other experts to demonstrate how and why certain body types might be drawn toward certain kinds of jobs, mates, hobbies and sports.

Dr. George Sheehan, director of Electrocardiology and Stress Taking at Riverview Hospital in New Jersey, worked out the chart here to show which body types might be attracted to which sports and why. One can understand, for example, that the competition in sports like tennis would appeal to the competitive nature of a mesomorph. Since mesomorphs have good muscular skills, they also tend to enjoy "hitting" sports where muscular skill and a certain aggression release are involved. Tennis, baseball and volleyball would be examples of this. The quiet, introverted ectomorph might far prefer the lonely pleasure of skiing down a mountain. She might also enjoy jogging, but not for the muscular activity involved, as the mesomorph would. The ectomorph might appreciate the privacy and noncompetitive side of jogging. Gregarious endomorphs are likely to be drawn to a sport for its social aspects. Swimming, for example, would be appealing if there were lots of people sitting around the pool. Golf with a group of friends would be enjoyable. Endomorphs can also get the most from a sport by playing it in a social situation such as a health club where other people are part of the fun.

If you want some professional examples of this theory, consider the mesomorphic build of skater Dorothy Hamill, whose skill and "cool" did so well in the highly competitive Olympics, or mesomorph Billie Jean King in the nerve-racking competition of professional tennis. Mickie Gorman, an ectomorph, is a champion

GHT FOR YOU . . .

marathon runner, while Olga Korbut and Nadia Comaneci, also predominately ectomorphs, are gymnasts, an activity that's inclined to be more solitary except in actual competition.

As a group, women tend to be more endo-morphic than men, which may account for some researchers saying that men are naturally more suited to sports than women. But women are challenging this idea. More and more women are taking up and becoming skilled at all kinds of sports, both on a professional and amateur basis. Most women seem to feel that they can participate in and become highly pro-ficient in almost any sport. The chief excep-tions, according to a survey of *Glamour* read-ers, are football and wrestling. Because of female cultural scripting, these sports would seem to diminish femininity and, therefore, women tend to avoid them.

When it comes right down to applying all these considerations to yourself, keep upper-most in your mind that almost no one is a per-fect endomorph, mesomorph or ectomorph; we are all mixtures. What doesn't appeal to the en-domorph in you might well appeal to the meso-morph. If you feel you're interested in a particu-lar sport, don't chalk it up as one you're temperamentally unsuited to; give it a try. On the other hand, if you've been trying to get in-terested in a sport, say tennis, and haven't been able to see what the big draw is, the chart may point you toward a sport that might work better. If you feel you're basically an ecto-morph, put your racket down and try jogging, or try swimming at a time and place that will let you enjoy a sense of solitude. No matter who you are and what your body type, there's a sport you can enjoy and benefit from.

MATCH-UP CHART
illustrating which sports best suit which body types

Body Type	Physical Traits	Temperament Traits	Sports Attitude	Might Enjoy
Endomorph	soft, smooth, rounded body, puts on weight easily, especially stomach	loves to eat, loves comfort, enjoys people, uninhibited expression of feelings	likes sports in company of others, likes team sports	swimming, volleyball, tennis—especially doubles, golf
Mesomorph	large-boned, firm, large muscles; not too much fatty tissue	loves power, loves muscular activity, is aggressive and competitive	likes competitive or hitting games, likes skill aspect of sport	tennis, volleyball, jogging
Ectomorph	slender, fragile, small-boned, often tall	loves privacy, hyperalert; shy, lots of nervous energy	prefers solitary sports or one that requires precision, interested in individual contest	jogging or running, sailing, cycling, yoga.

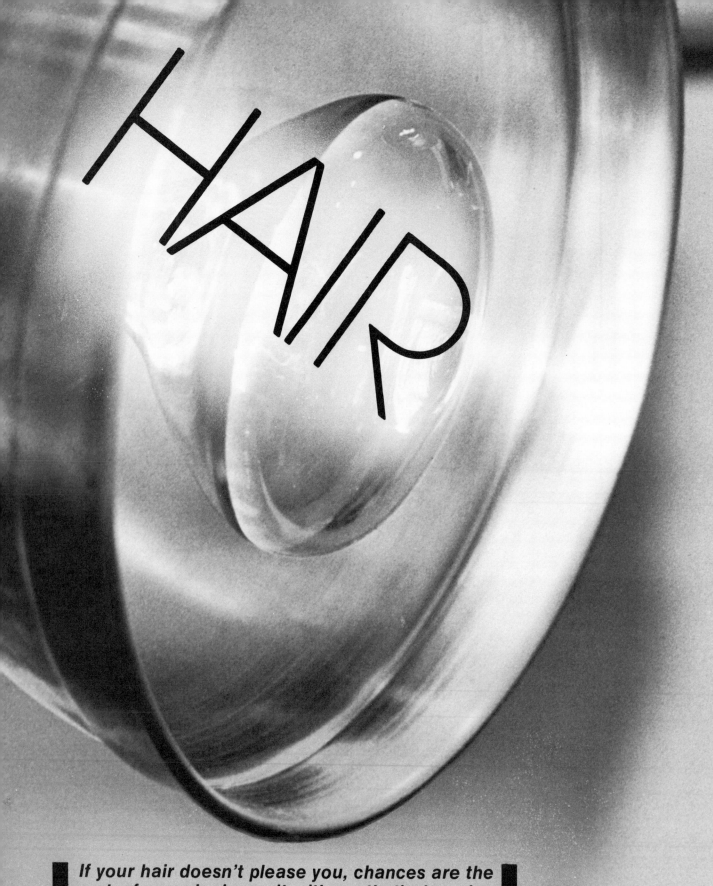

HAIR

If your hair doesn't please you, chances are the rest of your look won't either—that's how important hair is to most women in terms of a total beauty image. What follows in this chapter will help you learn to live realistically with your hair, maybe even to love it, certainly to improve its performance greatly.

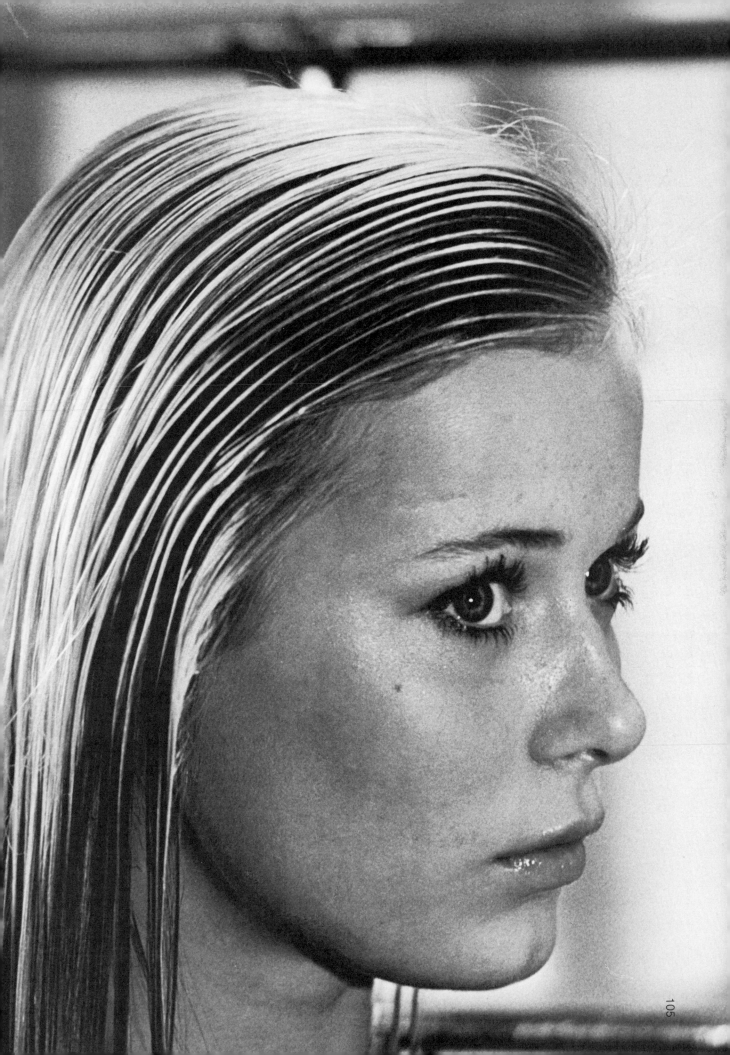

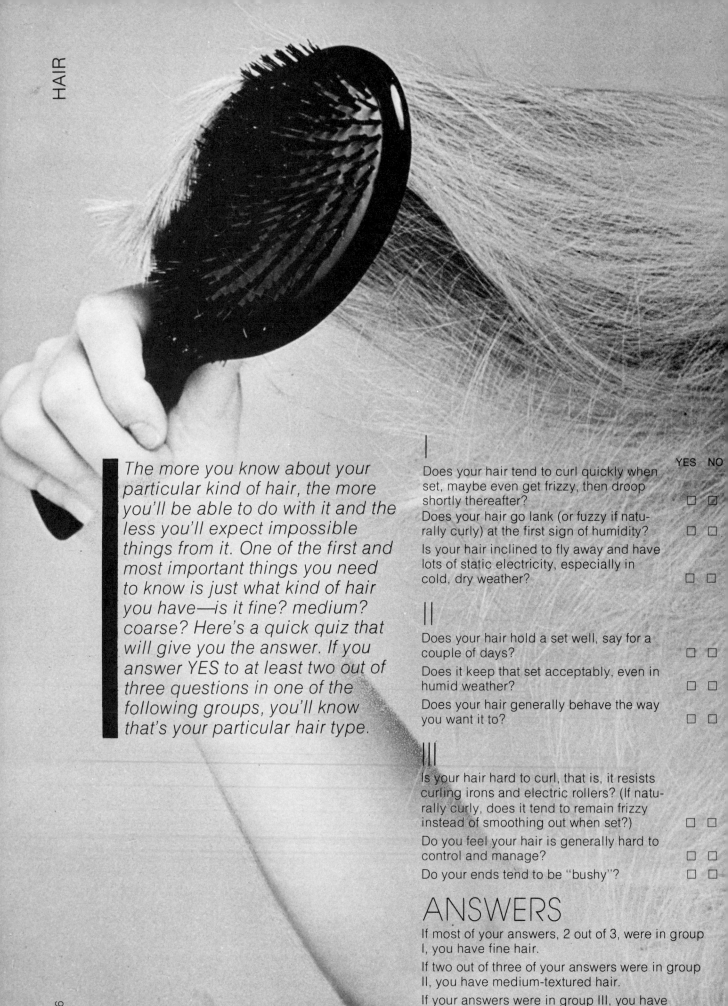

The more you know about your particular kind of hair, the more you'll be able to do with it and the less you'll expect impossible things from it. One of the first and most important things you need to know is just what kind of hair you have—is it fine? medium? coarse? Here's a quick quiz that will give you the answer. If you answer YES to at least two out of three questions in one of the following groups, you'll know that's your particular hair type.

I

	YES	NO
Does your hair tend to curl quickly when set, maybe even get frizzy, then droop shortly thereafter?	☐	☑
Does your hair go lank (or fuzzy if naturally curly) at the first sign of humidity?	☐	☐
Is your hair inclined to fly away and have lots of static electricity, especially in cold, dry weather?	☐	☐

II

	YES	NO
Does your hair hold a set well, say for a couple of days?	☐	☐
Does it keep that set acceptably, even in humid weather?	☐	☐
Does your hair generally behave the way you want it to?	☐	☐

III

	YES	NO
Is your hair hard to curl, that is, it resists curling irons and electric rollers? (If naturally curly, does it tend to remain frizzy instead of smoothing out when set?)	☐	☐
Do you feel your hair is generally hard to control and manage?	☐	☐
Do your ends tend to be "bushy"?	☐	☐

ANSWERS

If most of your answers, 2 out of 3, were in group I, you have fine hair.

If two out of three of your answers were in group II, you have medium-textured hair.

If your answers were in group III, you have coarse hair.

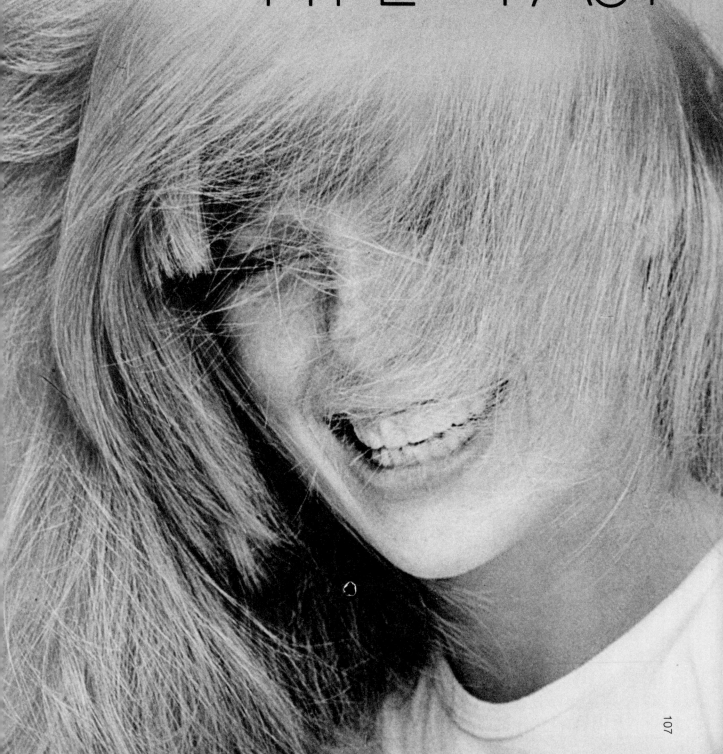

HOW TO FIND YOUR HAIR TYPE—FAST

GORGEOUS HEA

Ask any woman what beauty qualities she feels are most important and you're bound to hear some version of "gorgeous healthy hair" placed high on the list. Judging from what readers tell us, hair care accounts for the biggest expenditure of beauty time for most women, yet it's usually the thing that gives them most trouble. One reason may be a lack of basic information about hair, or conversely, an abundance of misinformation. Here are some straight answers to many of your most frequently asked questions about hair health. What you learn could "change your head."

1. What's the most important thing to know about your own hair?

Its limitations. Learn to live within them and you've got it made. But for a lot of girls, this is easier said than done because they don't really consider their hair's texture—is it fine, medium or coarse? The quiz on the preceding page helped you determine this.

You should also concern yourself with your hair's body or bulk. If the hairs on your head are massed and close together, your hair is thick. If they're sparse, hair is thin. And, of course, the amount of straightness or curliness imposes some limitations.

But first let's tackle just what you can and can't do with certain textures of hair. *Fine hair* is usually thin, looks fullest and best when it's blunt cut and not much longer than chin length. *Medium-textured hair* with medium body can take most any kind of style or length—it has the fewest limitations. *Coarse hair* often responds well to a longish blunt cut. The length tends to weigh the hair down and make it behave. Too short a cut is apt to leave you with hair that bushes and sticks out.

If your hair is curly, no matter what its texture, humidity will make it curl more. Chemical straightening, if it's done carefully, can be a solution if you insist on a straight look. But in gen-

eral, if you live in a relatively humid climate, you'll spend less time and energy and keep your hair in healthier condition if you work out a style that takes advantage of the curl—then just forget it and enjoy life.

Straight hair, especially if it's fine, will usually resist curling except under good weather conditions. So again, your best bet is to find a becoming style that doesn't rely too much on curl. Body waves and setting lotions will help fine hair hold a set, but when the weather is really difficult, you're still better off opting for a straightish look.

2. Does cutting make hair grow faster and healthier?

Although many people believe a haircut will "make hair grow like a weed," it just isn't so. The idea probably got started because after dry split ends are cut off, hair tends to break less and therefore loses less length through breakage. But cutting does not in any way affect hair's growth pattern. Regular trims do make hair look better. Removing dry brittle ends leaves the hair shafts glossy and healthy down the whole length to the very ends. To keep hair at its peak, experts recommend trimming long hair every two months. Shorter hair usually gets trimmed more frequently to maintain the short style.

3. Is there anything that will make hair grow faster?

No, unfortunately. There is nothing you can do that will make hair come out of the hair follicles any faster than nature intended. Hair grows, on the average, a half-inch a month or about six inches every year. It tends to grow faster in warm weather, but the average for a year is still about six inches for most people. Between the ages of fifteen and twenty-five, one's hair grows faster, then slows down gradually. Also, after hair reaches a length of ten inches, it slows down to about half the normal rate of growth.

4. Why is conditioning so important to hair health?

Hair reflects its history. When you consider that any single hair on your head can have a history of as many as six years of sunning, coloring, blow-drying, curling, brushing, swimming and whatever else you can think of to dry it out, it's no wonder hair needs all the help it can get. Actually, hair is dead the minute it leaves the hair follicles, so its care and feeding for the

THY HAIR how to get and keep it

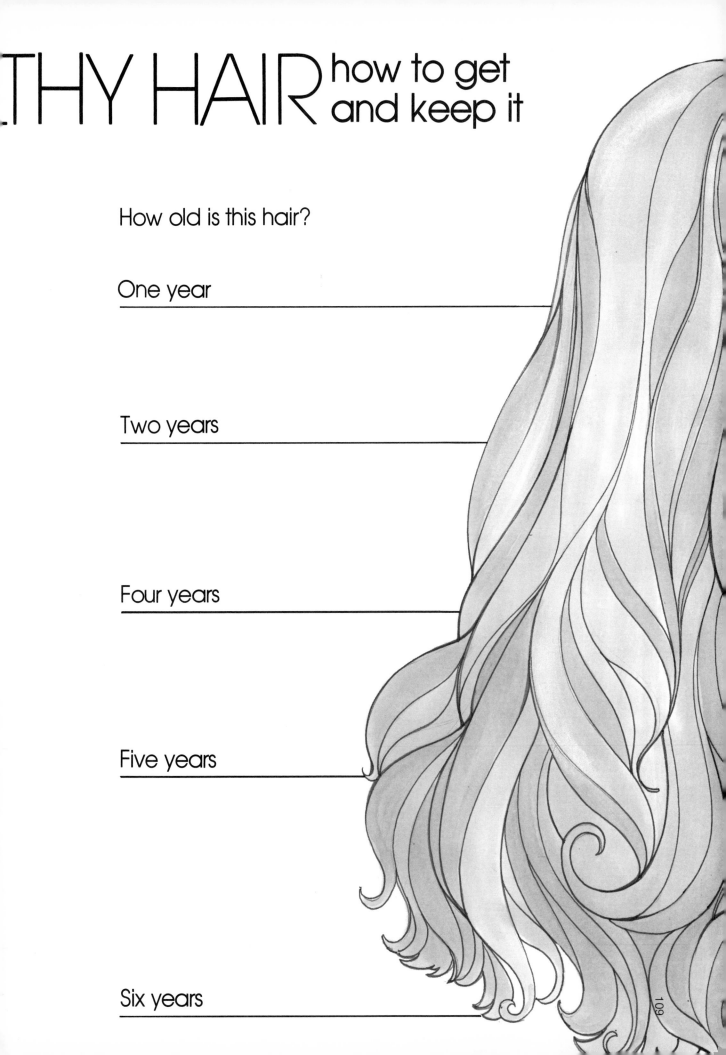

How old is this hair?

One year
_____

Two years
_____

Four years
_____

Five years
_____

Six years
_____

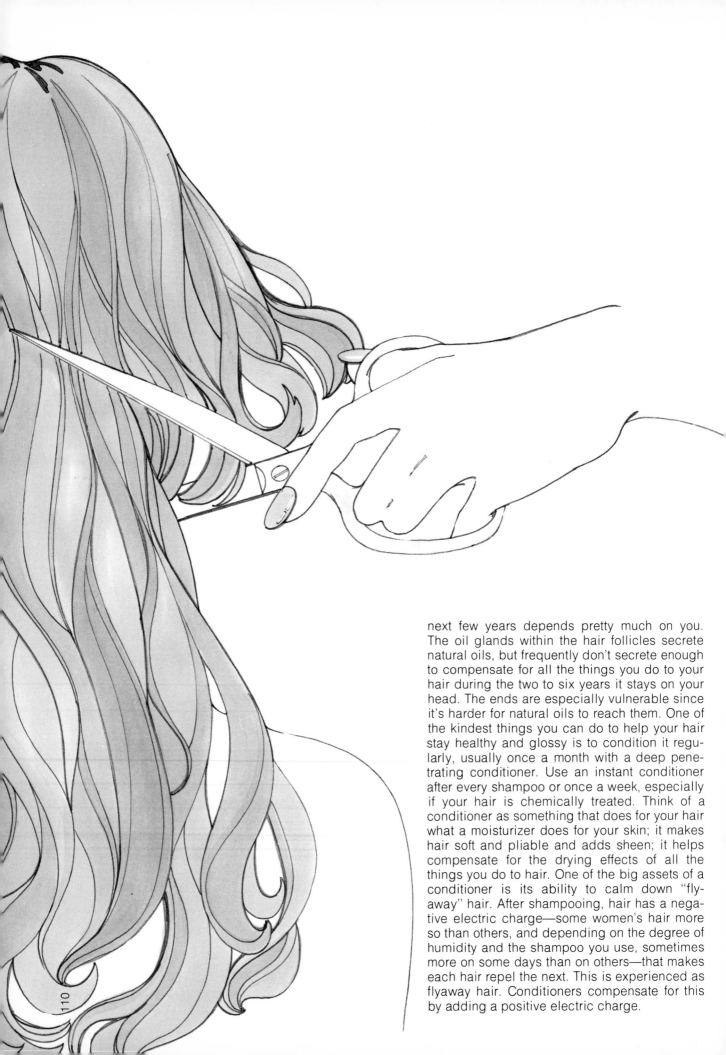

next few years depends pretty much on you. The oil glands within the hair follicles secrete natural oils, but frequently don't secrete enough to compensate for all the things you do to your hair during the two to six years it stays on your head. The ends are especially vulnerable since it's harder for natural oils to reach them. One of the kindest things you can do to help your hair stay healthy and glossy is to condition it regularly, usually once a month with a deep penetrating conditioner. Use an instant conditioner after every shampoo or once a week, especially if your hair is chemically treated. Think of a conditioner as something that does for your hair what a moisturizer does for your skin; it makes hair soft and pliable and adds sheen; it helps compensate for the drying effects of all the things you do to hair. One of the big assets of a conditioner is its ability to calm down "flyaway" hair. After shampooing, hair has a negative electric charge—some women's hair more so than others, and depending on the degree of humidity and the shampoo you use, sometimes more on some days than on others—that makes each hair repel the next. This is experienced as flyaway hair. Conditioners compensate for this by adding a positive electric charge.

5. What's all this business I keep reading about pH in various products?

In simplest terms, pH can be described as the measure of a liquid's acidity or alkalinity. Hair is surrounded by a liquid mantle of atmospheric moisture, perspiration and so forth. Ideally this liquid mantle should be slightly acid. But many of the things we routinely do to hair, such as coloring, permanent waving and straightening, even shampooing, can leave an alkaline residue on the hair. This alkalinity can weaken the hair's structure, making it less resilient or elastic and thus more prone to breaking and splitting. There are many products from shampoos to conditioners aimed at helping to restore or maintain the natural acid/alkaline balance of the hair's moisture mantle. Most will say something about pH on the label to help you recognize them. You may find using such a product especially useful after a coloring, waving or straightening treatment—all of which tend to leave alkaline residue on hair. But most important of all, don't abuse your hair by over-coloring, -waving, or whatever.

6. Is there any way to eliminate split ends, besides cutting?

Cutting is certainly the best, most effective way to eliminate split ends. Some hair salons, especially in Europe, use a process called singeing to remove split ends. A section of hair is twisted tightly so that the broken or split ends pop out. The splits are carefully singed off with a flame. This is a job for an expert in a salon. Many hairdressers find it time-consuming and ineffective for an entire head of hair. Preventing as many split ends as possible in the first place is the best solution. Although everyone gets some splits, hair that's not overprocessed chemically and that's conditioned and trimmed regularly will develop the fewest. The protein shampoos on the market now won't eliminate split ends, but they do help sleek hair ends by smoothing the outer surface of the hair shaft.

7. Is there any way to get rid of oily hair permanently?

There are many things you can do to help *control* oiliness, but nothing will permanently banish it. People with this problem usually notice it first in puberty. The oiliness lessens as you get older, usually with a noticeable decline somewhere between thirty-five and forty years of age. Hot weather stimulates the glands to secrete more oil; cold weather, less.

To help control this condition, shampoo hair as often as necessary with a shampoo for oily hair. Use a light hand with hairspray and setting lotions since they combine with the oily secretions in your hair and add to that "plastered-down" look. Stay away from cream rinses and use a noncream conditioner instead of an oil- or cream-based one. You may find it helpful to limit the amount of very fatty foods you eat. According to Dr. Cyril March, a well-known New York dermatologist, small amounts of fatty food substances, primarily cholesterols, can and do end up almost unchanged chemically on the scalp as well as facial skin. This doesn't mean that you shouldn't eat *any* fat, nor does it mean that a low-fat diet will cure acne if you have it. It simply means that if you are troubled by an extremely oily skin and scalp, an excess of fatty fried foods certainly is not going to help matters.

8. How does taking medication affect my hair?

Many drugs do affect hair. Exactly which ones and their specific effects are too lengthy to go into here, but for the most part, drugs that have a striking effect on hair are usually those connected with very serious illnesses and your doctor will warn you of their effect before you take them. Some women experience increased hair loss after stopping birth control pills. The loss is usually slight and only temporary. Hair growth patterns will return to normal in a very few months.

9. How about those 100 strokes a day?

Back in the days when your great-great-grand-mother had waist-length hair and there were no such things as conditioners to keep hair silky and pliant, there might have been some sense in this old adage, but not today. Dr. Edward Krull, a Detroit dermatologist, speaking at a recent dermatological seminar, states a rule that most dermatologists pass on to their patients: "Brush your hair enough to style and groom it, but not more." Excessive brushing can put stress on hair and cause it to break or split, especially if the hair has been chemically altered in any way. Wet hair is more prone to breakage from brushing than dry hair. Also, excessive brushing can aggravate an oily-scalp condition by both spreading the existing oil and stimulating the oil glands to produce more.

You should remember that brushing your hair to style it is better than combing. The bristles of the brush are flexible and give when they encounter a tangle; the teeth in a comb won't.

10. I keep hearing about proteins in hair products. Can they really penetrate the hair shaft and strengthen it?

Many protein products simply coat the hair shaft making it smoother and thicker temporarily. The result is more manageable hair—until you shampoo it again. Some protein products do actually deposit a small amount of protein in the hair shaft that gives the hair a smoother, more manageable feel. The results are beneficial, but temporary. You must continue to use the products if you are to continue to benefit.

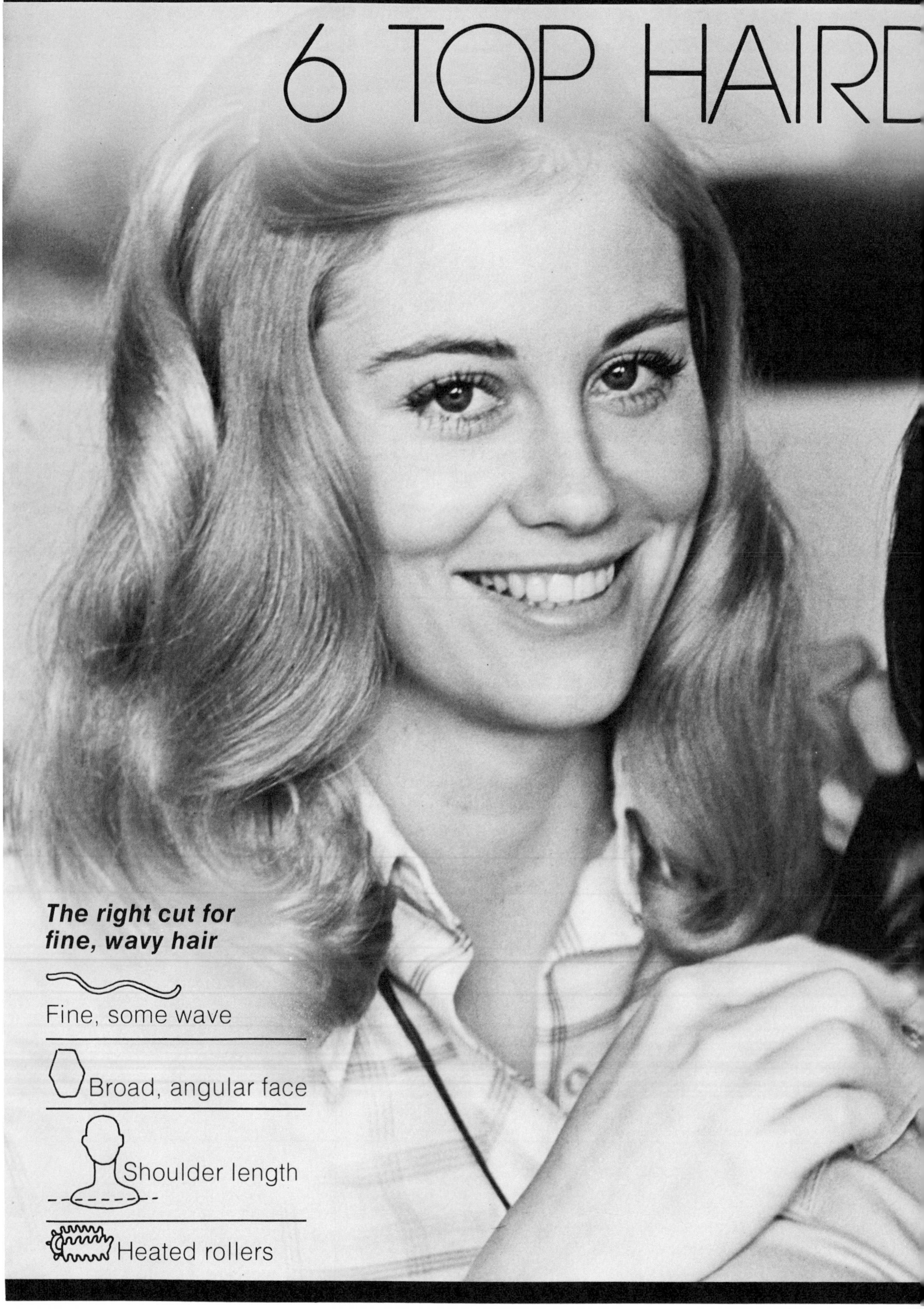

The right cut for fine, wavy hair

Fine, some wave

Broad, angular face

Shoulder length

Heated rollers

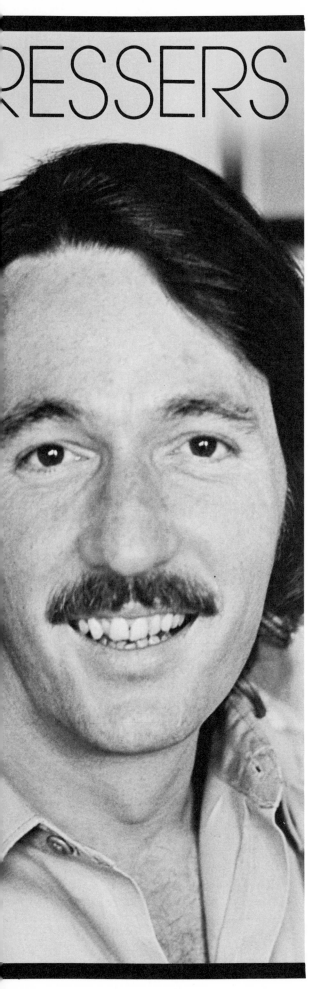

RESSERS tell you how to live with your kind of hair

Your hair, any hair, is only as good as its cut. That's the most important thing you can learn about living happily with it. But just what kind of cut is best for your hair and how do you get it? Here, six top New York hairdressers tell you all about it.

Maury Hopson

These days, almost no one tortures hair with daily settings, backcombing and other assorted means of getting hair to do what it stubbornly doesn't want to. But let's face it, we weren't all blessed with great or even good hair, and there has to be some way to control it. That's why cut is more important than ever. A good cut can make even the most reluctant hair fall happily into line. But part of the responsibility for getting that cut is yours. A hairdresser can tell whether you have fine, thick, wavy or straight hair, but *you* have to say how handy you are, how much time you can spend on it and so on. Hairdresser Maury Hopson, here, blunt cut this model's fine, slightly wavy hair because a blunt cut gives any style maximum fullness. Sides and front are a bit shorter than the back to add versatility and soften facial angles. Maury felt this hair type would be even more flexible if it were a little shorter, but the model preferred the bit of extra length. Fine hair bolstered with a little natural wave shouldn't be much more than shoulder length. You'll see in all the hair looks following, that hair type, face shape, etcetera, are all more important than the old clichés of age or role. To get the soft curl here, Maury set the hair on heated rollers, styling details, page 118. The key *left* shows hair type, face shape, length and styling method for this look.

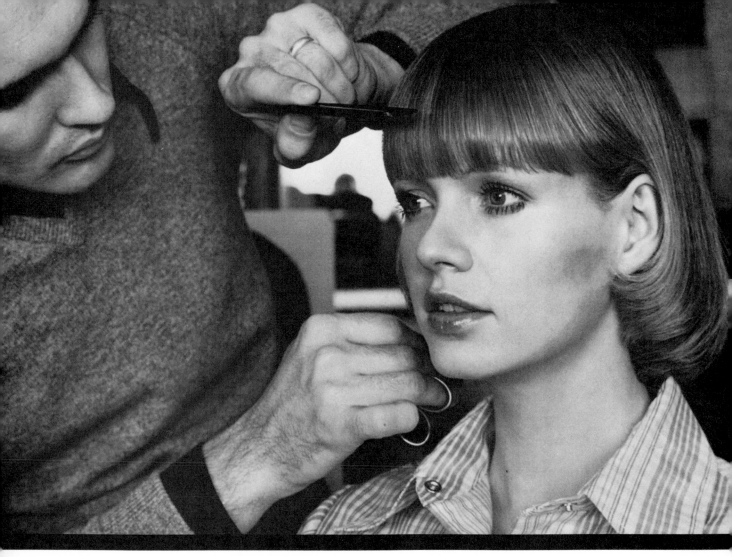

Roger Thompson

The right cut for superfine, straight hair

Straight, limp

Square face

Chin length

Blow dry

The model here has extremely fine straight hair, the kind that dies when the least sign of humidity appears. To live happily with this kind of hair, you should really keep it no longer than chin length, according to hairdresser Roger Thompson. And the best length for maximum control is about two-and-a-half to three inches all over the head—not a layered cut. This gives good control and lets you take advantage of even the slightest natural wave. Roger blunt cut the ends of the hair here to give it a full look. He believes that if the sides are cut too much longer or shorter than the back, fine hair loses its line. Roger has a very positive attitude about fine hair. "It's only bad when you try to make it do something not right for it," he says. Too curly a look, too long, or anything too complicated usually won't work. Fine hair also often has a lovely silky shine and texture that you should play up. Keeping the style smooth, just blowing it dry, as he did for this look, is the best way to show off this sheen. He rolled the ends of her hair around a round brush while they were just barely damp. This gives a soft turned-under look to the finished style. The same look, without the bangs, just a side or center part, is a good workable idea for this hair type. The bangs, here, are particularly good for this face shape. More about the styling, page 118.

The model here has lots of thick strawberry-blond hair. It's straight, but has so much body that she can do most anything with it. What she needs to avoid is a bushy look that could make her hair overpower her face. André at the Cinandre Salon cut her hair about chin length—a good length to keep it in proportion to her features, and to keep the bulk and body under control. It's not layered; most of the hair is about the same length, but the front and very crown are a little shorter—about an inch or so—to give it that soft look when it's blown dry. To give the sides their soft wind-ruffled look, André has a special blow-dry technique. See how to do it on page 118. One thing André cautions against for this kind of hair is too much setting. A real roller set on wet hair would usually give too much curl. If you want some curl, use electric rollers, but leave them in a very short time. Taking the first ones out as you finish rolling the last ones should be about right.

André of Cinandre

The right cut for coarse textured straight hair

Straight coarse

Heart shaped face

Chin length

Blow dry

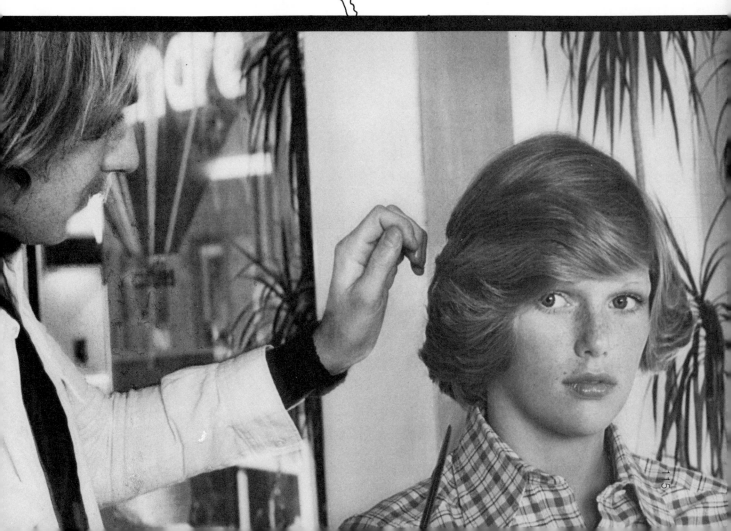

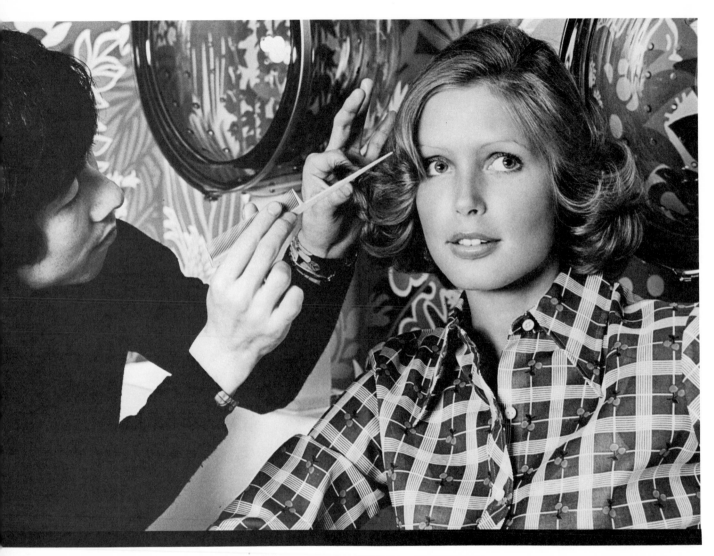

Suga
The right cut for medium textured straight hair

 Medium texture, straight

 Oval

Sharp-angled, chin to shoulder

 Heated rollers

The model here has medium textured straight hair, which is manageable—if she has the right cut. Otherwise the beautifully silky quality can be lost. Hairdresser Suga blunt cut the hair evenly all around but angled the cut so that hair is shortest at chin line, leaving it about shoulder length in back. This will give the hair a nice line when it's worn straight and it will also hold a curl well when it's set. If the hair were much longer, its weight would pull the curl out.

As pretty as the hair looks here after a set with heated rollers, it takes some common sense homework to keep it looking that way. Suga believes that too much dryness—from too-hot rollers or a hair dryer—can be damaging to most hair, and suggests regular conditioning. For the swing of this cut, hair must be superclean at all times, with ends trimmed every four to six weeks to keep the line of the cut neat. More about setting techniques, page 119.

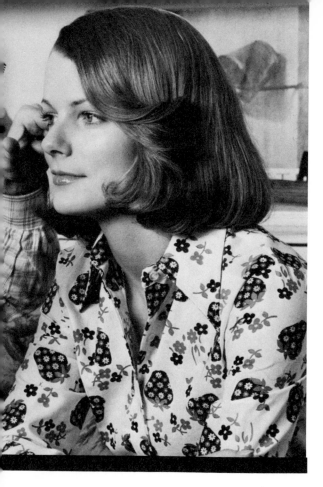

Alan Lewis
The right cut for medium textured curly hair

Naturally curly hair is a blessing only if it works *for*, not against, you. And the best insurance, if you want really manageable hair, is an expert cut. Alan Lewis brought the cool brunette good looks of the model's hair here under control with an even, all round blunt cut at shoulder length. Hair swinging across her cheeks softens a wide jawline. Alan blew the hair dry, then set it on large electric rollers for maximum smoothness. With hair like this you need a certain amount of length to insure a sleek look. An alternative would be a short, layered cut, which she could blow dry, let curl all over her head. More about the styling here is on page 119.

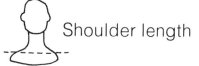 Medium texture, curly

☐ Square

Shoulder length

Blow dry, then heated rollers

Kenneth
The right cut for fine but thick hair

The model here has fine hair, but lots of it. The thickness could be a problem, advises Kenneth of the Kenneth Salon. A layered cut would make it too full and overpowering for her round face. Kenneth gave her an even blunt cut about chin length to flatter her face and bring out the maximum swing and shine. No cream rinses or creamy conditioners for this hair type, says Kenneth. They're too softening. Thick, fine hair like this takes to blow-drying beautifully—but hair must be kept very clean or it will tend to look stringy and lose its movement. More ideas on this look, page 119.

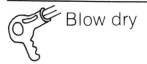
Fine texture, lots of it

◯ Round face

Above-chin length

Blow dry

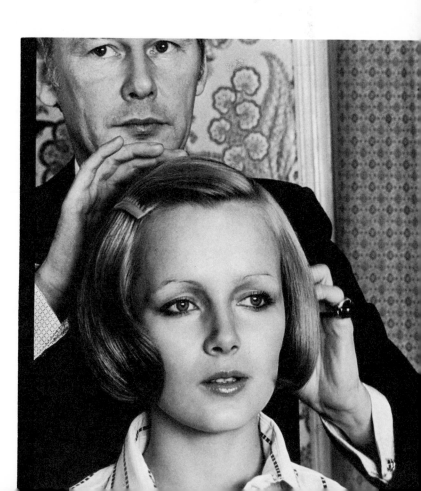

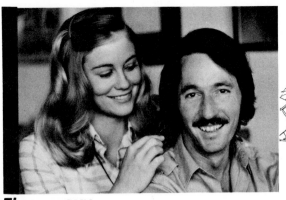

Fine, wavy

Try this little "comb trick" for a look like the one in the picture, above. Pull the hair you want to hold with the comb into place, stick a bobby pin in it, see sketch, right, then push comb in so that back flap of comb covers the bobby pin.

Hair as long as this, especially when it's fine, needs lots of conditioning. One good way to condition it would be while washing it in the shower. After rinsing shampoo out, conditioner is applied and combed through to the ends. Leave the conditioner on for a couple of minutes, then rinse again.

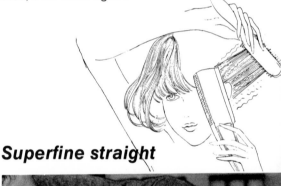

Superfine straight

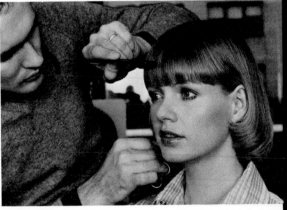

Very fine hair like this can get dry and brittle from too much blow-drying or electric roller setting. To prevent this, give yourself a good deep penetrating conditioning treatment. To use any deep conditioner, first apply conditioner, then put on a shower cap and sit under a warm dryer for about twenty minutes. The sketch, above, shows a blow-dry technique that gives fine hair extra fullness. While the hair is wet, brush it back, away from your face and blow it dry. The idea is to use your head as a giant roller. When the hair falls forward, it is luxuriously full. To finish, roll ends under, around a round brush.

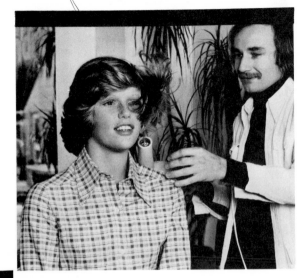

Coarse, straight

There's a trick to getting the soft "ruffled" look of the model's hair, page 118. The sketch, below, shows you how. Wrap slightly damp hair over and around brush, rolling away from your face. For a natural finish, spray on a fine mist of hairspray. Then comb through your hair lightly with your fingers. With this cut, you can also have a straight look, see sketch, below. If your hair is as thick as this model's, a blow dryer with a lot of power is essential.

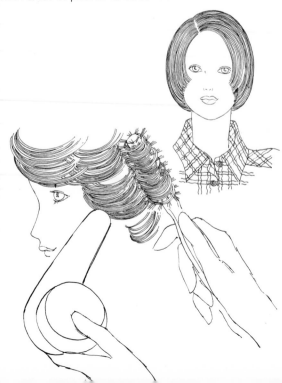

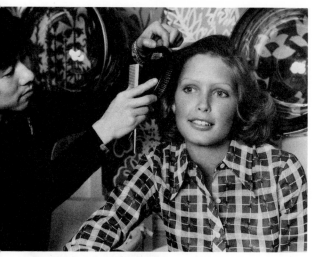

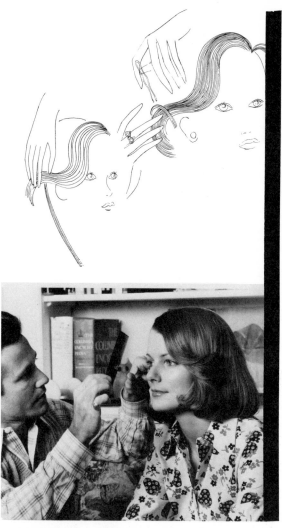

Medium straight

The curly look Suga gave the model here needs an electric roller setting to give it a full bouncy look. In the sketch, below, you see the position of the rollers with arrows showing the direction to wind them. All back rollers are rolled under. Anyone using electric rollers several times a week should condition hair regularly to protect hair from drying. Endpapers used when rolling the hair will help, too.

Medium curly

There's a trick to keeping the wave in this hair neatly in place and it's one you can learn. Pull a small strand of hair from behind the wave, see sketch, above, and wrap it around the wave. Then take a bobby- or hairpin and push it into the hair you've wrapped around so that only the very end will show. To blow hair dry quickly you might try a dryer with super drying power. It will speed up the blow-dry process.

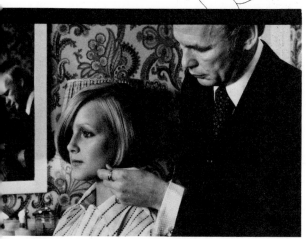

Fine but lots of it

The logistics of blowing-dry hair as thick as this model's could be a problem. That's why Kenneth showed her how to clip the top sections in fat pin curls to keep them out of the way as she blows the bottom sections dry. Anyone with thick hair knows how hard it can be to comb after a shampoo, too. An instant conditioner after the shampoo will help. To get the wave here, use a barrette to hold hair during the day. When you take out the barrette in the evening, you'll have this sexy wave.

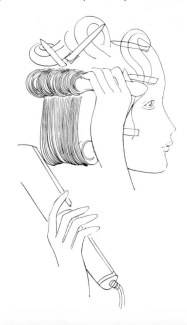

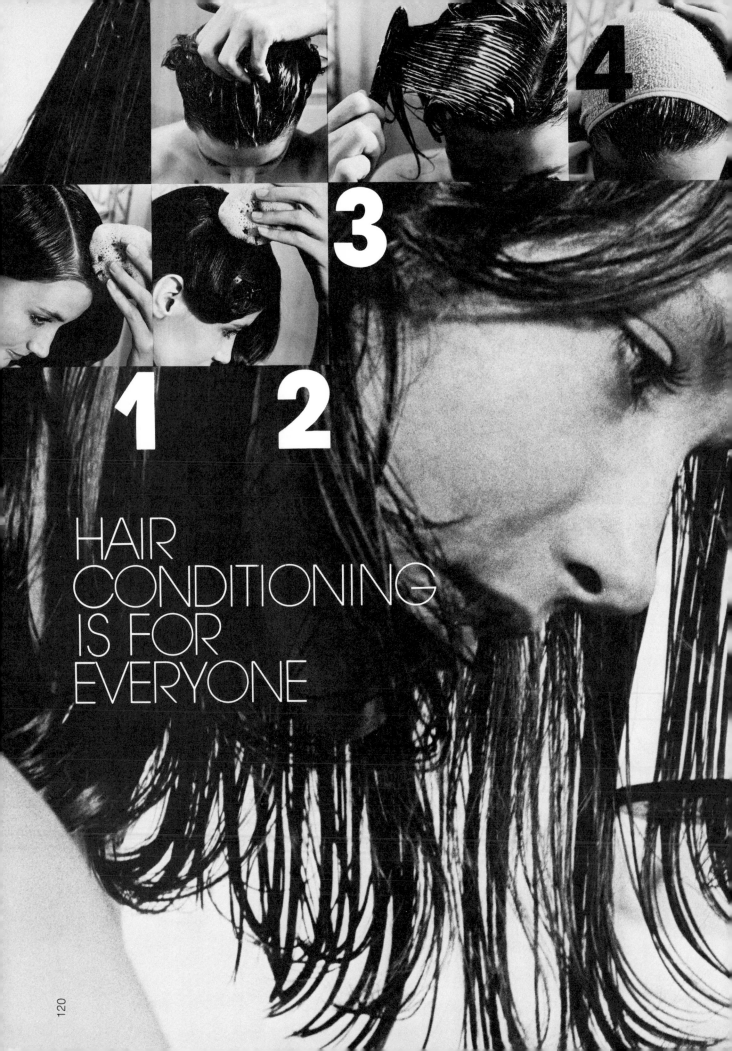

1

2

3

4

HAIR
CONDITIONING
IS FOR
EVERYONE

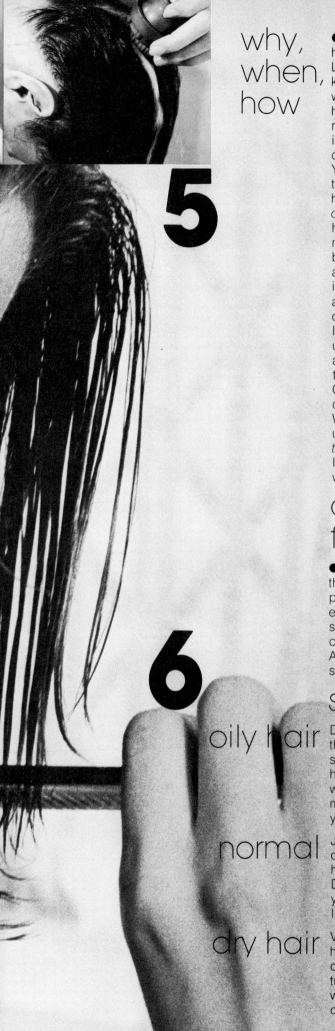

why, when, how

5

● "Every woman can do a lot to improve the health of her hair through conditioning," says Leslie Blanchard, one of New York's best-known hair health experts. Many of the things we do routinely to hair—coloring, straightening, heated rollers, and dryers—deplete hair of its natural oils and emollients, so it's especially important to condition regularly. Any good deep-penetrating conditioner will do the job. You can spot one by reading label directions— they will say the product should be left on the hair for at *least ten minutes* and that it is *rinsed out* before the hair is set. As a rule of thumb, hair that's *not* chemically treated (colored, permanented or chemically straightened) should be deep-conditioned every four weeks. Here are Mr. Blanchard's steps for a good conditioning treatment. ● 1, 2. Center-part hair and with a dry natural sponge rub through part to loosen dirt. If scalp is dry or scaly, moisten sponge lightly with mineral oil. Continue parting hair until you've covered entire head. Shampoo with a good mild shampoo. Towel dry. Apply conditioner according to product directions. ● 3. Comb through hair with fingers to distribute conditioner, then use a wide-tooth comb. ● 4. Wrap head with a warm moist towel for ten minutes. ● 5. Remove towel and rinse hair *very thoroughly* with warm water so no film will be left on hair. Towel dry again. ● 6. Comb hair with wide-tooth comb, blow dry.

an expert's ideas for healthy hair

● Be aware that there is such a thing as hair that's too squeaky clean. Overshampooing depletes hair of too much oil. You can wash it every night; just remember to choose a *mild* shampoo. ● Try finishing your shampoo with a cold water rinse; it helps make hair shinier. ● Always rinse salt, chlorinated water and perspiration out of hair after swimming or exercise.

6

special tips

oily hair Don't skip the sponge treatment described in the conditioning steps. Oily hair needs it most since it attracts so much dirt. Keep use of heated rollers and blowers down to twice a week. Heat stimulates oil glands to produce more oil. In general, the less you manipulate your hair, the less you stimulate the oil glands.

normal Just because your hair is "normal and healthy," don't skip conditioning. All hair needs it. Your hair gets split ends, too, so plan regular trims. Don't forget common sense things like keeping your hair covered if you're out in the sun for long hours, or rinsing it after swimming.

dry hair Very dry hair should be treated as gently as hair that's damaged by excessive use of chemicals. Both are fragile. This means use of electric rollers should be limited to once or twice a week as heat dries hair. Try using your blow dryer on gentler cool or medium settings.

How and why to
BRUSH your hair for beauty

what brush is right for you?

If you normally brush by flicking your wrist as you stroke, the half-round brush is best because the turning, flicking motion will wear down the side bristles of a flat brush. If you brush in a straight up-and-down motion, a flat oval brush is best, and it's best for long hair, too, because there's a lot of brushing surface and bristles are set in rubber for flexibility. The professional brush is better for short hair, since there isn't as much brushing surface. A full round brush is good for styling final stages of a blow dry. Remember that the thicker and coarser your hair, the stiffer the brush bristles should be. A firm bristle can penetrate the hair better. Fine hair needs a softer bristle.

why brush—and how

● To brush in order to stimulate circulation in the scalp and add extra fullness, bend from waist, throw hair over head, brush up from nape.
● A daily brushing helps distribute the natural oils over the entire hair shaft. If your hair is very long, brush once a day.
● A light daily brushing helps get rid of accumulated surface dust and dirt, but any manipulating tends to make hair more oily, so don't overdo it.
● Brush bristles give when they encounter a tangle, teeth on a comb are rigid and can break hair.
● Always brush hair gently. When your brush encounters a tangle, gently work it out with your fingers, then continue brushing.

brush care

Your brush should be washed when your hair gets shampooed so that you never brush clean hair with a dirty brush. Wash the brush by swishing it gently in tepid, soapy water. Don't use harsh detergents and don't soak the brush—this can loosen bristles and be harmful to a wooden handle. To loosen old hairs in a brush, comb through bristles gently or use a cleaning brush (one made especially for cleaning regular brushes). Rinse brush in lukewarm water, then cold, and shake off excess moisture. Dry brush bristle-side down on sink, never over a radiator or other heat source.

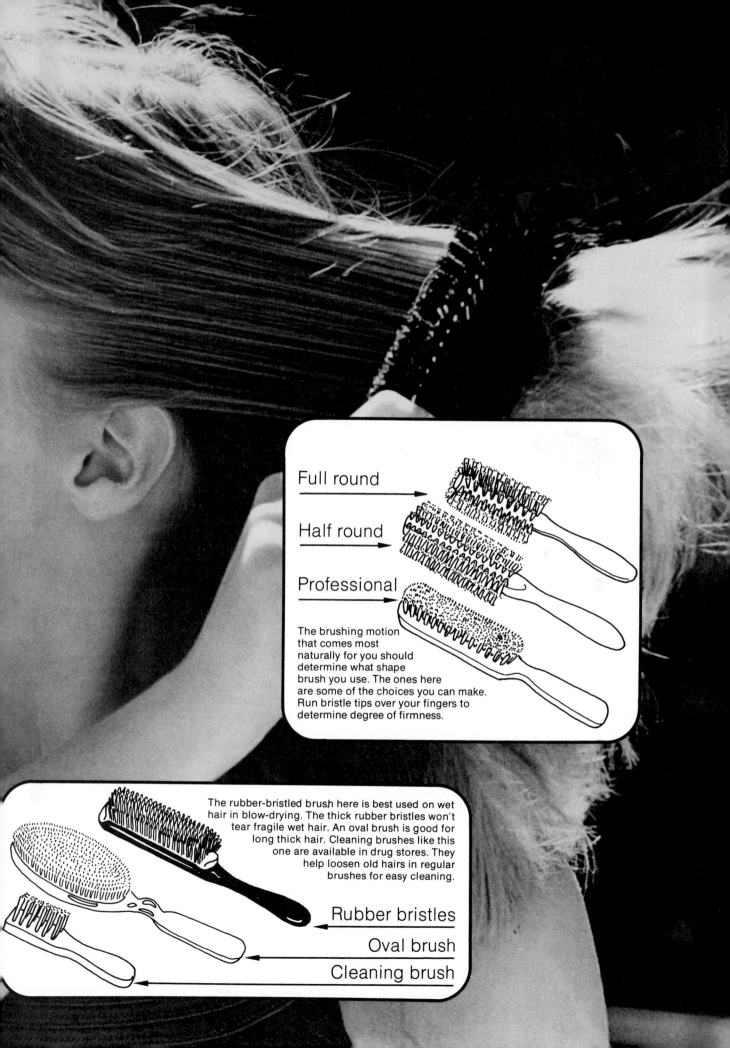

Full round

Half round

Professional

The brushing motion that comes most naturally for you should determine what shape brush you use. The ones here are some of the choices you can make. Run bristle tips over your fingers to determine degree of firmness.

The rubber-bristled brush here is best used on wet hair in blow-drying. The thick rubber bristles won't tear fragile wet hair. An oval brush is good for long thick hair. Cleaning brushes like this one are available in drug stores. They help loosen old hairs in regular brushes for easy cleaning.

Rubber bristles

Oval brush

Cleaning brush

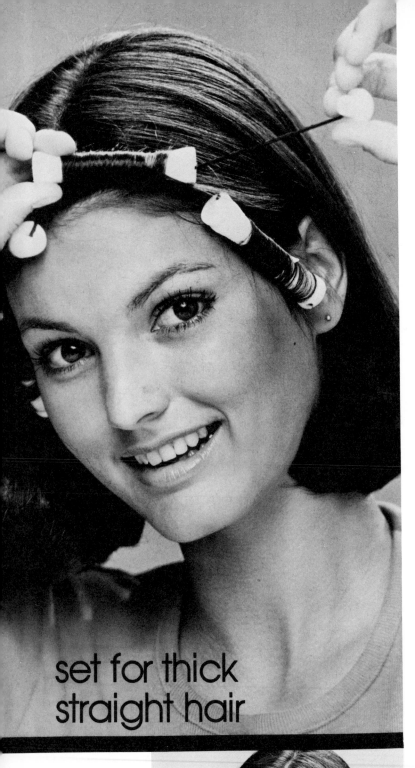

set for thick
straight hair

FOUR GREAT HAIRSETS YOU CAN DO IN MINUTES

These sets are especially good after a day of outdoor activity because they let you pull your hair together so fast. The results, however, are polished enough to be your regular routine. The one on this page is for straight, thick hair. You'll also find tips for common hair annoyances.

● For the fastest possible set, blow dry straight thick hair. You can curve ends up or under for a finished look. The only problem: The thickness of this kind of hair can make the front pieces fall forward and hang in your face.

● The solution: Four chunky rollers, the largest kind used for permanent waves (buy them in a beauty-supply store or some drug- or dime-stores), rolled away from the face. Dampen hair with setting lotion before rolling, for more control. You could also use medium-sized electric rollers for the same effect. ● Haircut tip: Since crown hair is apt to be short and wispy, it sometimes gets missed in a trim. To get rid of splits here, pull hair forward, see photo, below, and trim off ends.

● Do a quick "head wrap" set for curly or wavy hair, see opposite page. While hair is wet, roll down away from face on two big rollers. Center part the rest of your hair and use your head as a giant roller. Starting in back, comb and wrap left half of hair to the left, clipping and smoothing as you go. Then wrap the remaining side in the same direction, being sure you keep ends of hair smooth and flat where hair from opposite side overlaps. When hair dries, it will be straight. ● Use heated rollers to give hair just a little bend. ● Tip for ponytail wearers: If you've had hair back all day with an elastic band and want to remove the dent the band made, dampen brush, blow hair dry and the damp brush and warm dryer air will smooth hair, see bottom, opposite page.

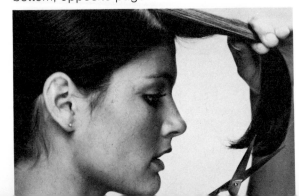

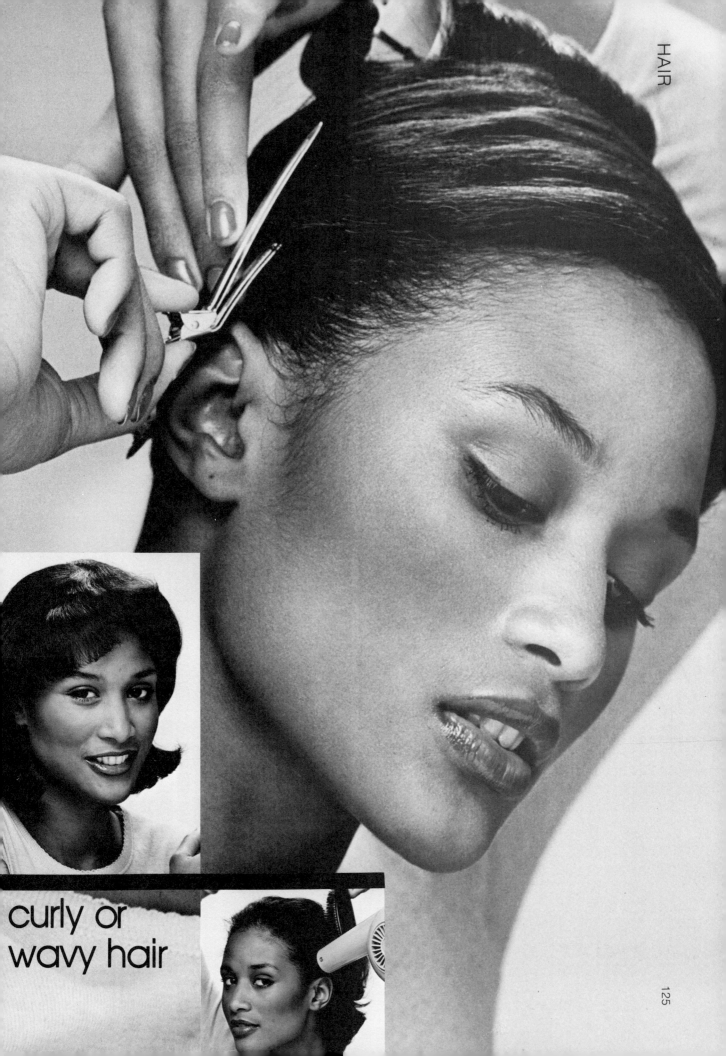

curly or
wavy hair

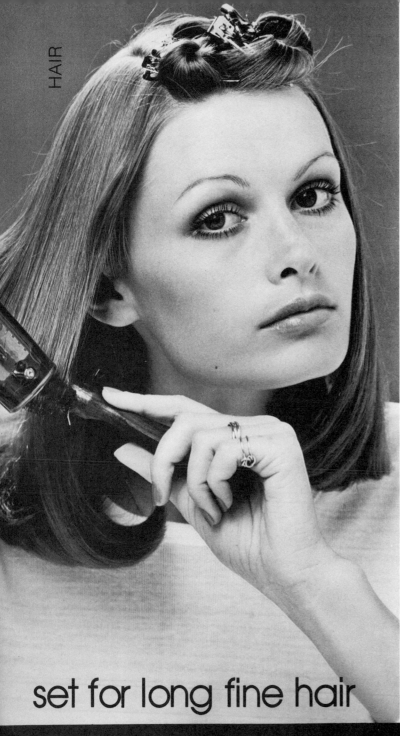

set for long fine hair

FOUR GREAT HAIRSETS

● Quick tricks: To control flyaway hair ends after blowing hair dry, spray a cotton ball with hairspray or setting lotion and gently smooth over the offending hairs. ● When too much electricity makes hair wispy and flyaway, spray your brush, opposite page, with hairspray and brush through hair.

● There's a trick to getting that incredible bounce and fullness to a pageboy. Here's how it's done: When hair is almost dry, roll it around a round brush, roll right to scalp and with dryer on high, move it back and forth across hair, see left. Now gently unroll hair from brush with dryer still moving back and forth as you unroll. Continue rolling and unrolling that piece of hair until it's dry. Then move on to the next section.

● To get the brushed-back bangs look, roll bangs over brush, rolling away from the face, and move dryer back-and-forth until they dry. You can hold them in place with clips until you finish drying rest of hair. ● For extra manageability for fine hair, you might try using a small amount of setting lotion on wet hair.

● A good quick set for thick, manageable hair that has only the slightest bend can be done with hairset tape, see opposite. Wait till hair is almost dry, letting it dry naturally or using a blower. Then tear off a piece of hairset tape about forty-eight inches long. Place the center of piece of tape on forehead, under bangs if you have them. Bring tape around behind your head, crisscross and bring to front under chin, as low as possible, then to back again, fastening by overlapping two ends. You'll get a smooth sleek look with ends turned up ever so slightly.

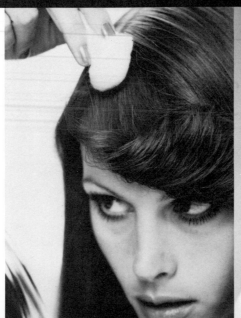

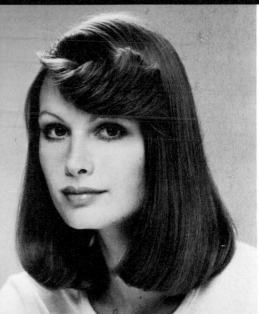

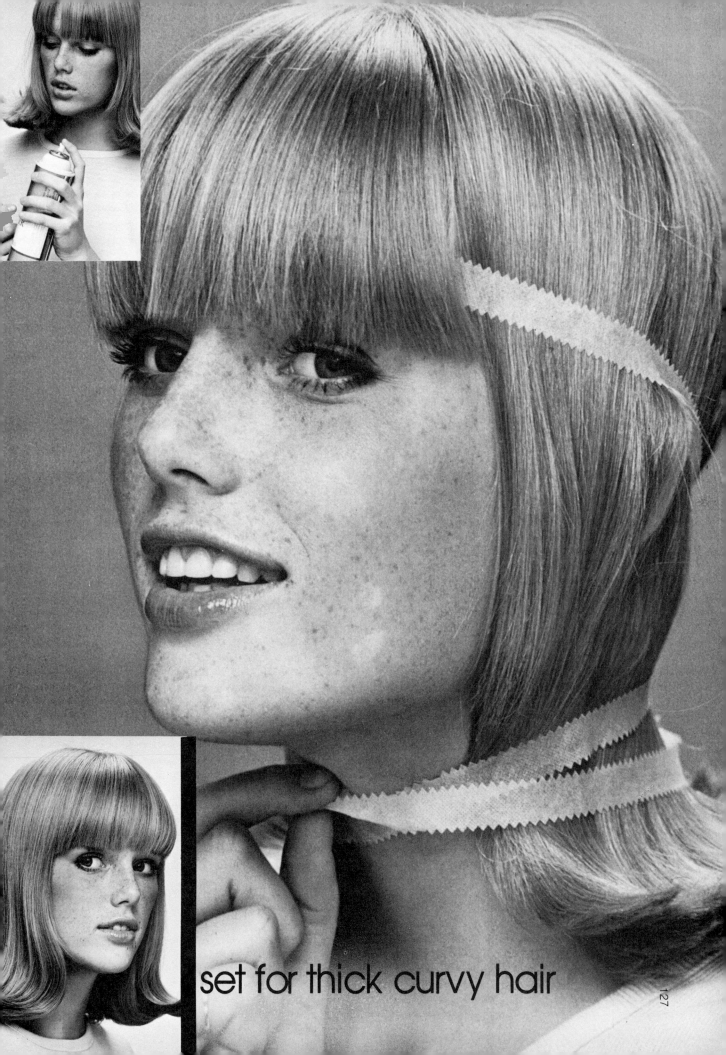

set for thick curvy hair

Everyone Can Wear BANGS

If you've always shied away from bangs because you weren't sure they'd work with your face shape, you're in for a surprise. Anyone can wear most any kind of bang; the trick is to have them cut to flatter your face. The sketches here will show you how.

STRAIGHT CHOP

- *A long face* can wear a straight chop bang if it's cut very long and very wide. The bang should be cut into the side hair. Cutting the bangs slightly longer in front is a second option. ● *A round face,* which often gives the illusion of largeness, can either have the straight bangs cut so side hair falls over cheeks to cut the width, or have them cut very wide and slightly shorter in front.
- *Square faces*—they also tend to appear large—should have the bangs cut above eyebrows, on the narrowish side, and aim for some fullness in side hair.
- *A heart-shaped face* should aim for a narrow bang with some width and fullness at the sides.
- Anyone with a *teardrop shape* should aim for the widest straight bang cut above brows.

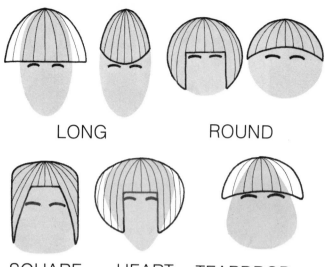

LONG   ROUND

SQUARE   HEART   TEARDROP

WISPY

- To wear wispy bangs, *a long face* should part them to one side, brushing hair away from the part. The bangs should be slightly shorter than brow length to compensate for face length.
- *A round face* should aim for shorter bangs and a center part with the wisps of the bangs separated next to part. Let side hair fall onto cheeks.
- *A square face* should also center-part bangs creating a definite separation in the center.
- *A heart-shaped face* should aim for brow-length bangs brushed to one side.
- *Teardrop shapes* need brow-length bangs parted to one side and away from part.

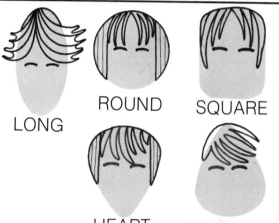

LONG   ROUND   SQUARE

HEART   TEARDROP

SIDE SWEPT

- To wear side-swept bangs, *a long face* should have a longer-than-brow-length bang brushed from the center of the forehead to one side.
- *A round face* should part the bangs at one side and brush hair away from part. Have them cut just below brow line.
- The same goes for *a square face.*
- *A heart-shaped face* will look best with bangs center-parted and brushed away from the part.
- *Teardrops* should aim for a full brow-length bang, parted slightly off-center and brushed away from the part.

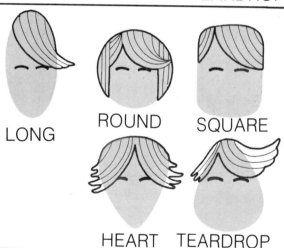

LONG   ROUND   SQUARE

HEART   TEARDROP

BEFORE YOU CUT

- Be sure you know your face shape. The best way to tell is to wrap your head turban-style with a towel so you can see nothing but your face. Then decide what shape it is.
- Don't cut bangs too short. Hair "shrinks" when it dries.
- Do be prepared for the new sensation of having something on your forehead. Be cool about it; don't develop into a fusser who's constantly pushing hair back.

- Do take advantage of dry shampoos if your hair is oily. Bangs lying on your forehead can get oily fast, so just spray with the dry shampoo, then brush out.

The young woman on the opposite page wears three kinds of bangs. A version of each will work for you, no matter what shape face you have. She happens to have an oval face—or what some people consider the perfect face shape—so she can wear most any kind of bang without having to compensate for extra roundness, squareness or other face irregularity.

10 THINGS YOU BEFORE YOU CC

1 COLOR CHOICE

Go only a few shades lighter or darker than your natural shade when you color. Either extreme is probably too much for the skin tone and eye color of this woman.

2

Take your skin tone into consideration when you pick a color. If you're very pale, very dark hair can look harsh. If you're sallow or dark complected, very blond hair will look unnatural. If you're in doubt, it's worth the effort to try on a couple of wigs in the color you're considering. You'll get an idea of how your coloring looks with the hair color in question.

3

Consider how much time you want to spend on your new color. The further from your natural color, the more time—and money—touch-ups will cost.

4

Think about highlighting, lightening tiny strands of hair, usually around the face, to give a blond illusion. Consider, too, "hair painting," lightening wider sections of hair but giving very subtle, almost tone-on-tone effect, as a flattering way to add a color glow. You can do highlighting yourself at home if all you want are a few strands next to your face. If you want a more all-over blond look, it's best to go to a salon. They can place the lights evenly and subtly. Golden and reddish highlights are another pretty idea, especially on light and medium brown hair. Henna is an exciting way to give dark brown hair subtle highlights. Henna and red highlights are best done in a salon. An inexperienced colorist—such as you—could end up with a brassy rather than a golden look.

PRODUCT CHOICE

5

If you want a lasting, noticeable change, pick a permanent hair-color produc rather than a rinse or semi-permanent, which won't make long-lasting or very noticeable changes (except on gray hair, which has a unique texture).

SHOULD KNOW
LOR YOUR HAIR

6 *If you're doing a permanent color job yourself, a shampoo-in product is easiest to use. When touch-up time comes, you just reshampoo with the product instead of doing difficult root touch-ups.*

7 *If you're changing hair color several shades, you might want a salon to do it the first time to work out the best color choice. If the color you want can only be achieved with a product that requires root touch-ups (very blond, some reds), do consider a salon process. It's very hard to do root touch-ups on your own hair.*

8 DOING THE JOB

If you've never used a color before, do a "strand test." Directions for this are always given with the product. It's the only way to see how the color looks on your hair. Color charts can be misleading.

9 *Follow the manufacturer's directions for coloring. If you take shortcuts, you may have to live with the results for a long time.*

10 UPKEEP

Highlighting or painting requires the least upkeep. Depending on how much highlighting you want and the natural color of your hair, once every three to six months is about it. If you're bleaching all over to go very light on medium or darker brown hair, expect touch-ups every three to four weeks. If you're lightening or darkening just a bit, you'll have to touch up every five to six weeks.

HOW TO CURL OR UNCURL YOUR HAIR SUCCESSFULLY

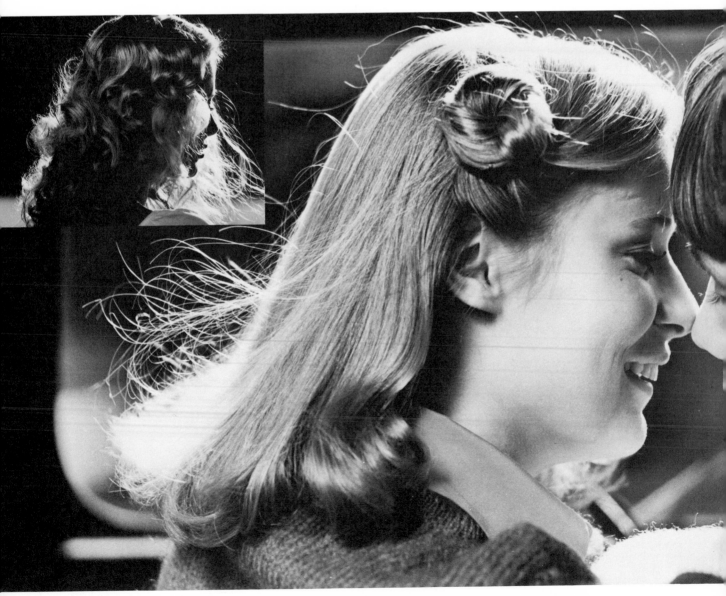

PERMANENTS

A permanent can be the basis of a great hair style, especially if you have fine, difficult hair. The only trick is getting the right kind of perm for your hair type and the kind of look you want.

What kind of perm do you need?

If you want one of the very curly looks around now, the kind that you just let dry naturally for a headful of curls, you want a real permanent, *not* a body wave. If you're doing the job yourself, look for a home permanent that says "curly" on the box or gives you some indication that it's intended for a very curly look.

If you just want to give more body to fine hair, you need a body wave. If you're doing the job yourself, pick a permanent that's labeled "body wave," or "gentle" or one that gives some indication that you'll get more body than curl. You can also determine the amount of curl you get by the size roller you use. The larger the roller, the less curl you'll get.

Always follow directions to the letter. You'll have to live with any mistake you make until the hair grows out or is cut off. Permanents are for keeps.

If you're having your permanent done in a salon, ask for their advice on what type would be best. Be sure you tell the stylist how much curl you're after and how you want to style your hair once you have the permanent. Very curly permanents don't blow dry well. You should either let them dry naturally or set them with regular or electric rollers. A body wave, if it's well done, can usually be blown dry. If your hair is very fine, you may have to use a few electric rollers to control the ends.

DO'S & DON'TS

Don't color *and* permanent your hair. The use of two chemical processes on your hair can damage it, causing split and broken ends. Depending on the kind of color and the permanent, the two can sometimes be done successfully in a salon—though never on the same day. If you feel you must combine a permanent and color, ask the advice of a competent stylist and follow it.

Don't have or give yourself a permanent more than every four months if your hair is short (if it's very short, every three months), and every six months if you wear it long.

Do condition your hair regularly if you permanent it. Conditioning will make your hair shinier and much more manageable. A deep condi-

tioner every three or four weeks is usually about right.

Do experiment with a new permanent a little to find the best way to handle it. Try different ways of setting it or of drying it. A heat lamp dries a curly permanent quickly and doesn't disturb the "natural curly" look you're after.

HAIR STRAIGHTENING

Hair straightening is probably the harshest thing you can do to your hair because the chemicals necessary to straighten hair must be fairly strong. It can be done safely and successfully if you follow these tips.

● Home straighteners are available, but they are successful only on hair that's moderately curly. If your hair is very curly, you should have the straightening done in a salon. If you do the job yourself, follow the product directions carefully.

● If you have the straightening done in a salon, tell the stylist how straight you want your hair. If you are envisioning dead straight hair, say so; if you want to leave a bit of bend in your hair, communicate this, too.

● Many women find that straightening their hair just before the summer months, when humidity can make curly hair difficult, is the best. They let the hair rest from the chemicals during the winter.

● If you want your hair as straight as possible all the time, it's worth your money to find the best salon around and pay for the best job. A good salon won't overprocess your hair. They will also take the time to straighten only the roots as new hair grows in instead of applying the straightener to all your hair, weakening the ends by overstraightening them.

● Don't have your hair straightened more than twice a year unless a reputable salon tells you it's safe. If you wear your hair short and have frequent trims, you may be able to have straightening done every four to five months if it's done carefully and if only new growth is done.

● Don't combine straightening with hair color.

● Be gentle with straightened hair. Deep condition it every three to four weeks. Limit the use of curling irons or heated rollers to twice a week. Use your dryer on gentle warm or cool settings as much as possible. Don't overbrush, and use a good quality brush with smooth-ended bristles.

LIMP AND STRINGY

After drying your hair, throw it forward as in the picture, opposite page, and brush hair forward. Throw hair back and, with your fingers, arrange it. A body wave will also pouf up hair and give it fullness.

Limp, drooping hair will take on more fullness if it's blown dry carefully. As you dry, lift each section of hair up and away from scalp, then wrap around a round brush. Now blow the section of hair dry. Taking lots of small sections instead of a few big ones will also add fullness and bounce to your hair. A few electric rollers in strategic spots will add more body. You might also try a light setting lotion.

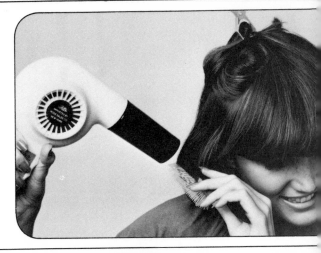

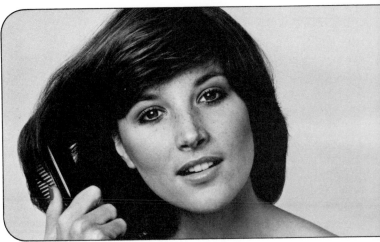

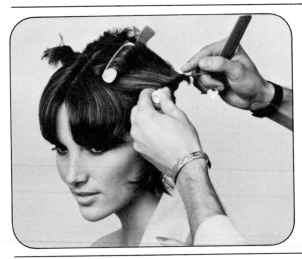

WON'T HOLD SET

A good cut helps solve this problem, too. If a good line is cut into the hair, you have that to fall back on when the curl fails. A body wave is another idea for this problem. It will give the hair a curve and direction that helps hold the set. Don't think that having a body wave necessarily means you won't have to set your hair. Depending on the amount of wave and your particular hair, you may still have to set, but your hair will hold that set much better. Aim for a simple style, since it will be easier to maintain than something more complicated.

DULL, LOSES SHINE

If your hair doesn't shine, try a different shampoo. Your present one may not agree with your hair type. Also, be certain you're rinsing all the shampoo from your hair. Any leftover traces will leave a dulling film on hair. Too much hairspray or setting lotion can also dull hair. If none of these seem to be your problem, try this: After washing, gently towel dry hair. Next, use your dryer on "cool" setting to finish drying. If your hair is dull and damaged by too many perms or coloring jobs, deep condition it every two weeks and try to let the hair "rest" for a couple of months to get it back in good shape.

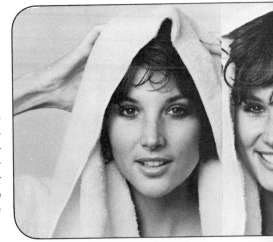

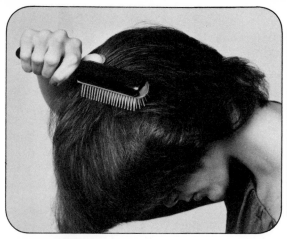

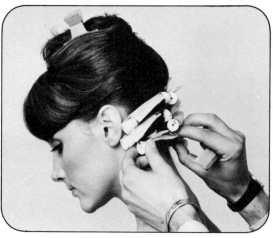

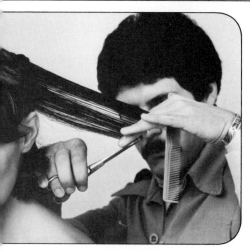

SEPARATES

Hair that separates into clumps instead of hanging like a smooth curtain is a problem many women fight. To solve it, get the best possible cut, so that hair is *cut* to fall smoothly. Don't wear your hair too long; it should be just *short* of shoulder length—or shorter—to keep it from catching and separating at your shoulders. After you blow your hair dry, brush each section up and out from your head to give more fullness, see picture, opposite page.

How to solve your biggest
HAIR PROBLEMS

"When my hair doesn't work, my looks don't work" is a complaint we hear a lot. Hair problems can be annoying, but are not unsolvable. We've taken some of the common ones and solved them for you here.

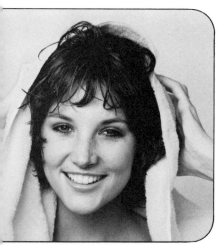

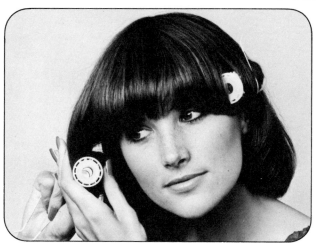

MORE HAIR PROBLEMS SOLVED

The great little cut here is one you should consider. The soft, brushed-back bangs, the chin-length sides and slightly longer back are very manageable and very contemporary looking. Worn center-parted or with straight bangs for versatility. Having the ends of the hair blunt cut will give the style the most body. This is a good cut for fine- or medium-texture hair since there's not too much length to pull curl out.

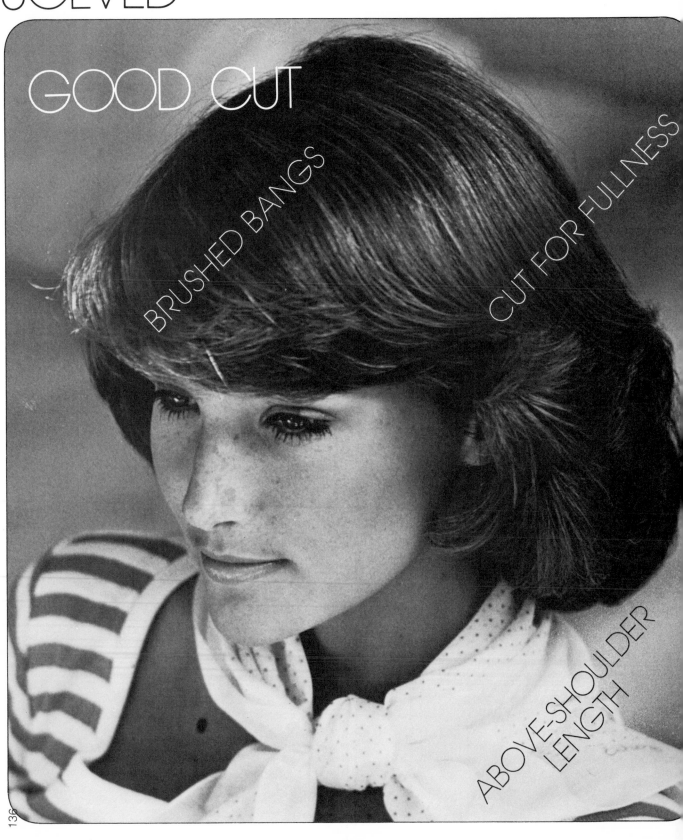

GOOD CUT

BRUSHED BANGS

CUT FOR FULLNESS

ABOVE-SHOULDER LENGTH

This is the same cut as shown on the opposite page but the hair here has had a body wave—a good idea for very fine hair. The wave gives the hair extra fullness and manageability. The bangs are worn straight across to show you how versatile this cut is. To get this look with a body wave, first blow hair dry, then set it on a few medium- to large-size electric rollers.

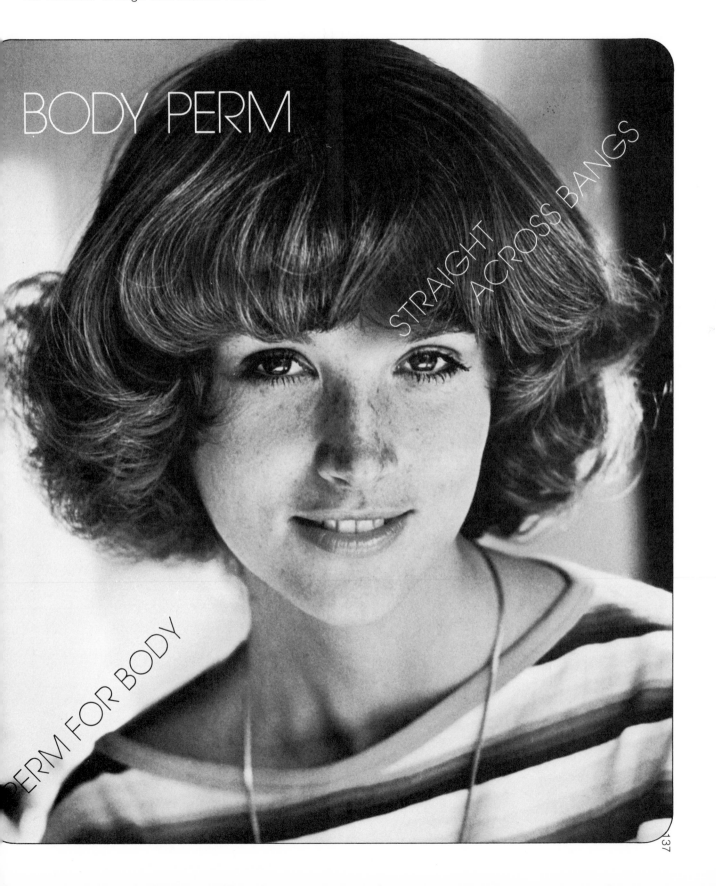

BODY PERM

STRAIGHT ACROSS BANGS

PERM FOR BODY

IS IT TIME TO CHANGE TH

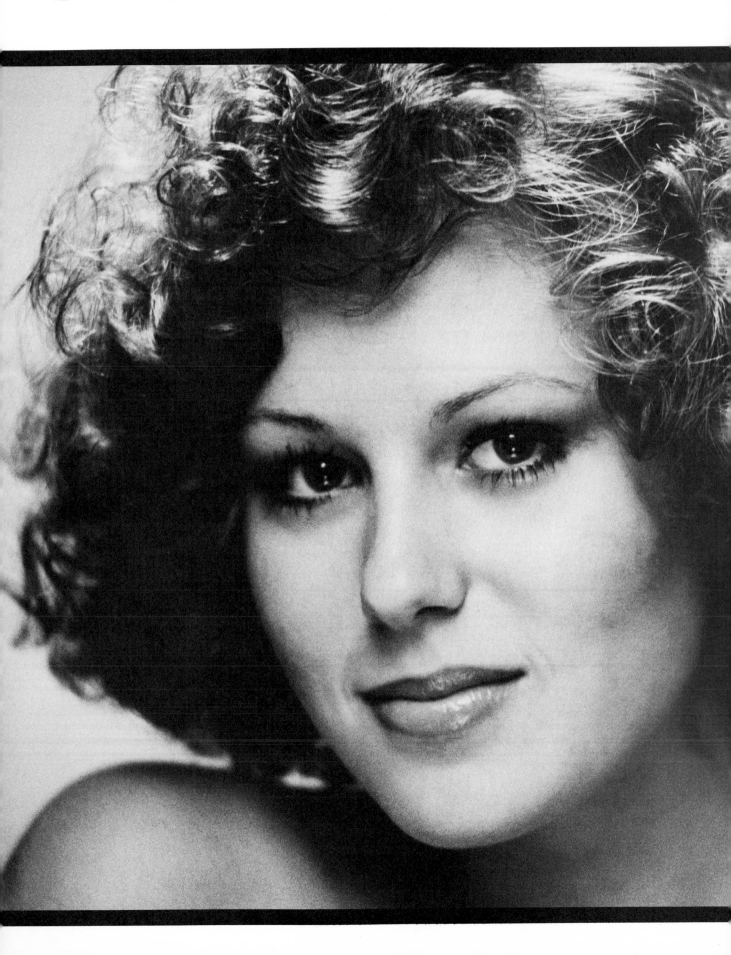

LOOK OF YOUR HAIR?

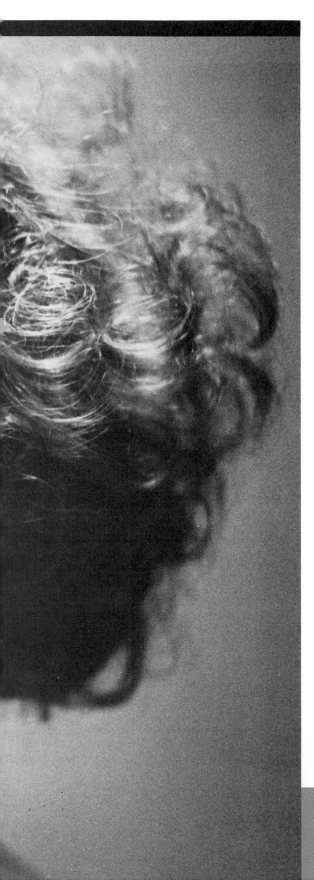

Versatility in a hairstyle is second only to compatibility—with your features and your hair type. No matter how becoming a hairstyle is for you, if it looks out of proportion to most of your clothes or if you just can't vary its look, it's time to change to something more flexible. Take the quiz that follows to see if you should be thinking about a new hairstyle, and then have a look at some of the fresh, contemporary haircuts that follow. We've shown what kind of necklines each style works best with because that's one of the areas often neglected in picking a new look.

How versatile is your hairstyle?

If your hairstyle is really versatile, it not only works with several kinds of necklines, but in a lot of other ways too. To check out your present style, answer the questions below. If you answer NO to three or more, you should think of changing your style to something a bit more versatile.

	YES	NO
1. Does your hairstyle look well with most of the necklines you like to wear—it's not so long that it catches in turtle- or cowlnecks, so short it looks bare and out of proportion to your favorite shirts or dresses?	☐	☐
2. Have you changed your cut or style in the last three years?	☐	☐
3. Can your cut stand up to humidity and bad weather?	☐	☐
4. Can you wear your hair at least two different ways with your present cut?	☐	☐
5. Does your hair work for both casual and dressy looks—or can you vary the look so it does?	☐	☐
6. Are you satisfied with the amount of time you have to spend maintaining your look?	☐	☐

Versatile curls

The hair here is just below chin-length. Hair is slightly shorter at the top and sides, ends are tapered a bit all over for fullness. This look is great for high necks—the hair won't catch in collars—and it's a nice balance to the new asymmetrical or one-shoulder neckline for party clothes. You can also wear it with combs, in a loose ponytail or chignon.

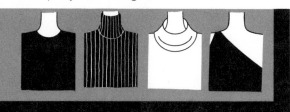

TIME TO CHANGE YOUR

A lot of factors are involved when you pick a hairstyle—your features, hair type, and what kind of necklines you wear most often. There are enough styles, right, to include one that's perfect for you. We grouped them according to the necklines that work best with them to help you. All hairstyles to the right of sketch go with that neckline. Before you decide, here are some tips to keep in mind:

Tips for hair and necklines

● Plan to spend more time maintaining a curly style if your hair is straight, unless you have a permanent.

● Plan on more time for longer looks—the drying time, if nothing else, is longer.

● A really short look will have to be cut every four or five weeks to maintain a neat line.

● A permanent, if you plan on one, will add body or curl. In most cases, you'll still have to set a body wave and let a curly perm dry naturally for the most curl and fullness.

● If you want to change the look of your hair a lot, a longish look offers most versatility. Wear it up, down, pulled back, whatever.

● If you want to expend a minimum of care, a short look is best, but with some shortcuts, you sacrifice a lot of versatility.

● Make sure your hair clears your neckline neatly and doesn't catch inside a turtle- or cowlneck.

● The asymmetrical neckline, bottom, is a great evening look and is easy to wear. Hair should be simple, not too long. Hair that hangs into the neckline will spoil the simple, uncluttered look.

● If you wear a lot of turtlenecks or cowlnecks but like long hair, pull hair back into a chignon, braids or something that will give you a neat line in back. See picture to the far right of cowlneck for an idea.

● If you like very short hair but have trouble "dressing it up" for evening, try a knockout pair of earrings, a decorative haircomb or a flower on a comb to add interest.

Versatile cut

If you want a cut that works with many necklines—say, all those sketched, right— and many hair types, try this. It's short but not extreme, can be worn softly waved as here, or straight for a more casual look.

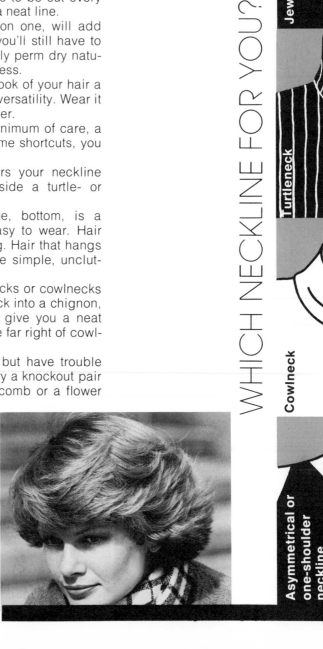

WHICH NECKLINE FOR YOU?

Jewel neck

Turtleneck

Cowlneck

Asymmetrical or one-shoulder neckline

HAIRSTYLE?

| Short, straight | Short, wavy | Longish, straight | Long, curly |

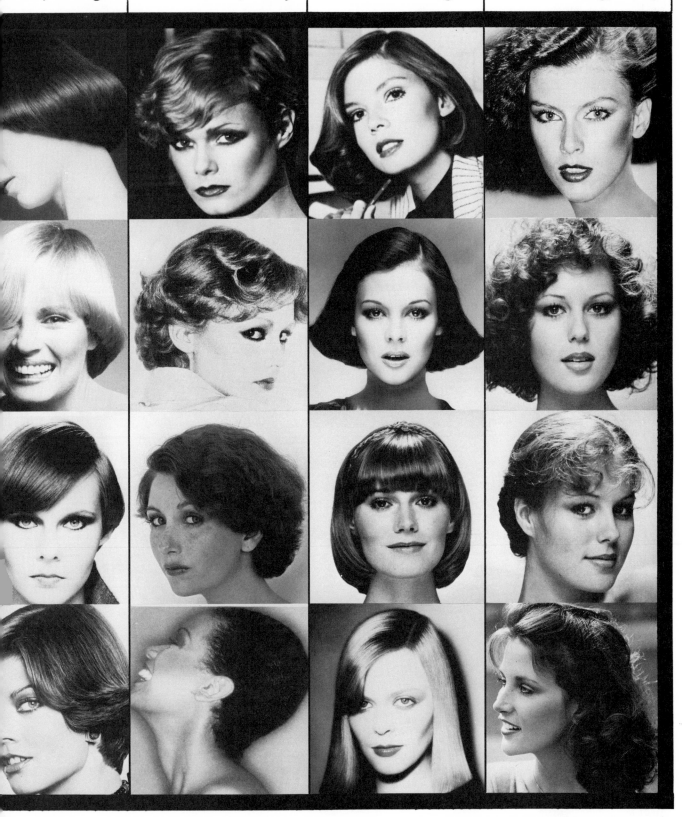

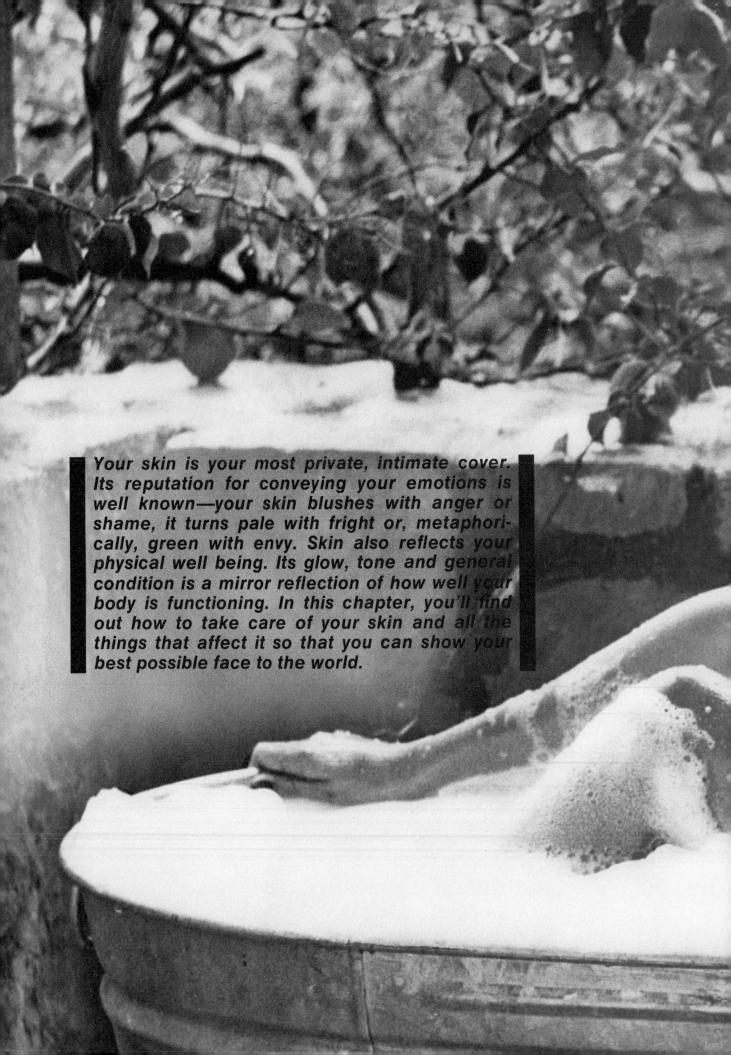

Your skin is your most private, intimate cover. Its reputation for conveying your emotions is well known—your skin blushes with anger or shame, it turns pale with fright or, metaphorically, green with envy. Skin also reflects your physical well being. Its glow, tone and general condition is a mirror reflection of how well your body is functioning. In this chapter, you'll find out how to take care of your skin and all the things that affect it so that you can show your best possible face to the world.

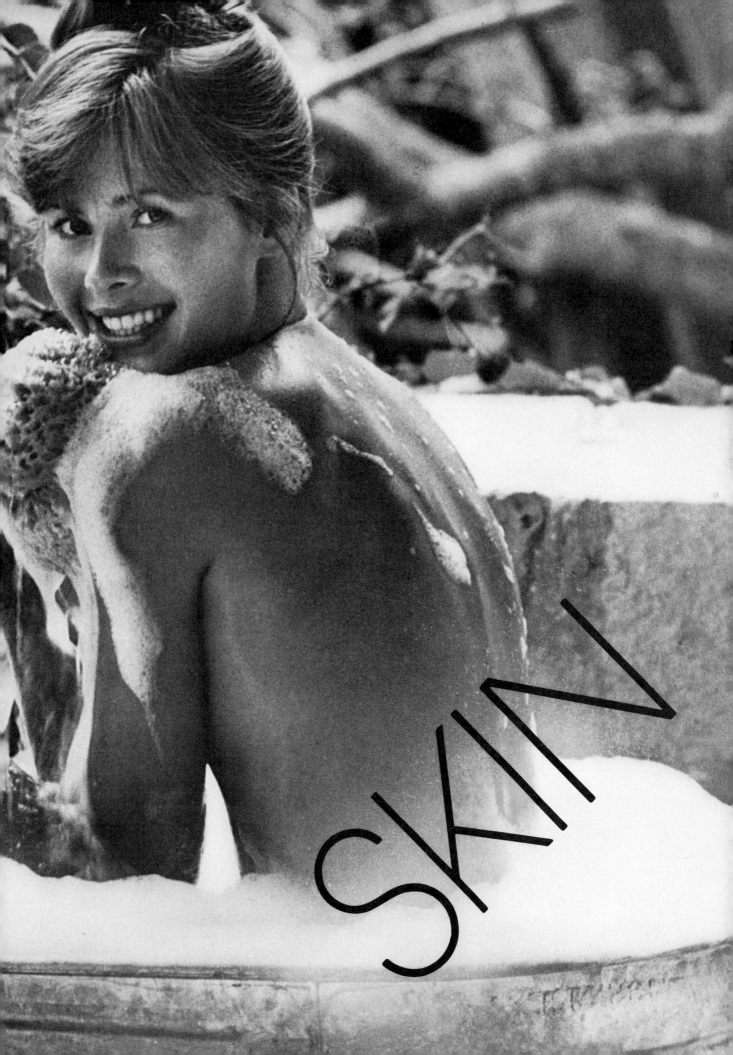

SKIN

How to be your own
SKIN EXPERT

Anyone who's ever shopped for skin-care products knows the choice is overwhelming—moisturizers, astringents, toners, zillions of cleansers and soaps and what have you. But with something as important as the looks of your skin at stake, you can't afford to make mistakes. You don't have to. Take our skin quiz, which follows, to find out exactly what kind of skin you have—dry, oily or a combination of both. Then find the section following that corresponds to your kind of skin and get a rundown on exactly what you need to make it healthy and glowing. You'll discover it's as easy as ABC to be your skin expert and to take care of one of your most important beauty assets like a real pro.

SKIN QUIZ

	1	2	3
My pores are 1. Almost invisible. 2. Visible. 3. Very obvious.	☐	☐	☐
My skin breaks out 1. Never or seldom. 2. Occasionally or in monthly cycles. 3. Frequently.	☐	☐	☐
My skin is 1. Dry and flaky. 2. Oily down the center T-zone of forehead, nose, chin. 3. Shiny most of the time.	☐	☐	☐
After I put on makeup in the morning, my face gets an oily shine: 1. It doesn't really get shiny. 2. About noon. 3. Within an hour.	☐	☐	☐
After shampooing, my hair gets oily and sticks together 1. In about a week's time. 2. In about three to four days. 3. In a day or two.	☐	☐	☐
My age is 1. Over 30. 2. 20 to 30. 3. Under 20.	☐	☐	☐

RATE YOURSELF

DRY SKIN TYPE:
If at least four out of six of your answers were number 1, you're a dry-skin type and should follow the routine for that kind of skin.

OILY SKIN TYPE:
If at least four out of six of your answers were 3, you're an oily-skin type and should follow that routine.

COMBINATION SKIN TYPE:
If your answers don't fit into either the oily- or dry-skin categories above, you're a combination skin type with both oily and dry areas and should follow that routine.

EXPERT CARE FOR
dry skin

To keep dry skin at its delicate best, give it a good cleansing night and morning. The night cleansing is very important since you have a day's accumulation of dirt and makeup to remove. A mild soap, cleansing lotion or cleansing cream is especially good for dry skin. If you prefer a soap rather than a lotion or cream, look for a mild, superfatted complexion soap or a glycerine soap. You might also try using a cream or lotion in the morning and a soap at night. Stay away from astringents, they're too drying for you. Instead, use a good skin toner to remove any last traces of oil or makeup and to give skin a nice smooth feel. If your skin is extra dry or sensitive, wet a cotton ball with water, squeeze out the excess, then wet with toner to dilute its strength. Night or morning, always finish with a good moisturizer on face and neck. You might also like to try a super-rich lubricant around eyes. Any good eye cream will do. This is an especially good idea in winter, when cold weather and central heating make skin especially dry.

ESSENTIALS

- Gentle but thorough cleanser
- Toner lotion, diluted with water if necessary
- Extra-rich moisturizer

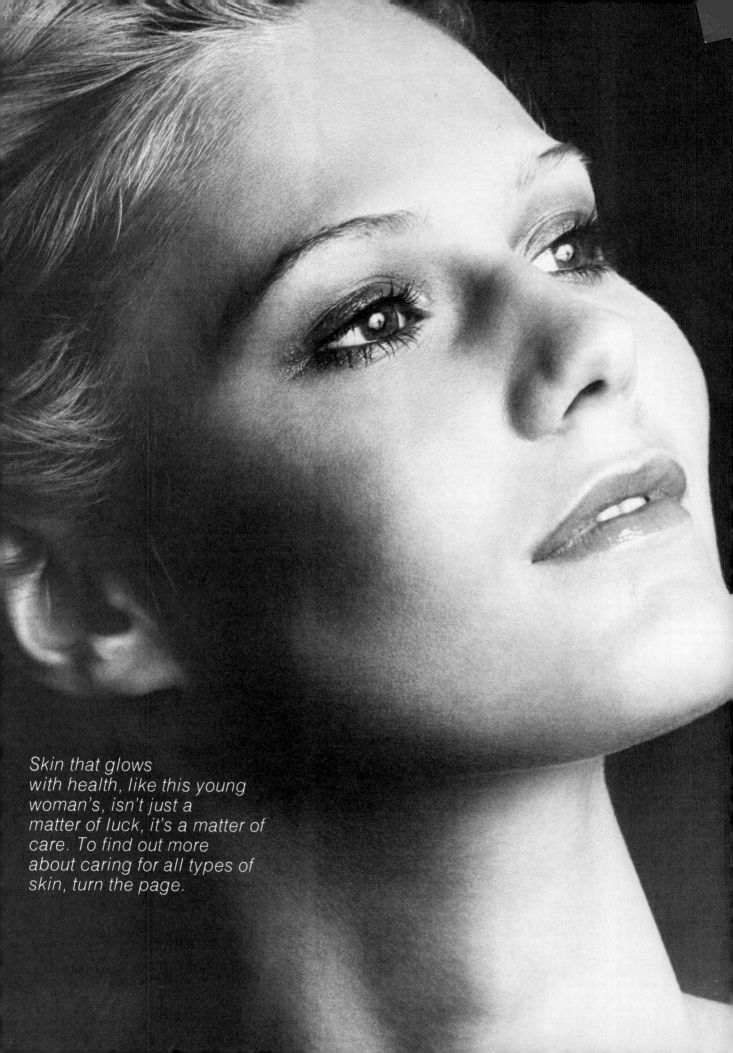

Skin that glows
with health, like this young
woman's, isn't just a
matter of luck, it's a matter of
care. To find out more
about caring for all types of
skin, turn the page.

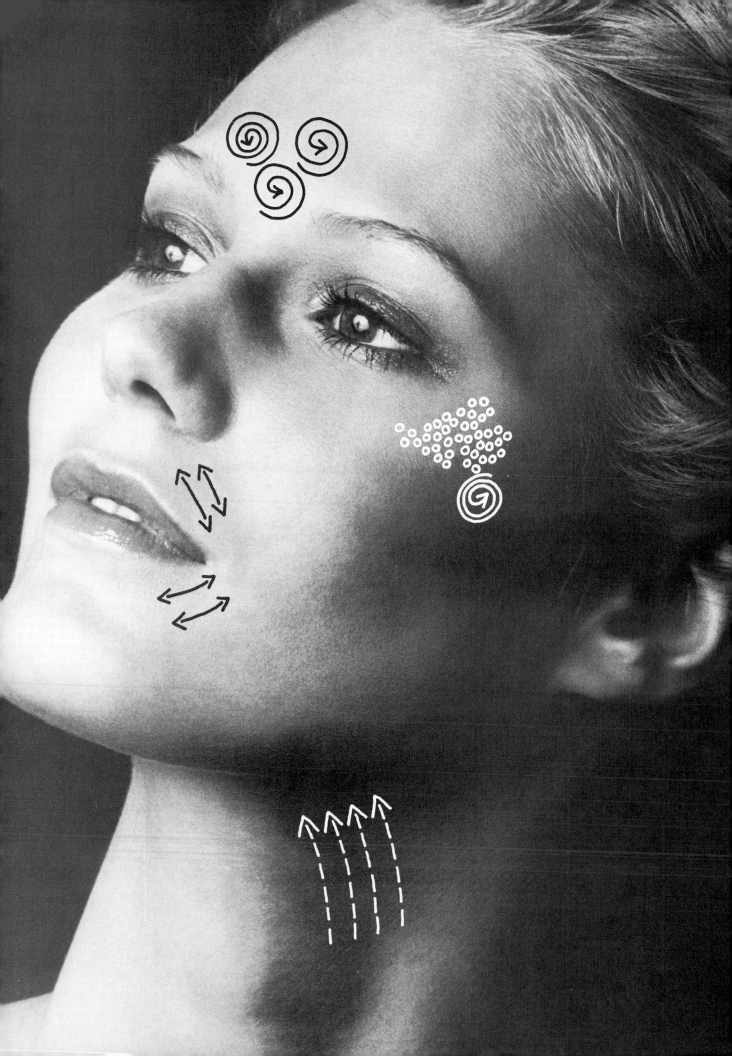

CLEAN your skin like a pro

No skin can look its best without being scrupulously clean. This means the right technique as well as the right cleanser for your skin. The guide that follows shows you how to work on each area of your face for proper cleansing. The massaging motion also helps stimulate circulation.

FOREHEAD, CHEEKS

When you've applied cleanser to your face, you're ready to give your skin a gentle massage to loosen dirt and stimulate circulation. On forehead and cheeks, use a three-part circular motion massaging with tips of fingers; arrows in photo opposite show you how. Work your way across forehead and cheeks, massaging gently as you go.

EYES

This area gets the gentlest treatment because the skin is extremely sensitive. Start by patting the upper lid lightly, starting at inner corner and moving out, using fingertips. Be sure to keep eyes closed so soap or lotion won't get in. Use same motion on lower eye area, working from inner corner out. Keeping your elbows raised as high as possible while you work will help take pressure off fingertips and give your fingers a light touch.

MOUTH

Keep your mouth relaxed and slightly open; massage in a back-and-forth motion over upper lip, then in a full circle. Repeat circle in opposite direction. Keep elbows high so pressure is off fingertips.

CHIN, NECK

This is one area to give extra effort to. Massaging around chin area can help stimulate circulation. Keep chin level, begin at base of neck using an upward motion and stroke with fingertips up and over chin and to ear line at sides of neck.

EXPERT CARE FOR oily skin

Oily skin, with its tendency to shine and break out, needs the most efficient deep-down cleansing. The best idea is to use a cleanser formulated especially for this skin type. Since oily skin should be cleansed midday as well as night and morning if you can manage it, pick a cleanser that's effective but not harsh. An astringent is also an essential for oily skin. It helps remove any last trace of oil and has a slight drying effect. Many have an antibacterial ingredient that's useful for skin that tends to break out. All skins need moisturizing, even oily skin. The moisturizer helps keep your own natural moisture from evaporating too fast. If you use a product that's light it will help keep skin moist without adding to your oil problem. If you wish, just apply moisturizer to eye area and neck.

ESSENTIALS

- Deep cleanser especially formulated for oily skin
- Astringent for oily skin
- Light-weight moisturizer

EXPERT CARE FOR dry/oily skin

You might have both dry and oily patches that need to be dealt with separately. This is not an uncommon situation since the natural concentration of oil glands is heavier in some parts of the face than in others—namely in a T-shaped area across forehead and down the nose. In some people these oily areas are quite oily in contrast to the rest of the skin. If this is you, try using a soap with real cleansing potential and concentrate on the oiliest areas. Another good idea is some kind of scrub product, a gentle abrasive or grainy cleanser, used weekly. You might want to use an astringent on the oiliest part of your face and a toner on the rest. A good moisturizer morning and night is essential for you, too. Concentrate on dry patches and around the eye and neck.

ESSENTIALS

- Effective but gentle cleanser
- Good toner, probably two, one a little milder than the other
- Good light-weight moisturizer

Questions and answers about
ACNE

Most young women have acne, true or false? False, right? Actually that statement is more true than false, but if your answer is wrong, don't feel bad. Most people would answer as you did because acne is one of the most misunderstood terms around.

Acne is not a single disease limited just to teenagers. In its mildest form it consists of only a few blackheads and random small breakouts. In its severest form, there are many deep boil-like blemishes. Anyone who has this kind of acne should be treated by a dermatologist. Actually, anyone with oily skin that's inclined to break out would benefit by a visit to a dermatologist to get his or her suggestions on overall care. In addition, you can help yourself by sorting out some of the facts and fictions about acne.

What causes acne?

You may have been told that you didn't wash your face enough and that's why you have breakouts. Doctors know that's usually nonsense. Acne occurs when the sebaceous glands become overactive, causing excess skin oiliness. This in turn stops up pores and eventually can cause the increased infectious boillike breakouts. The glandular activity has to do with increased hormonal production during puberty, rather than with uncleanliness. A clean skin does, however, help prevent a surface oil build-up. Doctors are still not absolutely certain why some individuals have such hyperactive sebaceous glands and why this overactivity results in acne, but they are learning some interesting new things. Dr. Ruth Freinkel, a professor of dermatology at Northwestern University, says that it seems those who come down with acne, unlike those who don't, seem to have receptors in their cells that accept the male sex-hormones that are present in both sexes.

Does lack of sleep cause acne?

Like cleanliness, sleep has been thrown into the "cure-all" basket for acne. "Get eight hours of sleep and your skin will be clearer" is advice we've heard, but unfortunately, it doesn't usually pay off. Habitual lack of sleep can cause illness, but eight hours doesn't guarantee clear skin. Sleep as much as *you* need to.

Does food cause trouble?

How much effect certain foods have on acne is still under debate. Fatty or fried foods, even chocolate, used to be thought of as culprits in acne cases, later as innocent bystanders. Recently some researchers have found evidence that certain ingested fatty substances found their way to the oily secretions of the face relatively unchanged from their original form. It would seem, then, that the oil in the food was contributing to the excess facial oil. Some doctors still don't accept this theory and research is still being done. About the only sensible thing you can do is follow your own doctor's advice and watch to see how your skin reacts after this kind of food. Iodides and bromides do irritate acne. They occur in iodized salt, saltwater fish and shellfish.

What can you do about it all?

It can't be emphasized enough that a dermatologist can be a great help in the treatment of acne. There are many medicines—like antibiotics, steroids and the correct dosages of supplementary vitamins, especially vitamin A—that only a doctor can recommend. But he or she can also prescribe treatment products like a special skin astringent or soap. If your breakouts are not severe, it is possible to buy over-the-counter remedies that will really help, if you choose carefully. Dermatologists tell us that there are four medications that are valuable: Benzoyl peroxide, sulfur, resorcinol and salicylic acid. They all inflame the skin and cause it to peel, which is beneficial. In essence, the skin peeling "dries out" the pimples and helps remove part of the inflamed and hardened skin. Benzoyl peroxide is the strongest of the group. Any effective acne product should list one or more of these ingredients on its label.

Acne and sun

Although dermatologists constantly warn patients about sun damage, acne treatment is an exception. Many doctors advise patients to get moderate amounts of sun (depending on how fair-skinned they are) because slight peeling is beneficial, along with the overall benefits of fresh air.

What else helps?

What helps is a list of don'ts that are easy to live with: don't pick; it spreads infection and increases the chance of scarring. Don't use gooey creams. Your skin doesn't need more oil. If your hair is oily, avoid on-the-face hair styles. Do get plenty of exercise, it's good for you in many ways.

Aftereffects

If a bad case has left you with a lot of scars, don't feel you must live with them. Dermabrasion, the mechanical peeling of the outer skin layer, and chemabrasion, the chemical peeling, can, in certain cases, greatly improve the looks of your skin. A visit to a good dermatologist can familiarize you with the pros and cons of each.

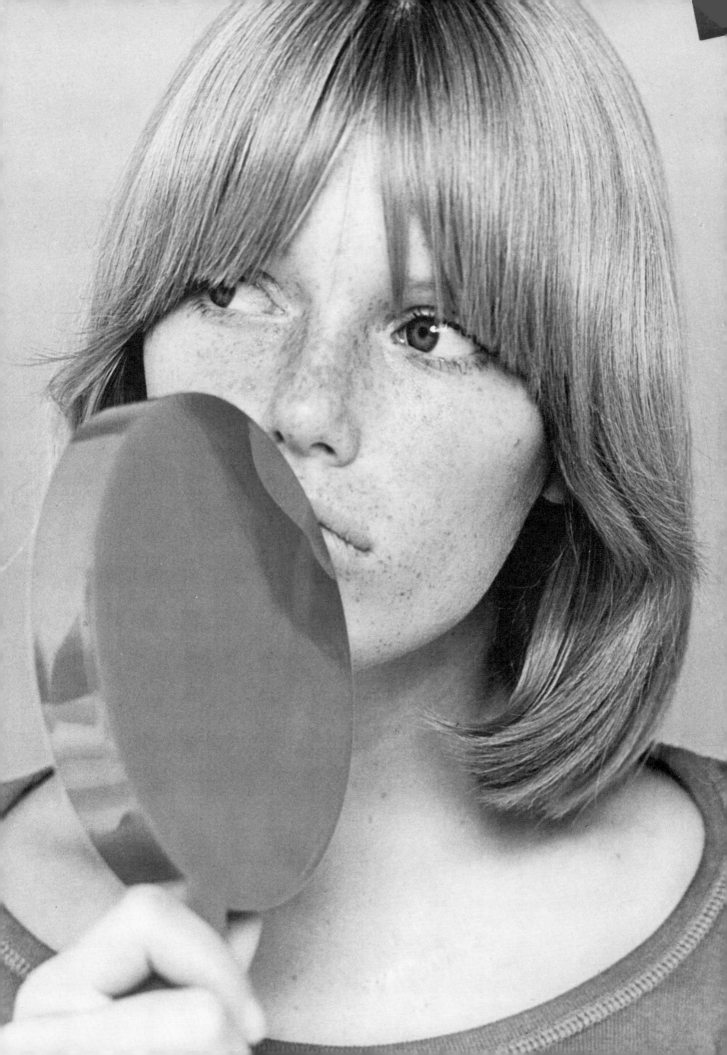

UNMASK FOR BEAUTY

One of the smartest beauty moves you can make—especially before any special evening or day— is to use a facial mask. There's absolutely nothing like one for putting a smooth polish and extra glow on a woman's cheeks.

There are almost as many different kinds of masks as there are women who use them, so if you aren't happy with the first one you try, do experiment with others. There's bound to be one that will give you the look and feel you're after. Basically, masks provide stimulation and cleansing action. They do this by bringing more blood into the tiny blood vessels of the skin. This increased circulation gives you that familiar glow and it also helps flush the impurities from pores. Depending on your skin type, you'll also want a mask to moisturize or remove some of the excess oil. Masks do this by temporarily altering the outer layers of your skin. By removing the dead, dry outer skin, a mask leaves your skin in better condition to soak up a moisturizer. Some even have moisturizers in them. If your skin is oily, removing this outer layer helps skin to breathe, helps make it less likely to trap oil secretions that can turn into breakouts and blackheads. Run through our list of masks here to see which one might work best for you. Then unmask a beautiful new skin for yourself.

CLEANSING MASKS

All of these masks do a bang-up job of getting skin super clean and most have several other benefits, too. If you're not certain whether a mask is a cleansing mask, ask and/or read the label. You can also often identify them by their slightly grainy texture or by their mudlike consistency. Most "mud" and grainy masks are cleansing masks. These masks are recommended for oily skin and can be used weekly. Use depends on the individual mask you select; use your judgment; if once a week seems adequate, fine. If not, try twice a week. In general, a mask shouldn't be used more than twice a week.

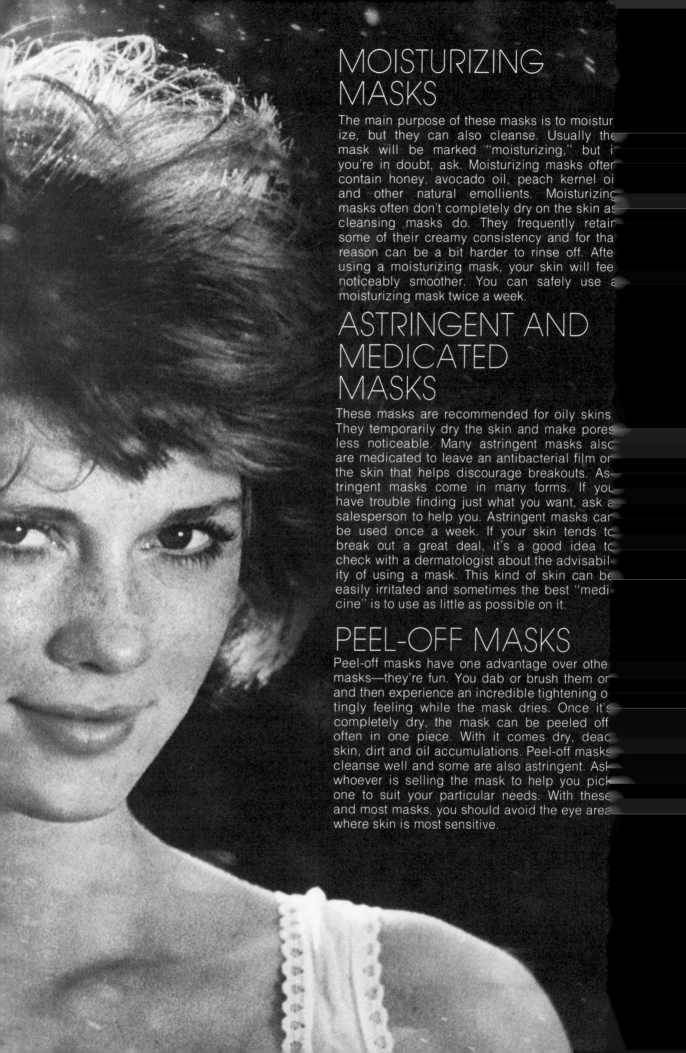

MOISTURIZING MASKS

The main purpose of these masks is to moisturize, but they can also cleanse. Usually the mask will be marked "moisturizing," but if you're in doubt, ask. Moisturizing masks often contain honey, avocado oil, peach kernel oil and other natural emollients. Moisturizing masks often don't completely dry on the skin as cleansing masks do. They frequently retain some of their creamy consistency and for that reason can be a bit harder to rinse off. After using a moisturizing mask, your skin will feel noticeably smoother. You can safely use a moisturizing mask twice a week.

ASTRINGENT AND MEDICATED MASKS

These masks are recommended for oily skins. They temporarily dry the skin and make pores less noticeable. Many astringent masks also are medicated to leave an antibacterial film on the skin that helps discourage breakouts. Astringent masks come in many forms. If you have trouble finding just what you want, ask a salesperson to help you. Astringent masks can be used once a week. If your skin tends to break out a great deal, it's a good idea to check with a dermatologist about the advisability of using a mask. This kind of skin can be easily irritated and sometimes the best "medicine" is to use as little as possible on it.

PEEL-OFF MASKS

Peel-off masks have one advantage over other masks—they're fun. You dab or brush them on and then experience an incredible tightening or tingly feeling while the mask dries. Once it's completely dry, the mask can be peeled off often in one piece. With it comes dry, dead skin, dirt and oil accumulations. Peel-off masks cleanse well and some are also astringent. Ask whoever is selling the mask to help you pick one to suit your particular needs. With these and most masks, you should avoid the eye area where skin is most sensitive.

WINTER
skin care

The condition of your skin is affected by your skin type—dry, oily, or normal—and by your environment—heat, cold, humidity, etcetera. In order to work out a really effective care routine, you must take both of these factors into consideration. We've worked out a special plan to help you find the most effective way to solve skin problems based on the effects of these two important factors.

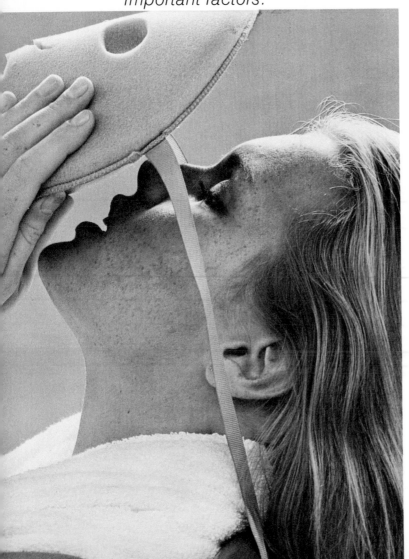

Cold weather problem

One of the special problems of this time of year is the combination of cold, dry outdoor air and hot, dry indoor air. This combination is especially hard on dry skin and can cause all skin types to chap and develop an uneven texture. The solution is a very rich moisturizer used morning and evening. If chapping occurs, ask a pharmacist to recommend a mild medicated lotion to help soothe the chapped skin. Do invest in a humidifier for indoors. It's especially important to have one in the room where you sleep. You'll notice a difference in your skin and you won't wake up with that dry feeling in your nose and throat.

Skin care ideas

● Be consistent. Don't use your cleanser, moisturizer, etcetera only when you remember. To see results, you must develop a daily routine and follow it everyday.
● Be aware that the condition of your skin will change as your environment changes. A cleanser or moisturizer that works in summer may not be rich enough in winter.
● Never wash your face immediately before going out into the cold; it's too drying and you risk chapping. Do it at least a half-hour before and moisturize well.

City pollution can cause eye irritations

● Winter or summer, big city air with its pollution can cause eye irritations that give you a puffy, red-eyed look. One solution is a mask especially designed to reduce eye puffiness caused by irritation. (To locate one, ask at a cosmetic counter.) Another idea is to use a good eyedrop preparation designed to reduce redness, and then to lie down and apply cotton pads saturated with witch hazel on your eyes. If you put the witch hazel in the refrigerator to cool it, it's especially refreshing.
● If you're troubled by breakouts on chest and back, the culprit just might be city air. Doctors don't know why, but periods of heavy pollution seem to bring more complaints about this problem. In winter, when dry skin patches can clog pores, the problem can be aggravated. Try using your facial toner or astringent on your back and chest and use a medicated breakout cream on any pimples.

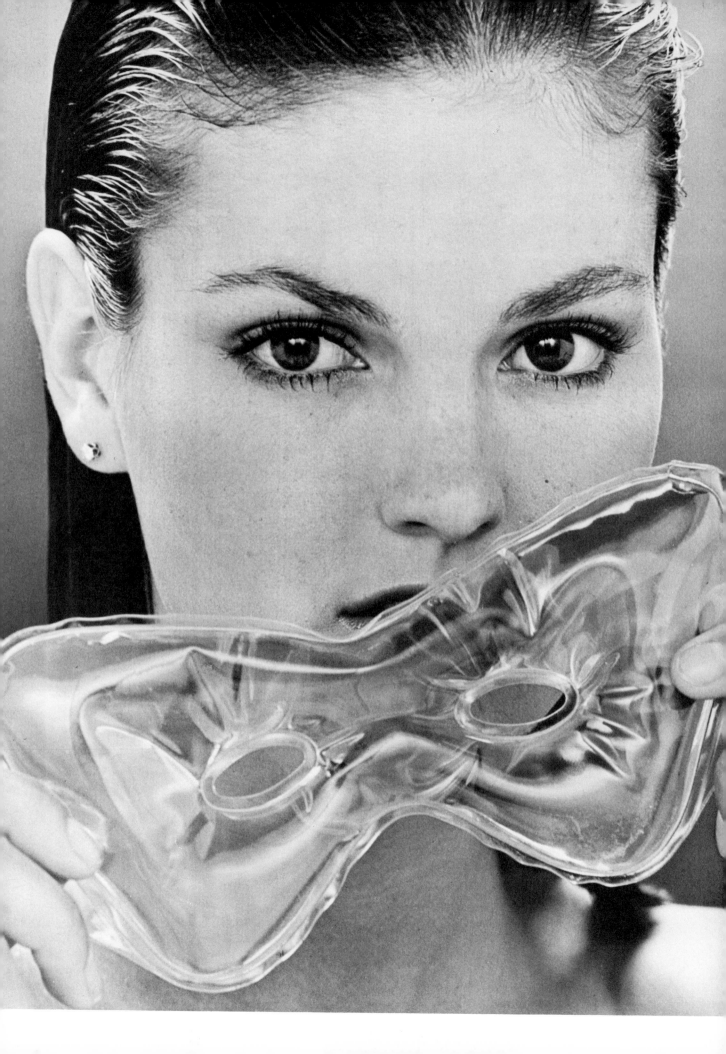

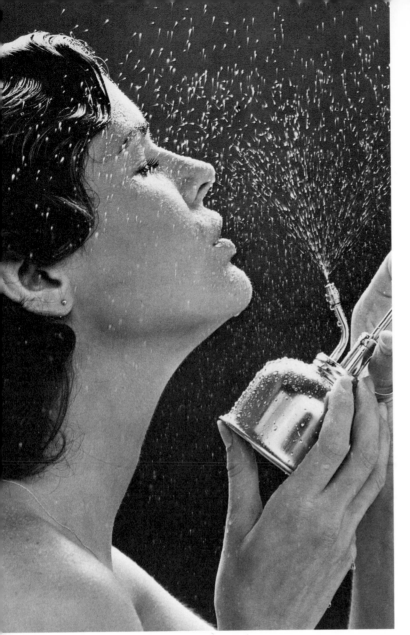

WINTER SKIN CARE

Tips for cold-weather activities

Most of us are inclined to forget that even in cold weather, the sun can be a beauty spoiler. Don't put your sunglasses away now; squinting into bright sun, especially if it's reflected on snow, can be hard on eyes and skin—where else do squint lines come from? Sunglasses plus a good protective moisturizer, preferably one containing a sunscreen, are musts for cold-weather outdoor activities. Any activity that works up a sweat—skiing, skating, even a good hike—will increase your chances of chapping. Don't forget to protect lips and the area around your mouth and chin with a moisturizer. A lip-protection stick used alone or under lipstick is a sound idea. When you come indoors after several hours of outdoor activity, resist the urge to run to a heater or fireplace. Warm up slowly; it's much easier on skin, causes less drying and shock to your skin owing to sudden temperature changes. When you want to do a supergood moisturizing job, try the trick in the picture here. Spray face lightly with water (or pat on water) and then moisturize. Moisturizer works best on slightly damp skin.

Winter travel tips

Unless you're going skiing, a winter trip usually means warm weather. The quick change from cold to warm, especially warm and humid, can make skin act up. To cope:
● Cleanse face often (even three times daily) with a gentle cleanser. A good mask would also help—pick a cleansing mask or a cleansing moisturizing mask combined.
● Wear a minimum of makeup where skin that's probably become more oily may develop clogged pores and break out. You can make yourself look terrific by concentrating makeup on eyes and lips.

Winter in warm places

Winter may mean snow and cold to most of the country, but there are places where it never really gets cold and you still have to cope with hot, humid weather. If you live in one of them, you have your problems, too. Here are some ideas:
● Though it may still be possible to get a tan, lifestyles usually change with the calendar and you're not out as much as usual. Try using a bronze-tinted moisturizer to give skin a sunny glow.
● If your climate is not cold, but cool enough to require some heat in winter, remember your skin will react to the drying heat and you should compensate by using a little moisturizer in dry areas, especially around eyes.
● Consider changing your skin cleanser now. You might need something more gentle than what you used when it was really hot and your skin was at its oiliest. A mild soap formulated for normal to oily skin would be good.

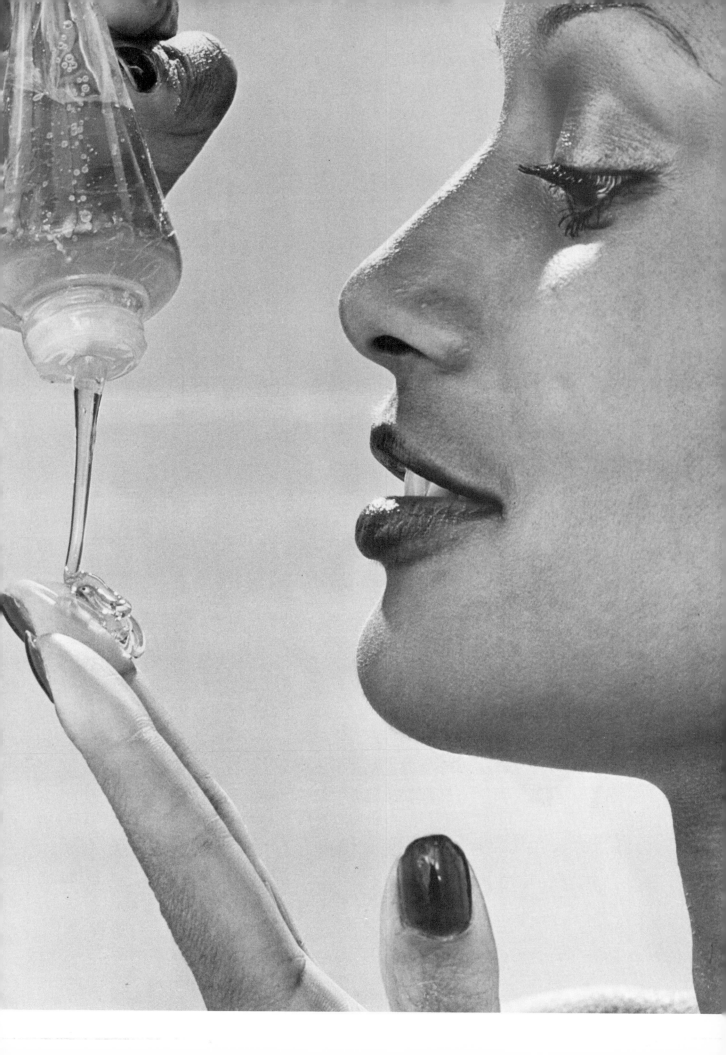

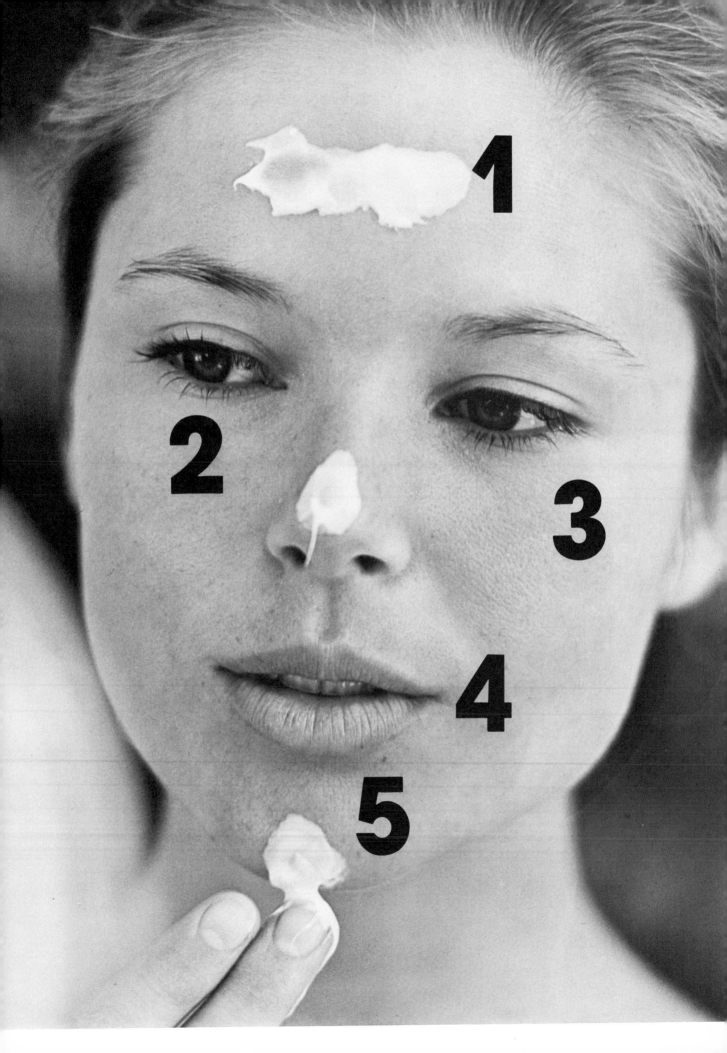

5 steps to
SUMMER-PROOF YOUR SKIN

Summer gives skin a fresh new color, a melting, moist glow— and for most of us, some special summer skin problems, too. The five changes in skin care recommended here won't guarantee a breakout free summer or less oiliness, but they will help you cope with these summer annoyances better than you've coped before.

1. Change moisturizers

Heat speeds up your metabolism, which means more active oil glands and oily skin. Humidity, by slowing down evaporation, holds this excess oil on the skin. If your skin is already oily, this can be a nuisance that eventually leads to clogged pores and breakouts. Cope by changing your winter moisturizer to something light. You may find moisturizing around eyes only is sufficient. If your skin is basically dry, you'll probably find the extra oiliness a help, but you might also need a lighter moisturizer. Remember, tanning will dry skin, so don't skip a moisturizer altogether.

2. Use masks more often

Sun exposure thickens and toughens the outer layer of skin and tends to trap excess oils and dirt in pore openings. This is a problem for dry or oily skin. A good mask will help loosen and remove this dead surface layer and let skin "breathe." Use a mask twice a week if necessary. You'll have to experiment to find just the right mask and the right number of times per week to use it.

3. Add a sunscreen

Apply the sunscreen every morning when you makeup. Dermatologists tell us the sun exposure you get taking a walk has cumulative effect that can damage skin, especially with a lot of outdoor sports activity. If you worry about adding the oil in a sunscreen to an already oily skin, there are many nongreasy screens to choose from. Some contain a fair amount of alcohol and help dry out skin a bit.

4. Cleanse more often

If you work, have some travel-size products in a desk drawer to use at noon. Presaturated astringent pads do a good, fast job of ridding oily skin of accumulated grime. Drier skin would probably like a cleansing lotion rather than a soap. If you prefer the soap, use a mild, superfatted one.

5. Add an oil blotter

There are many good ones around in either lotion, gel or powder form. Use it in the morning and during the day if your skin gets terribly oily.

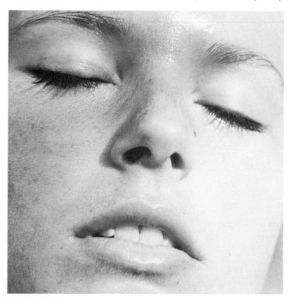

how to be your own beauty
TROUBLE-SHOOTER

They're not the same for everybody, but everybody has them—beauty trouble spots, those annoying bugaboos in your beauty life you thought you'd never get rid of: a downy mustache above your lip, a breakout when you least expect it. The troubleshooting campaign here will help banish them and start you on the road to a trouble-free beauty life.

Help for those unexpected breakouts

Here's a three-step plan to help you cope with breakouts. First, discourage their arrival by using a supplemental cleanser designed to get and keep oily skin really clean. (Ask your pharmacist to recommend an acne scrub.) These cleansers help unclog pores and get rid of the dead skin cells that do some of the clogging. After cleansing, use an astringent or oil-blotting lotion. Finally, have a good medicated breakout stick or cream handy. At the very first sign of a breakout, apply it according to directions.

To fight dark circles, tiny eye lines

Everyone has dark circles once in a while, and they do nothing for your good looks. Try a good circle cover-up cream or stick to conceal them. Look for a sheer, creamy consistency so you don't get a masklike effect. If you gently dot moisturizer under eyes, blend, and then use the concealer you'll get the best effect. Never pick a coverup more than a shade lighter than your skin, it won't look natural. If you're bothered by fine lines around your eyes, a rich eye stick will soften them and give a flattering sheen to eye area.

Mustache banisher

No one's looks are improved by that shadowy down over the upper lip. To take away the shadow, try a good facial bleach. Have a look at your jawline, too. People who tend toward facial hair usually have peach fuzz around the jaw and up to hairline as well as a mustache. The bleach can be used on any unwanted facial hair.

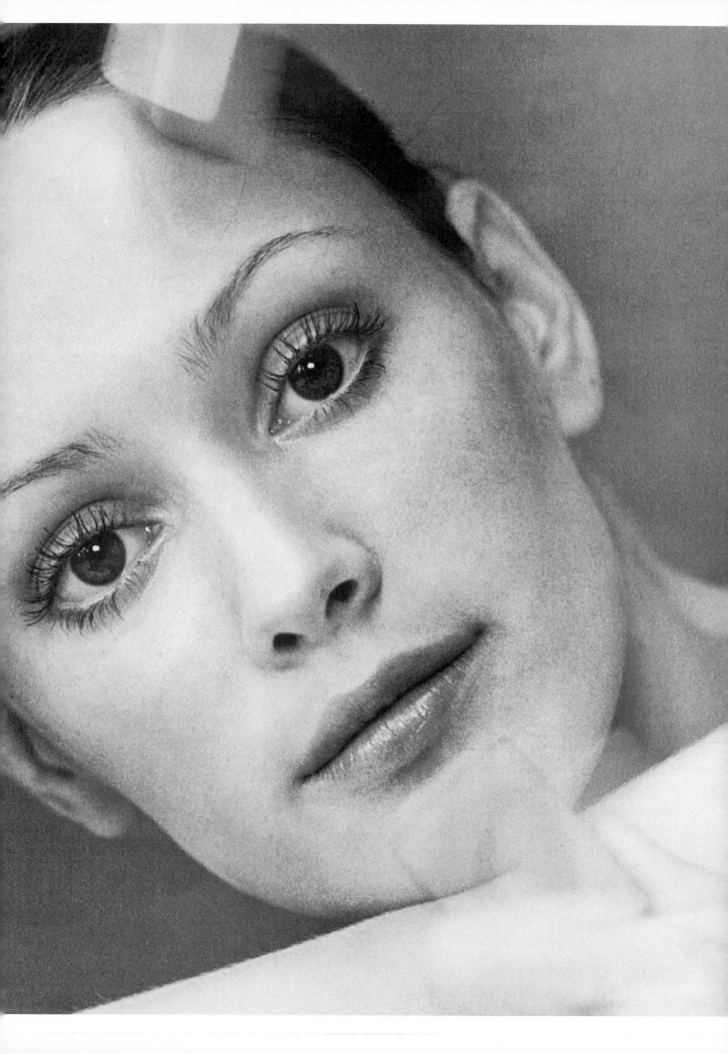

how to get rid of the HAIR you don't want

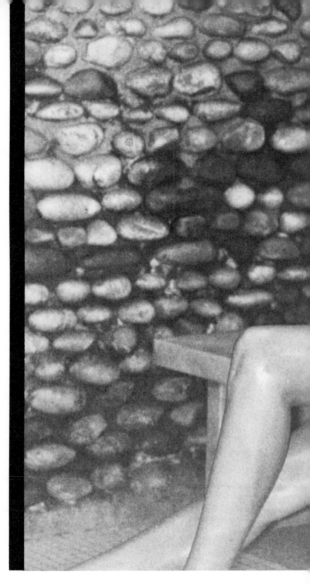

Hair on the head, in thick shining masses, is something everyone wants. Hair in profusion most anywhere else is a beauty worry that no one needs. Here is a rundown of the most effective and practical means of removing all kinds of excess hair.

PLUCKING

This is a sound method for removing scattered hairs on the face and breast, but obviously impractical if the hair is dense. Although some people find it uncomfortable, it has no adverse effects. Anyone who finds the discomfort acute might consider clipping breast hairs close with a sharp, small scissors. Regrowth will be noticeable sooner than if you'd plucked, however.

SHAVING

This is a very efficient way to remove excess hair from legs and underarms. It causes no change in the texture or growth of hair. Shaving is not a satisfactory solution for arm, facial and other body hair. The stubbly regrowth is much more of a problem there than on legs, which are not seen at such close range or touched as often.

Some women with coarse curly hair complain of ingrown hair as a result of shaving. The best way to handle this is not to shave as closely as you ordinarily would and try never to pull or stretch the skin to get at hair from a better shaving angle. Using an electric razor to shave hair in some hidden places like the upper thigh and armpit is a good way to cut down on the itching that usually results from blade shaving. Using a good medicated powder after shaving should also help.

BLEACHING

This is a most satisfactory way to make hair on arms, face, stomach and inner upper thighs (bikini area) appear less conspicuous. You can buy a commercial bleach made for facial hair.

DEPILATION

You'll find this an effective hair-removal method for arms, legs and bikini-exposed hair on stomach and thighs. Follow the directions on the label carefully and test the depilatory on a small area first to be sure no irritation will occur. If your hair is coarse, the time needed for the depilatory to work may be a disadvantage, especially since it has to be done as often as shaving. The regrowth of hair after a depilatory is used tends not to feel so stubby as the regrowth that appears after shaving. Depilatories should never be used on the face unless the directions specifically state that it is safe for this kind of use.

WAXING

Excess hair from arms, legs, stomach, inner

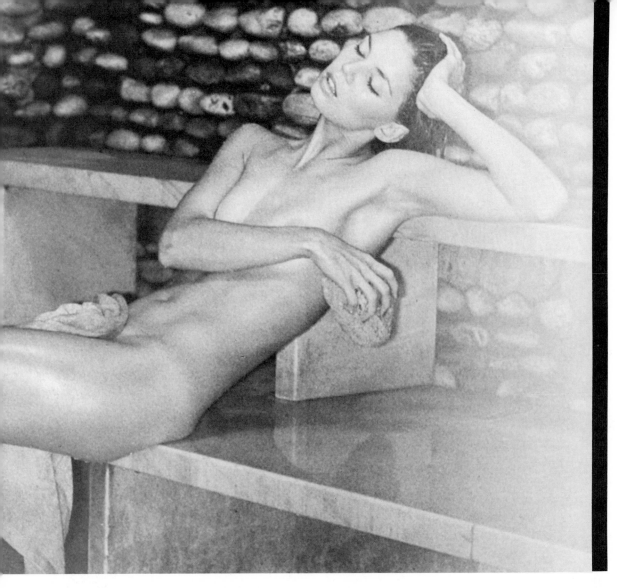

thigh tops and small areas of the face, upper lip, sides of cheeks is easily removed by waxing. The wax is heated first, then applied in strips. A cloth is pressed against the wax, which when dry is pulled off with the cloth against the direction the hair grows. The advantage of waxing is that it lasts a longer time than depilation or shaving since hair is removed below the surface of the skin and regrowth is not particularly stubby. The main disadvantage is that it is uncomfortable and there is also a risk of getting the wax too hot if you're doing the job yourself. Hair must also be fairly long to be waxed successfully, so you must endure a period of hairiness before rewaxing is possible. The regrowth is usually soft and not stubbly, however. People who are prone to ingrown hair may have more of a problem with waxing. If there seems to be an increase in the number of ingrown hairs, bleaching is probably a better solution than waxing.

ELECTROLYSIS

If you are really self-conscious about body hair and feel you have a great deal of it, you should probably consider electrolysis. But you should also know what you're getting into. First of all,

there's the time involved. Although removing a single hair takes only a few seconds, clearing large areas on arms and legs can take a couple of years of weekly or twice-weekly sessions. Then there's the expense. Fees vary, but you can expect to spend about five dollars for fifteen minutes or ten dollars for a half-hour. If you go to a posh salon, you'll spend more. There are also certain risks to electrolysis. Even the most skilled technician can't guarantee that there won't be some regrowth. Although electrolysis is permanent, sometimes it takes more than one treatment to completely destroy a hair. There is also the risk of scarring, depending on the area to be treated. A good technician is your best insurance against this, but certain areas of the face—the upper lip, for example—carry more risk no matter how good the technician is. Lastly, electrolysis is somewhat uncomfortable, especially if you're undergoing prolonged treatment to clear large areas.

Home electrolysis devices do exist. Those with a retractable needle are relatively safe and they do work, but they require manual dexterity and a lot of patience in order to be successful. A professional electrologist can remove several hundred hairs in a session while an inexperienced person at home may only be able to remove thirty to forty hairs in an hour.

SKIN AND BODY

Many women meticulously care for their facial skin
but never give their body skin a second thought.
This is a big mistake. If you're interested in
maintaining a youthful appearance indefinitely, the
skin on your body can give you away long before
it's necessary, if you neglect it. The next pages will
show you how to polish and protect every inch of
your precious skin so it remains a beauty asset
for as long as you care for it.

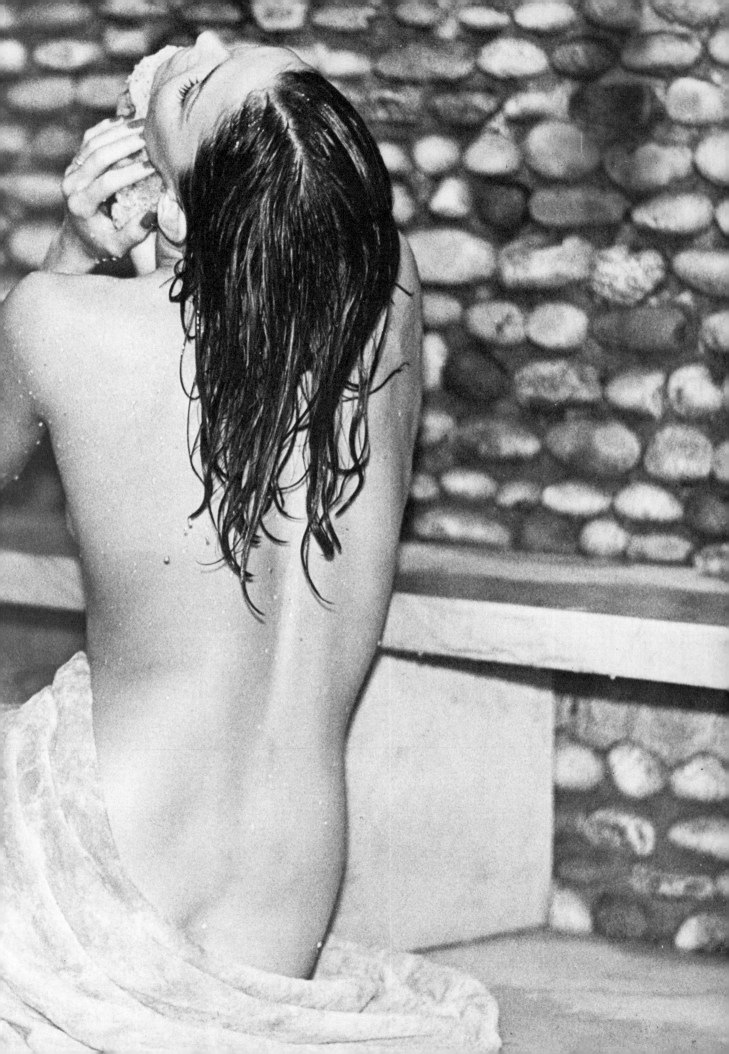

Freckles, strap marks

While some people find freckles appealing, others do not. They are caused by uneven skin pigmentation, and come out in full glory under the sun. You can't completely prevent them if you're a freckler, but a really good sunscreen or even better a sunblock product will help minimize them. Be sure you reapply the product after swimming or every couple of hours if you're perspiring a lot. The best cure for strap marks is to get them the same color as the surrounding skin with some carefully plotted sun exposure. A bit of bronzing gel or a deep tan foundation applied over strap marks will help.

Stretch marks, stomach scars

Stretch marks occur when skin stretches drastically, then relaxes, usually as a result of pregnancy or a great deal of rapid weight loss. A one-piece maillot—becoming very classy again—will hide stretch marks and other stomach scars and will probably make you feel the most secure emotionally. Recently, plastic surgeons have developed a technique for removing severe stretch marks. It's expensive and probably too drastic unless you're really disturbed by these marks. If you want to investigate, check with your state or county medical association for the names of local plastic surgeons.

Fresh scars from abdominal operations are best covered with one-piece suits. You'll find most of these scars tend to fade with time.

Psoriasis

If you have problems with the scaly, itchy patches of psoriasis, ask your dermatologist about the new high-intensity black-light treatment. The patient is given medication to swallow, then put under the special light, and in most cases, dramatic improvement is seen. Without this treatment, dermatologists often prescribe some sun exposure to help.

Acne and bareness

Many dermatologists suggest controlled sun exposure for acne patients. The drying, peeling effect of sun helps clear skin, keeping breakouts at a minimum. Large acne cysts, especially those that frequently appear on the back, can be injected with cortisone. If you're taking antibiotics for acne, be sure to check with your doctor to see if the one you're taking predisposes you to sunburn.

Body scars

If a cut or other injury has resulted in a keloid scar (a raised lump of scar tissue), there is a good possibility a dermatologist can make it less noticeable by injecting it with steroids. Check with your doctor.

Moles, birthmarks

Many moles can be successfully and relatively inexpensively removed by a dermatologist. Birthmarks sometimes can be removed, but they're trickier so check with your doctor. A cover cream or stick can help camouflage small marks.

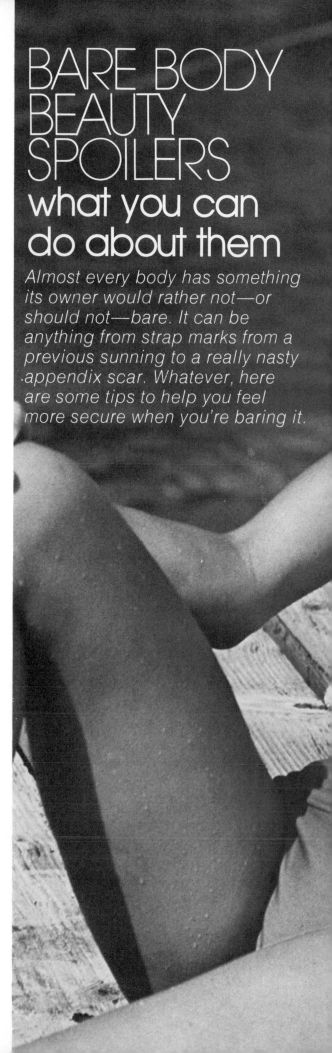

BARE BODY BEAUTY SPOILERS
what you can do about them

Almost every body has something its owner would rather not—or should not—bare. It can be anything from strap marks from a previous sunning to a really nasty appendix scar. Whatever, here are some tips to help you feel more secure when you're baring it.

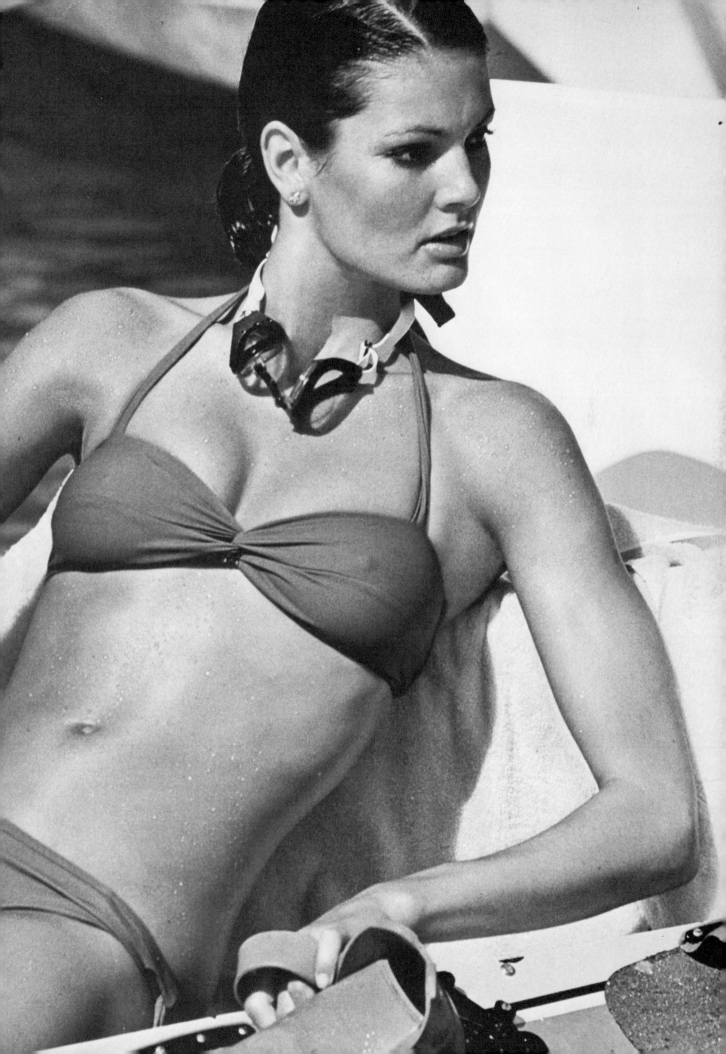

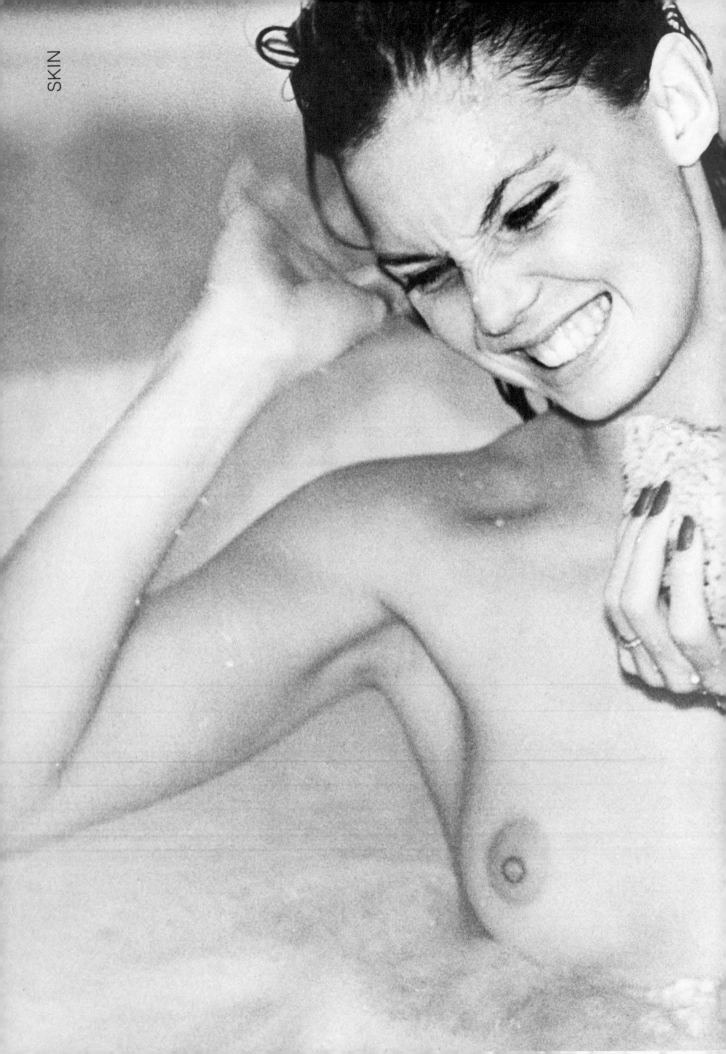

how much bathing is good for SKIN?

We Americans come in for a lot of criticism about our "clean" hang-ups, and some of it may be justified. If your skin, especially in winter—or if you've been sunning a lot in summer—is showing any of the three endangered species signals listed here, you may be overdoing the washing up. Fortunately, you don't have to stop; all you have to do is add some perfectly delightful ingredients to counter the irritants of weather.

SNAKESKIN PATCHES

A lack of moisture is one of the chief causes of rough, dry snakeskin patches. Cold weather and central heating are the main culprits that deplete skin's natural moisture in cold weather. Sun is usually the cause in warm. Dermatologists tell us that using emollients on moist skin, rather than on dry, or while you're actually bathing makes them most effective. A bath oil used in your tub water can be very effective as well as pleasant. If you shower most of the time, buy a product that can be used in the shower. Many are available. You might also try some premoistened towelettes that coat your body with a bath-oil like substance.

Although the whole point here is not to overdo cleansing, dry flaky skin can use some *gentle* abrasive action to get rid of the flaky patches. You might try a natural sponge to gently sponge away roughness or buy one of the body-sloughing lotions available now. A cosmetic salesperson or your druggist can recommend one. Don't use it too often, about once a week should be enough.

NO GLOW SKIN

Women frequently complain that their skin loses its soft sheen in winter. The explanation is simple enough. When skin is dry, tiny scales stand up on its surface and prevent normal light reflection. What you see is "no glow" skin. The solution is to slip on some body polishers that will help smooth and add a sheen. Pick any good body moisturizer and apply it liberally after every bath or shower. If you're especially troubled by dry skin, pick a product that contains some urea, an ingredient that helps skin retain moisture. Check product labels or ask your druggist to recommend something that contains it.

WRONG CLEANSER SYMPTOMS

If your skin is taut and dry and it feels a size too small for your body, you may be using too strong a bath soap. It may take some experimenting to find the right one, but it's worth it. Look for a superfatted soap or one that's recommended for dry skin. Your local drugstore has a selection of special soaps that are gentle yet effective. Some of the new "natural" soaps with natural oils such as avocado might work for you. If your skin is so taut and dry that you notice small itchy red patches, you may have developed a kind of dermatitis or allergy to a particular soap. A visit to a dermatologist would be worthwhile. Ask the doctor to recommend a gentle soap and something to soothe your skin in the meantime.

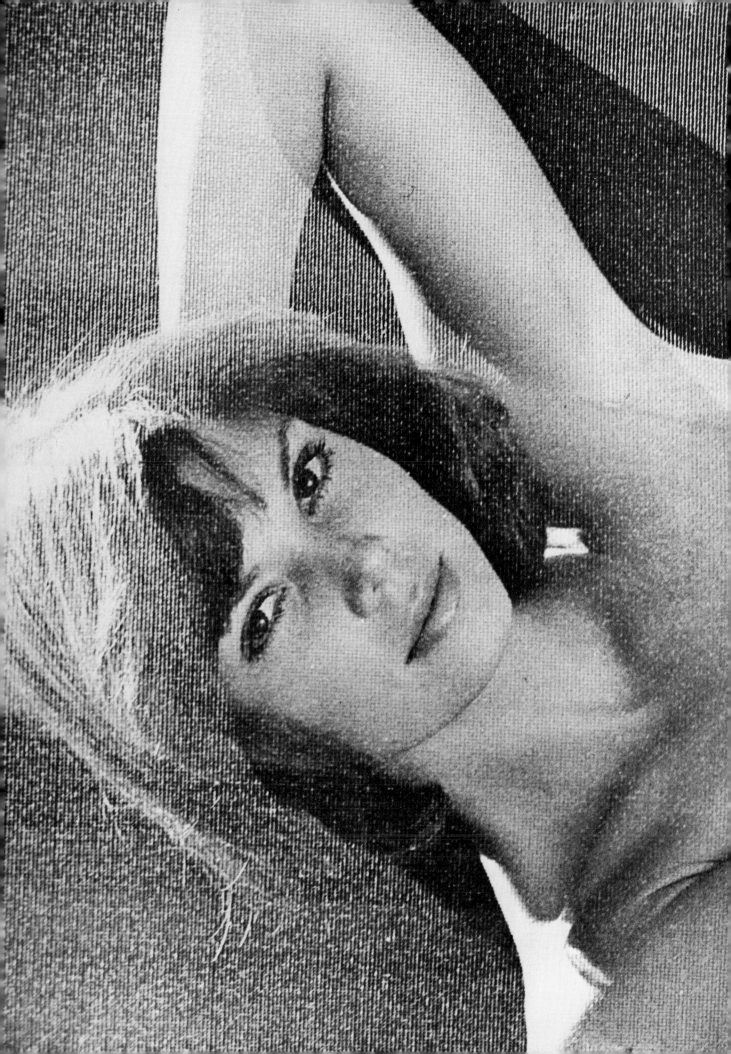

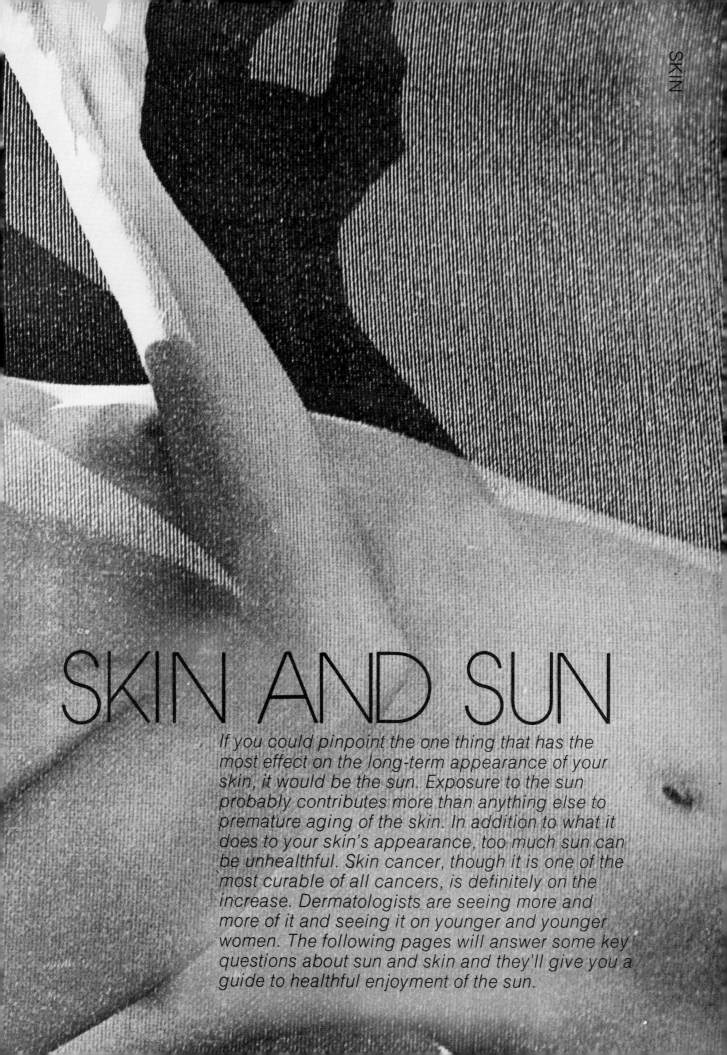

SKIN AND SUN

If you could pinpoint the one thing that has the most effect on the long-term appearance of your skin, it would be the sun. Exposure to the sun probably contributes more than anything else to premature aging of the skin. In addition to what it does to your skin's appearance, too much sun can be unhealthful. Skin cancer, though it is one of the most curable of all cancers, is definitely on the increase. Dermatologists are seeing more and more of it and seeing it on younger and younger women. The following pages will answer some key questions about sun and skin and they'll give you a guide to healthful enjoyment of the sun.

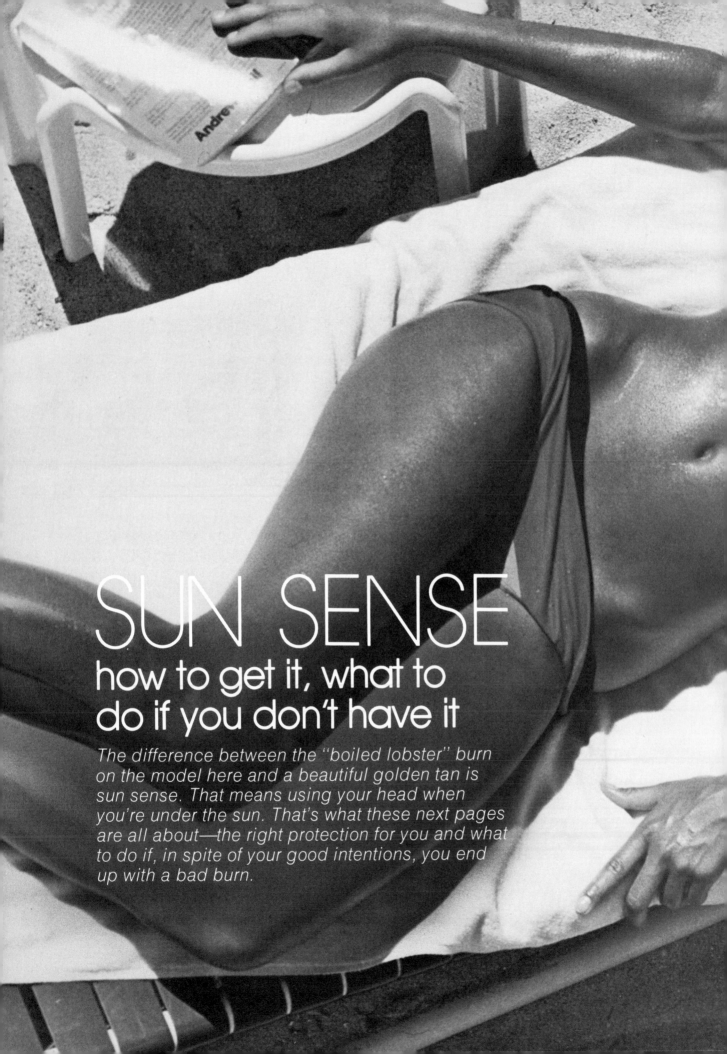

SUN SENSE

how to get it, what to do if you don't have it

The difference between the "boiled lobster" burn on the model here and a beautiful golden tan is sun sense. That means using your head when you're under the sun. That's what these next pages are all about—the right protection for you and what to do if, in spite of your good intentions, you end up with a bad burn.

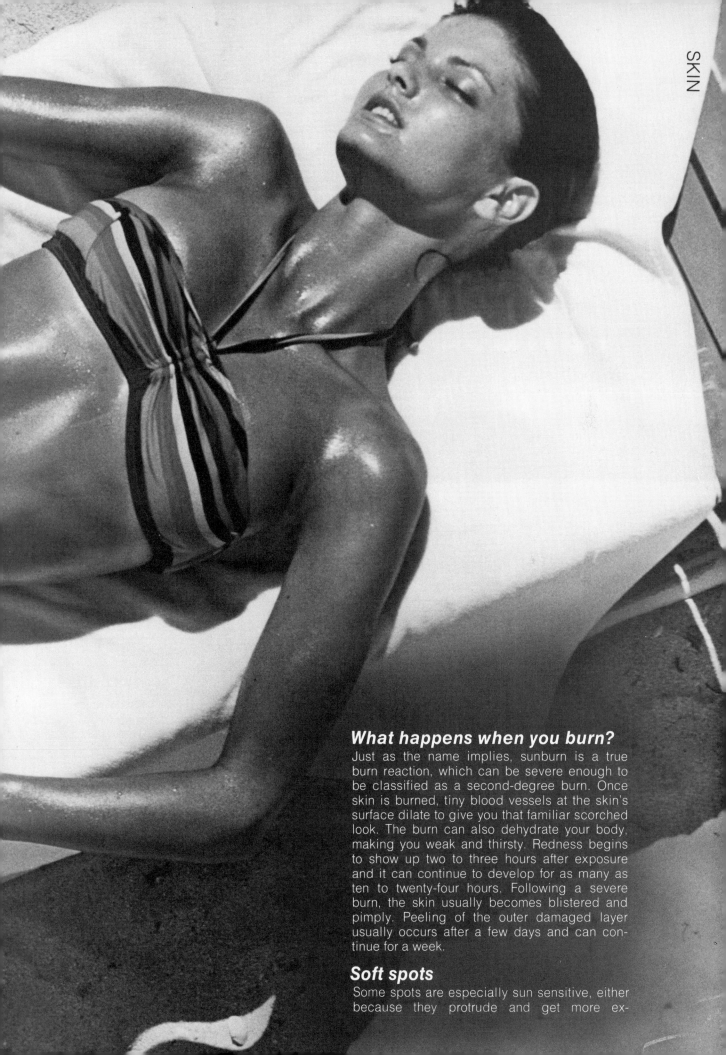

What happens when you burn?

Just as the name implies, sunburn is a true burn reaction, which can be severe enough to be classified as a second-degree burn. Once skin is burned, tiny blood vessels at the skin's surface dilate to give you that familiar scorched look. The burn can also dehydrate your body, making you weak and thirsty. Redness begins to show up two to three hours after exposure and it can continue to develop for as many as ten to twenty-four hours. Following a severe burn, the skin usually becomes blistered and pimply. Peeling of the outer damaged layer usually occurs after a few days and can continue for a week.

Soft spots

Some spots are especially sun sensitive, either because they protrude and get more exposure—like nose and knees—or because the skin is very tender, like neck and behind knees.

How important is protection?

The only way to enjoy the sun and be sensible at the same time is to protect your skin. Protection can be in the form of a good sunblocking or screening lotion or in the form of protective clothing. Usually, a combination of both is best. You must always remember that no sun product, even the best one, can totally protect you if you remain outdoors for long, long hours, especially at midday. You must also remember to reapply the product frequently, especially after swimming and when you're perspiring profusely.

When is a doctor necessary?

If you've really gotten a severe sunburn with more than a third of your body blistered and if you have chills and feel feverish, see a doctor. The chills and fever are signs that your body is experiencing some shock reaction and medical attention is necessary. If the burn is not severe enough to cause chills and fever, but you're still very uncomfortable, Dr. Robert Auerbach, a New York dermatologist, recommends cold compresses. Use a large, cool, wet towel, first on the lower front of your body, then the top half, then your back so that your entire body isn't chilled at once. If you prefer the convenience of a tub instead of compresses, don't plunge into a cold tub. Have the water cool, not cold. Don't doctor it up with vinegar, tea or other mythical sunburn remedies. If you want some lubrication for that dry feeling, put a glass of milk in the bath water. Also, be certain you drink plenty of fluids; eat salty crackers to help replace the salt you've lost from dehydration.

Dr. Auerbach also discourages using spray-on preparations with local skin anesthetics in them as skin damaged by sunburn is more sensitive than normal skin and more likely to develop an allergic reaction.

Since a sunburn usually makes you feel warm and uncomfortable, it's a good idea not to rush around and exhaust yourself. This only makes you warmer and increases the chance of feeling downright sick as a result of the burn. Keep relatively quiet and try to stay as cool as possible for the eight hours immediately following a burn. As we stressed earlier, continue to drink a lot of fluids—water, fruit juices or whatever appeals to you—since the burn has proba-

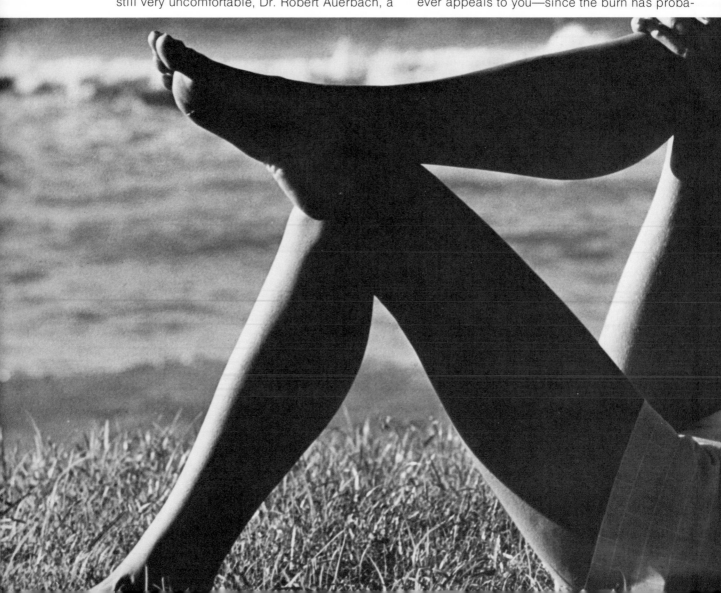

bly dehydrated you. You should also try to eat lightly, as a big heavy meal can cause you to feel sick and increase your discomfort.

A certain degree of swelling usually accompanies a bad burn and gravity makes the swelling settle in the ankles. Many women ask if they can take a diuretic to relieve swollen ankles. Dr. Auerbach cautions that since a bad burn dehydrates the body, causing the loss of certain essential minerals, it can be risky to take a diuretic, which could cause excessive fluid and mineral loss. A better idea is to put your feet up on a pillow while you lie down for an hour and let the fluid move away from your ankles. Once the accumulated fluids—which by the way are produced whenever tissue is injured—get moving in your system, the kidneys usually take over and eliminate them.

Many women hate the after-burn peeling as much as the burn itself. Dr. Auerbach points out that nothing will stop you from peeling; it's nature's way of getting rid of the damaged skin, but you can make the peeling less of a beauty problem by using body moisturizers frequently to diminish the scaly look. Don't hurry the peeling process by pulling off dry skin. If the skin underneath isn't completely healed, you'll have a very sore tender area to cope with and probably a scab—which is worse than the peeling!

Remember that skin that has recently been badly burned is even more sensitive to sun than normal skin, especially if there's been extensive peeling. If you allow yourself to get burned again, you're going to suffer even more than you did the first time because of that sensitive skin. Take sun exposure very slowly after a burn, protect skin with sunscreens and don't forget to reapply them after a swim or at least every couple of hours.

SUN EXPOSURE GUIDE

These times refer to your first exposure of the season, with unprotected skin. Never take your sun at noon. Dr. Robert Auerbach, who worked out this guide for us, cautions not to exceed these times, and points out that even cautious sun exposure is not really good for skin. Very fair skinned, light-eyed people should never go in the sun unprotected. Medium to fair skins can follow these times, then use sunscreens for the rest of their exposure. If you tan, you'll get results in a week following these exposures. Never exceed your maximum exposure time without the protection of a sunscreen, even after you're tan.

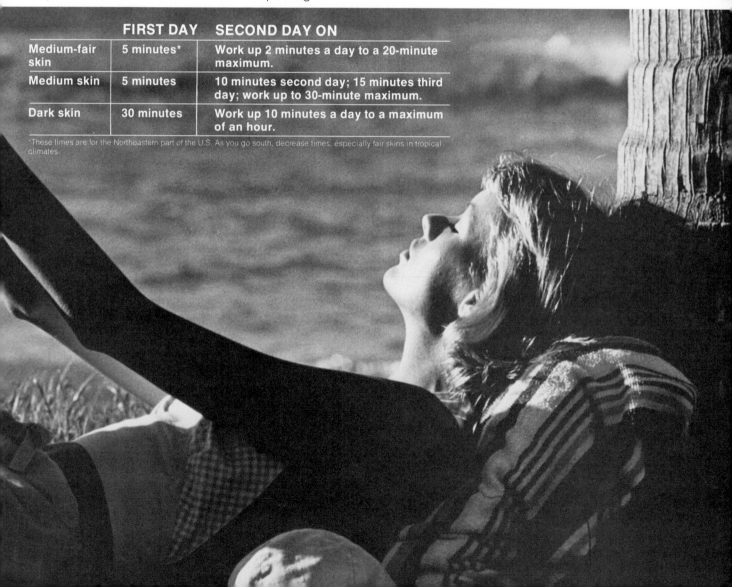

	FIRST DAY	SECOND DAY ON
Medium-fair skin	5 minutes*	Work up 2 minutes a day to a 20-minute maximum.
Medium skin	5 minutes	10 minutes second day; 15 minutes third day; work up to 30-minute maximum.
Dark skin	30 minutes	Work up 10 minutes a day to a maximum of an hour.

*These times are for the Northeastern part of the U.S. As you go south, decrease times, especially fair skins in tropical climates.

SUNNING FOR BEAUTY

The sun has enormous potential to make or break summer looks. Whether your skin looks like tan crepe paper or a glowing bit of silk depends on how well you protect it. The chart and tips here tell you how to play sun smart.

GUIDE TO SUNTANNING PRODUCTS

Minimum protection:

Products that provide no real sun protection usually just lubricate the skin. You can identify them frequently by the words "oil" or "butter" in the product name. Such products usually list no active ingredients on their label. They are cosmetic rather than protective.

Medium protection:

These products usually contain some sunscreening ingredients, which will be listed on the label as "active ingredients." Some of the most effective sunscreens are para-aminobenzoic acid (sometimes called PABA), the salicylates and benzophenone. These products will usually be in lotion or cream form, and the label will be worded to inform you that the product screens out *some* of the burning rays.

Maximum protection:

These are the true sunblocks. Product labels will also include active ingredients (usually one of the above listed). The label will usually say the product blocks out *most* of the sun's burning rays.

   Note: Total physical blocks to the sun's rays are available in such preparations as zinc oxide.

Artificial tanners:

These products will *temporarily* stain skin.

SUN CAUTIONS

Don't think sun lotions are for other people. Everyone needs some protection and/or lubrication. You have to let experience guide you, but here is a rough breakdown on who needs what.

● Fair, extremely sun-sensitive skin: Look for products with maximum filtering and reapply often.

● Medium complexion: Look for products offering medium filtering, usually those whose labels say product will let you tan with minimum risk of burning.

● Dark complexions: Start with a medium filter, then go to a minimum filter.

● Watch out for "reflected" sunlight—from sand under beach umbrellas, white boat decks, etcetera. It can give you a nasty burn.

● Remember that water absorbs ultraviolet rays—while swimming or wading, you are exposed to the sun's rays and you can burn.

● Don't feel you're home-free as soon as you have a little tan. You should still keep applying sun protective lotions to prevent burn or too deep a tan and to keep your skin lubricated. Remember, you may need more than one sun lotion—one for extrasensitive areas, another for the rest of you.

● Some medications—for example, antibiotics and certain tranquilizers—can increase the skin's sun sensitivity. So check with your doctor to be sure you'll have no problems.

SKIN TEST

You may think the sun hasn't changed your skin at all, but chances are it has already made some visible and tactile differences—all the more reason to follow the advice in this sun-sense section. Look at the skin on your bosom, run your fingers over it. Then look at the skin on your chest, that part *not* covered by a swimsuit; run your fingers over this. The skin on your bosom will probably be noticeably finer-grained and smoother unless you've been sunning nude. Although this difference may seem slight now, how slight will it be ten summers from now if you don't protect yourself?

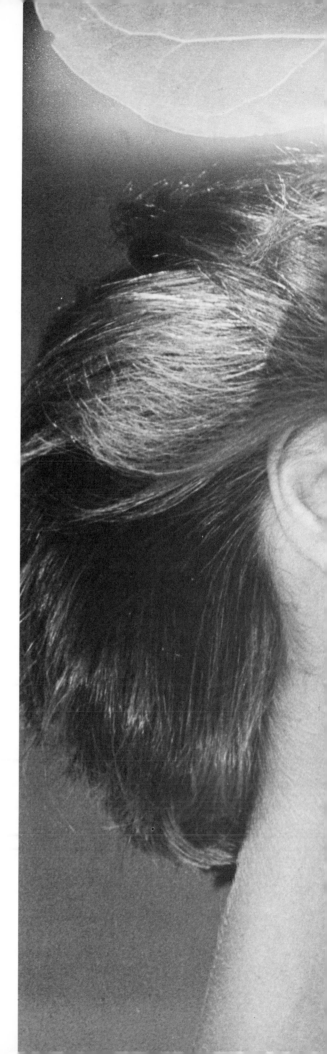

What some of the usual sun/ beauty talk misses is the fact that sun can be a beauty ally as well as an enemy. The questions and answers here give you the straight facts about sun and your looks and health. Respect the advice and you'll not only avoid sun problems, you'll discover how to turn the sun into a strong beauty ally, too.

Does sun help clear up breakouts?

Many women find their breakouts less trouble-some in summer. This is because sun exposure stimulates cell growth in the outer skin layer. This accelerated growth results in a peeling process that helps keep pore openings freer and therefore less vulnerable to infection. Although sun exposure does help acne, and many dermatologists recommend *limited* exposure, don't overdo.

Does sun bring out freckles? Will they fade later?

Sun exposure causes the pigmentation present in everyone's skin to darken. This is what happens when you tan. Many people have clumps of unevenly distributed pigment. When exposed to sun, some clumps darken more than the surrounding, less pigmented skin. These darker spots are freckles. They do tend to fade in winter but next summer they'll return. If you want to make freckles less noticeable, use a good sunscreening product. You may want to use a maximum protection product on your face and something less screening on the rest of your body where freckles aren't as noticeable.

Does a woman have to add anything to her skin care routine in summer besides sun protectors?

Many women find their skin gets oilier in hot weather. If so, add a skin toner after your cleansing routine. If you already use a toner, change to an astringent—it's stronger. An oil-based makeup may need to be traded in for a water-based one, and you should consider changing from a heavy-weight nighttime moisturizer to a light-weight undermakeup moisturizer for both day and night use. You might also find a deep cleansing mask a help.

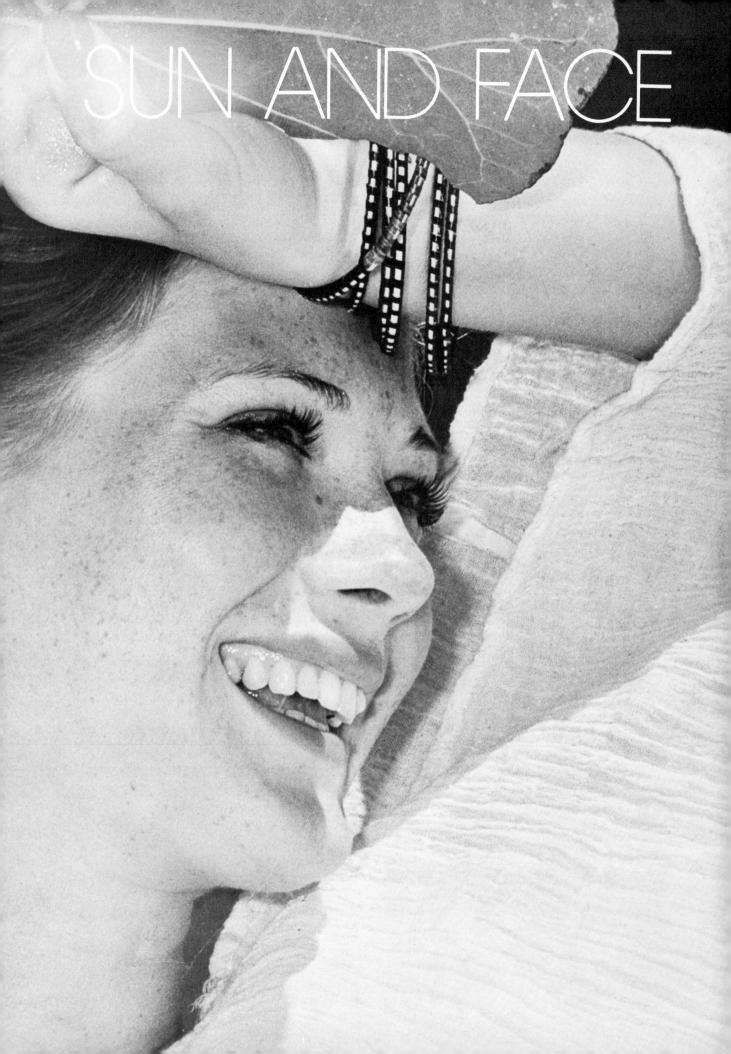

SUN AND FACE

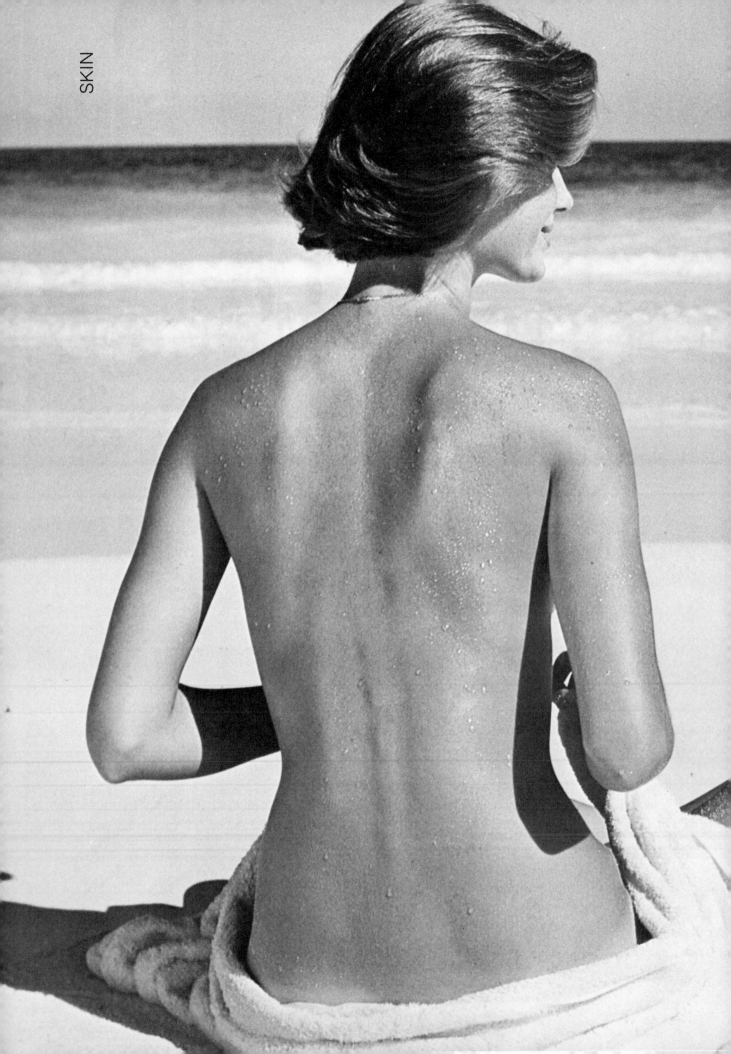

SUN AND BODY
the big questions and answers

Does the sun actually help any skin problems?

Dermatologists frequently tell patients with psoriasis to get some sun exposure. It seems to help heal the itchy, flaky patches. Sun also seems to help some other types of dermatitis, but you should never treat any skin condition by self-medicating with sun exposure. You may overdo and you may sun when it could be the worst thing for whatever is causing the dermatitis. The best idea is to check with your doctor for recommendations.

Does sun make acne on the back worse?

Many women complain that they get an increase of large boillike acne infections on their backs during sun exposure. This is probably because heat increases the oily secretions of the body and these, combined with perspiration, can clog pores and cause breakouts. The best solution is to treat the breakouts with some kind of acne cream or lotions. If you have an occasional breakout that seems to get out of hand, your dermatologist may be able to inject it with cortisone to speed the healing.

What are those large "frecklelike" spots some people get over the shoulders?

The big brownish splotches that spread across your shoulders are really pretty much the same as freckles anywhere else. Some people have more irregular pigmentation here than in other spots, in fact, this can be the only place some people have it. The pigment darkens with sun exposure and you notice the freckling. As with other freckles, they tend to fade during winter, but they will return when you sun again.

Does a tan affect the way my figure looks?

Most women find that a healthy-looking light tan seems to make their body look slimmer and more compact. It's an illusion, of course, but a flattering one. Some women feel more comfortable with their extra pounds if they can get a start on a tan before they have to appear in public in a bikini. You might try one of the products that "tans" without sun if you're slightly overweight and need the emotional support of a tan before baring it on the beach.

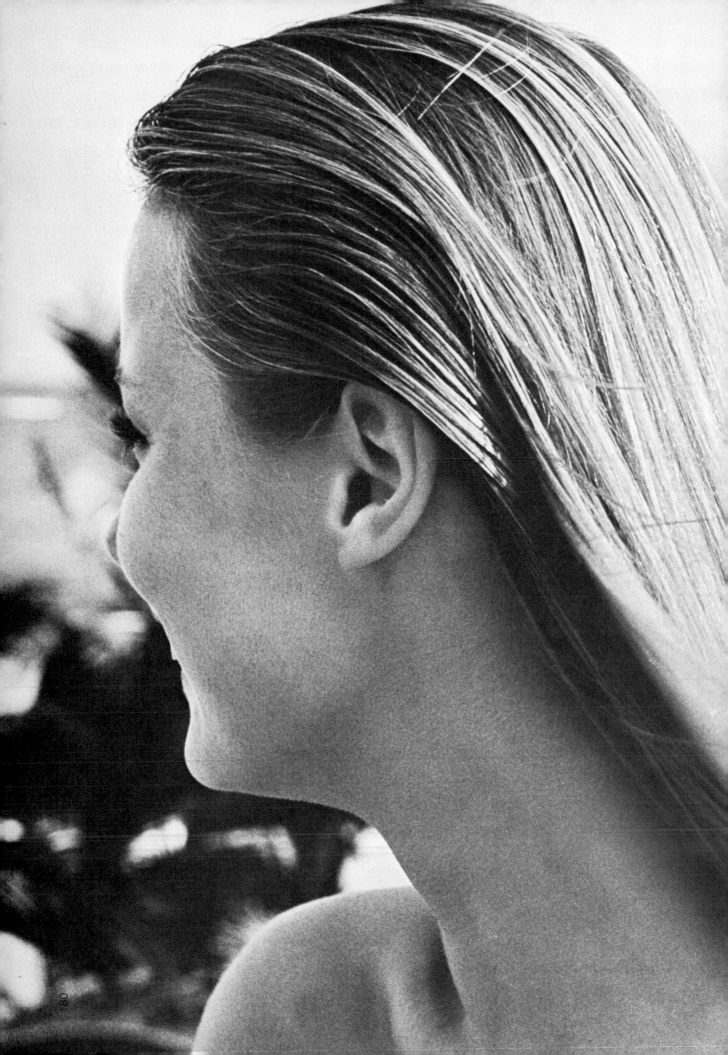

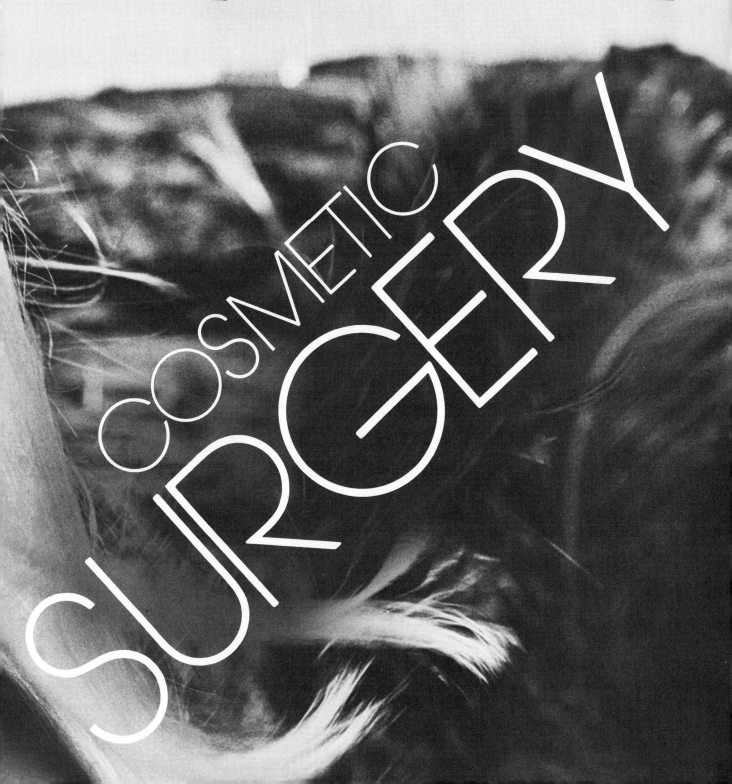

Cosmetic surgery is probably the most drastic beauty move you can make; it can also be the most important and successful one. Before you take the plunge, give careful thought to your decision and familiarize yourself with what cosmetic surgery can and can't do. This chapter will help you do this. Finally, if you decide cosmetic surgery is the answer for you, don't approach it fearfully; instead be confident, treat it as one of the most exciting adventures you're ever going to have.

COSMETIC
SURGERY

Who should have
COSMETIC SURGERY

Provided you can afford it, anyone who really wants *it should have it. The important thing is to examine just why you want it to be sure your motives—and your expectations—are realistic.*

Cosmetic surgery is quite safe. Most operations are performed under local anesthetic so the major risk of anesthetic complications is greatly reduced. Since safety isn't a big consideration here, what is? Your motives should be the prime consideration. It can be difficult to assess just why you feel you need surgery, but if you are generally happy with your appearance and not preoccupied with your looks in total, and if you have one *particular feature or flaw that you've been very dissatisfied with for* a long time, *chances are you're a good candidate for surgery.*

HOW DO YOU BEGIN?

Once you've decided to investigate cosmetic surgery seriously, your first step should be to find a doctor. Most women find that with something this important, they don't necessarily want to settle on the first and only doctor they see. Consultations are standard procedure in cosmetic surgery. The usual practice is to call your county or state medical society and ask for the names of accredited plastic surgeons in your area, or ask your family doctor for recommendations. The county medical society can usually tell you where the doctor went to school, when, and how long he or she has been accredited if you'd like to consider these factors in making your final decision. Pick one doctor and make an appointment for a consultation. You'll be billed for the consultation in one of two ways. Some doctors charge a flat fee for the consultation and you're billed for that. Others have a fee that is deductible from the cost of your surgery, should you decide on it. Otherwise you pay the fee. In the latter case, the fee is apt to be more than in the former. Both are fairly common and considered fair.

SEEING THE DOCTOR

Once you have an appointment, don't go in cold. Make a list of questions you'd like to have answers to so that you use your time wisely. We give you suggested questions for some of the most common operations later in this chapter, but you'll undoubtedly have some of your own. Don't be timid. It's your face and body and your money, so ask all the questions you want, no matter how silly they may seem to you. The doctor has heard sillier! Try to get a fix on how you feel about the doctor—whether you could develop a rapport or not, whether you think he or she understands or cares about what you want. If you have questions or doubts as to whether this doctor is for you, see another one. Most women see at least two before making a decision and we recommend that you do also.

Don't be surprised if the doctor asks you a few questions, too. Most plastic surgeons are very particular about whom they operate on since a patient with unrealistic expectations can be a problem later on. The doctor will probably ask why you feel you need the operation and how long you've been thinking about it. The doctor will probably question you in detail about exactly what it is about your nose, ears, eyes or whatever, that bothers you, especially on a second visit if you've decided to have the surgery.

After your visit, even if you like the doctor and feel you'll go ahead with the surgery, it's a good idea to go home and give it some more thought. You'll have to make another appointment anyway, so you may as well give yourself some free thinking time in between.

One final word on what to expect when you actually see a doctor. You may have heard a lot about "before" and "after" pictures. If your doctor is either reluctant or refuses to show you such pictures, don't feel this is a bad sign. It has more and more become the practice not to show such pictures. First of all, it's difficult to get pictures to show. Many people don't want to advertise the fact that they've had cosmetic surgery by having their pictures shown to strangers. Also, you may not understand what the medical limitations of a particular operation for a particular patient are, and you can be disappointed or misled by looking at someone else's pictures. Most doctors have a few pictures, often textbook photos from books or papers they've written, that give you an idea of what can be accomplished by certain operations, but don't expect to see a parade of before and after pictures. A much more successful idea is to have the doctor explain in detail what he or she thinks should be done in your case and what the results for you will be.

HOW MUCH DOES IT COST?

Cosmetic surgery is expensive. It should be, it's very painstaking work. In fact, some of the procedures, especially on the eye, are said to be some of the most delicate of all surgery. The results are for life, so that should help you pay the price emotionally. Financially, a relatively new income tax law now allows you to take the standard medical deduction for cosmetic surgery. This is a big help for most people. Also, hospitalization does sometimes cover some of your hospital stay. It depends on the kind of medical policy you have, and, to some extent, your doctor. If there is any other small work that can be done while you're having your surgery, say the removal of a mole or polyps, your hospital insurance may cover most expenses. Some doctors are more inclined to "find" these extras than others. This is something you should discuss with your doctor. Fees vary from city to city and doctor to doctor so it is hard to get a range. In general, the longer the doctor has been practicing and the more well known he or she is, the higher the fees will be. You'll get an idea of the going rate by asking the two doctors you consult what they charge and comparing them.

Fees for cosmetic surgery are almost always due in advance of the operation. Don't feel that your doctor is strange or unethical in asking for payment as much as two weeks ahead. Almost without exception, all plastic surgeons do this for several reasons. Patients often get frightened at the last minute and cancel out. Having you pay for your surgery in advance usually gives your doctor a good idea that you are serious and will turn up for the operation. If you don't, your doctor is in for trouble. An operating room and certain of the hospital's personnel have been engaged, and if the patient doesn't show up, it ties up the hospital facilities. It also damages the doctor's reputation.

RHINOPLASTY OR NOSE SURGERY

Nasal surgery or, more medically correct, rhinoplasty, is probably the most common type of cosmetic surgery, especially among young women. It is a comparatively simple procedure and is usually highly successful.

What can rhinoplasty do for you?

This type of surgery can make a dramatic change in your appearance. It can completely get rid of a hump or bump in the bridge of the nose. It can straighten a crooked nose, it can shorten a too-long one. Narrowing the width of the nose bridge is also possible. It is sometimes possible to change thick, fleshy or flaring nostrils, but usually it's a tricky, difficult task and it's usually not advisable.

One of the biggest hurdles for most women is visualizing how they will look with a "new" nose. Here is one trick that will help you get an idea of how surgery might change your nose. You'll need black or dark brown eyeliner, a hand mirror and a black or very dark piece of fabric to hang behind you. With the eyeliner, "paint" out what you don't like about your nose, say, a bit of the sides of nose bridge if you feel it's too wide or the tip if you feel it's too long. Now go to a bathroom mirror and hang the black cloth behind you so that when you hold the hand mirror and look into it, you see your profile outlined against the dark cloth. The dark liner you've drawn on your nose will make that part of it fade away and you'll get the illusion of what a new nose will look like.

What is the surgery like?

Once you've decided on surgery and actually gotten to the hospital, here, briefly, is what will happen.

You will be given a general physical and will have some blood tests taken and probably an X ray or two. You will be able to eat and drink normally until about midnight when you'll be told not to eat or drink anything (if surgery is scheduled for early morning). You will also be given a mild antibacterial soap to wash your face with—some surgeons ask that you sham-

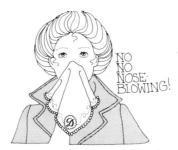

NO NO NOSE BLOWING!

Your doctor will probably tell you not to blow your nose for a certain period of time following nose surgery.

poo your hair, too. At bedtime, you'll be given some medication to help you relax and go to sleep. You'll be given more medication early in the morning and just as you go into surgery. The idea is to progressively relax you so that by the time you're actually in the operating room you're completely at ease and heavily sedated. Most patients report feeling or remembering almost nothing about the operation itself. The operation takes from one to two hours, depending on what's to be done. You'll be pleasantly drowsy for the remainder of the day. You will awake to find your nose bandaged, usually with some sort of splint in place to protect the new contours. You may also have packing inside your nose. It sounds terribly uncomfortable. Breathing through your mouth soon becomes routine and you get used to the bandages. You

When you bend, bend from your knees and don't hang your head forward. This reduces any chances of bleeding following nose surgery.

will probably be asked to keep your head elevated for your stay in the hospital and you're usually told not to lower your head to a level below your waist for about two weeks to reduce any chance of bleeding. You'll also be instructed not to blow your nose for about a week. Approximately three days after surgery, the original dressing is changed for something much smaller. You'll usually be able to go home at this point. This small dressing will be kept on from seven to fourteen days, depending on what was done and how rapidly you're healing.

You'll see your surgeon in his office several times during this period for further instructions.

In about three weeks, your nose will be solidly healed in position so that it need no longer be considered a delicate structure. There may still be some swelling, but it will probably not be noticeable to anyone but you. Actually, most patients find their new nose looks great when the final bandage or splint is removed. It can be as much as six months before all the swelling is gone and the subtle contours of the new nose are revealed, but again, no one but you will notice this and you may not even be aware of it.

Surgery is usually performed entirely inside the nose so you'll have no scars.

SUGGESTED QUESTIONS TO ASK DURING YOUR PRESURGERY CONSULTATION

When you're having a consultation with your surgeon, it's a good idea to make yourself a list of questions so you don't forget to ask anything. Here are some you may want answers to.

● **What do you recommend doing to my nose to get the effect I want?**
● **Exactly how will the new nose look?**
● **How long will I have to be in the hospital?**
● **How long will I have bandages on?**
● **When can I expect to get back to work or school?**
● **When will I be able to wear my glasses again?**

(Some surgeons recommend taping glasses to your forehead for a couple of weeks so that the pressure of the glasses won't damage the nose bridge.)

● **Will my nose feel normal afterward or should I expect some numbness or stuffiness for a while?**
● **How long must I refrain from shampooing my hair after surgery?**
● **How much will surgery cost?**
● **Will my medical insurance cover any of it?**
● **When is the fee due?**

EAR SURGERY

Ears that stick out Dumbo fashion can be as much of a trial as a large nose. Hair can sometimes help conceal the problem, but who wants to go through life having to wear a hairstyle that will conceal stick-out ears?

Believe it or not, many of the patients who undergo this surgery are children. The ear reaches its full size when a child is about five and because children can be so unkind to each other about defects like big or protruding ears, many doctors strongly recommend that parents have children's ears fixed as early as possible. They can, of course, be repaired at anytime in life.

What's the surgery like?

Surgery to flatten protruding ears is quite simple. Adults are usually given local anesthetic; children usually given light general anesthetic. If you are given local anesthetic, you will be given medication over a period of hours to be sure you're relaxed and properly sedated for the actual surgery. The surgery takes from an hour to two hours, depending on what's being done. Following surgery, the head is bandaged so that the patient looks as though she's wearing a football helmet. Children should always be told they will awaken bandaged so they won't be frightened. This bandage remains in place for about two days. Patients can usually go home after two days. No further bandaging is necessary during the day, but a stocking cap of some kind is worn to protect the ears at night. Stitches are usually removed in ten days or two weeks and the nightcap is worn for about two weeks.

There are small scars that are well hidden in the fold behind the ear. The scars tend to fade with time so that they become invisible, even if you look for them. It may take as long as two to three months for the ears to assume their permanent position because swelling must go down and the cartilage must settle in its new position. For all intents and purposes, however, the ears look normal and much improved as soon as the helmet bandage is removed.

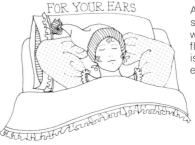

FOR YOUR EARS

A stocking cap, or some kind of cap that will keep ears flat to your head, is necessary following ear surgery.

186

BLEPHAROPLASTY OR EYELID SURGERY

Blepharoplasty is the medical term for eyelid surgery. This is a common cosmetic surgery operation, mainly for older women, but sometimes it's desired by young women. In this case, it's usually to remove the hereditary fat pouches from underneath the eye. This problem, which manifests itself in what are commonly known as "bags" under the eye, can frequently be seen in young children. The condition is not usually operable in children, but when it is pronounced, a woman in her late twenties or thirties may well be advised to have these bags removed surgically. When they are extreme, they give a tired, sometimes dissipated look to the face even in young women. This condition is usually hereditary and caused by an underlying weakness in the tissue that normally holds these fatty deposits in place. In young women, it's usually only the undereye area that causes the trouble.

To correct this problem, a small incision is made just under each eye and some of the fat is removed. Sometimes a portion of the skin is also removed, but in young women, this usually isn't necessary. Once the fat is removed, tiny stitches close the incision. The remaining hairline scar is concealed in the eyelash line and finally disappears altogether.

As with other cosmetic surgery procedures, eyelid surgery is usually done under local anesthetic. By the time the patient reaches the operating room, she is sedated so much that she is unaware of the proceedings. Following surgery, the patient is usually asked to apply cold compresses to the eyes to reduce swelling and discoloration. Hospitalization is usually overnight. Stitches are removed from three to five days later in the surgeon's office. Most of the swelling and discoloration disappears within ten days to two weeks following surgery. The faint scar will be almost invisible shortly after surgery.

QUESTIONS YOU MAY WANT TO ASK

- **How long will I have to stay in the hospital?**
- **How long will the stitches stay in?**
- **How long before I can wear contact lenses?**
- **How long before I can wear eye makeup?**
- **What is the fee?**
- **When is it payable?**

BREASTS
what doctors can and can't do to reshape them *

When breasts are too small or need lifting

Many people think that too much attention is given to the size and shape of a woman's breasts. But in considering cosmetic surgery for the area, the only opinion that really matters is the attitude of the woman herself about her self-image. . . .

Reshaping and correcting the size and contours of the breasts has become increasingly popular with women in the past ten years. This is owing primarily to great advances in techniques and satisfactory results. Most earlier hazards have been reduced or eliminated.

The general term for breast surgery is *mammaplasty*, derived from the Latin *mamma* for breast. "Augmentation mammaplasty," or "breast augmentation," refers to enlarging the breast, as contrasted with "breast reduction" or "reduction mammaplasty." The procedures involve primarily enlarging, reducing, or equalizing the breasts, including lifting the sagging or drooping bosom. Cosmetic surgeons agree that no correction is more eagerly sought, and none gives greater gratification to the patient. . . .

In spite of the rise in popularity, there is probably more confusion, misunderstanding, and misinformation about breast surgery than most other phases of plastic surgery. As in every type of surgery or medical treatment, it is imperative for satisfactory results to seek out qualified, experienced specialists. . . .

Statistics on the number of women who have had plastic surgery of the breasts in recent years are understandably vague, but there is general agreement that there have been well over 50,000 augmentations—with the numbers rising rapidly. Patients range in age from about sixteen (earlier in some cases) into the sixties, and occasionally beyond.

Mammaplasty, like all other cosmetic surgery, is not necessarily a cure-all, or the perfect solution for every individual or situation. . . . [But] by transforming a woman's self-image from depressive to upbeat, along with her improved physical aspect, the "right" patient can experience good results.

* Samm Sinclair Baker, and Dr. James W. Smith, *Doctor, Make Me Beautiful*, David McKay Co., New York, 1973. Reprinted by arrangement with the publishers.

Should YOU have augmentation mammaplasty?

Your interview with a cosmetic surgeon will probably cover such questions as those which follow. Take a piece of paper and a pencil and jot down your replies. If practically all your answers are in the affirmative—along with detailed positive information on your health—then you are probably a good candidate. . . .

QUESTIONS ABOUT BREAST ENLARGEMENT

1. Do you wear brassiere inserts almost all the time to give others the impression that your breasts are larger than they are?
2. Are you constantly annoyed by this?
3. Do you feel your physical activities are severely restricted by the constant use of these inserts?
4. Do you feel yourself "less of a woman" than others who are more endowed?
5. Do you feel that your self-confidence as a woman would increase if your breasts were in better proportion to the rest of you?
6. Have you long wished for this operation but never had the time or opportunity to pursue it?
7. Would you be willing to see a psychiatrist before the surgery if your plastic surgeon suggested it?
8. Would you be willing to accept small scars beneath your breasts?
9. If you are small-breasted or one breast is noticeably smaller than the other, does this limit your degree of social involvement (physical or emotional) with men or with other women?
10. Do you hide yourself in locker rooms or in bathing accommodations so that other women will not realize your breast size?
11. Have you broken engagements to be married one or more times because you decided that you would not be enough of a woman for your future husband?
12. Do you shun the thought of physical contact because of feelings of insecurity about the

size of your breasts or the feeling of inadequacy about sex?

13. Does it cause you to hesitate to dance with a man or to have him embrace you?

14. Has your husband ever embarrassed you by comparing your smallness to the larger breasts of other women?

15. Are you having domestic problems that you think would be lessened or solved by the operation?

16. Do you get hysterical easily?

17. Do you get depressed frequently?

18. Is your husband maintaining his attractiveness and youthful appearance while you feel that you are aging prematurely?

19. Do you often wish your breast size were the same as when you were pregnant?

20. Does your husband frequently refer to that time during your pregnancy when your breasts were fuller?

21. Have you some degree of frigidity?

22. Do you think that "frigidity" could be related to your breast size?

23. Have you required repeated breast biopsies, and live in fear of breast cancer or of new breast tumors?

If most (not necessarily all) of your answers to the preceding questions are "yes," then it probably would be worthwhile for you to arrange a consultation with a specialist to discuss breast enlargement.

When breasts are too big or unequal in size

Enormous breasts are a *burden* to the woman who must carry them—physically as well as psychologically. . . . It becomes difficult for many girls and women toting the weight of an immense bosom to participate in athletics, games, dancing, and many other activities.

Many of the young girls who seek reduction mammaplasty have become extremely shy, often owing to unfortunate experiences at school. They are taunted by whistles, hoots, and calls . . . and try to hide as much as possible of their overdeveloped breasts, binding them too tightly, and wearing loose-fitting clothing.

With 80 percent of those afflicted, the problem of excessively large breasts begins at puberty, in the early teens or before. Such girls have an estrogen sensitivity stemming from any of several steroid hormones in the body. When checked by the physician, the patient may have a normal estrogen level, yet the breast responds more sensitively than usual, and the result is sizable breast enlargement.

By contrast, the girl with very small breasts may have a "normal" estrogen level which, in her case, *does not* stimulate the breasts to grow. In any case, with very oversized breasts, breast feeding may not be possible either before or after reduction surgery. . . .

Modern surgical techniques make it possible to reduce the oversize breast in the great majority of instances. . . . The simple operation is all that is required in 95 to 98 percent of the cases, as the breasts do not enlarge again. There should be no concern about the surgery inducing cancer in the young girl since cancer of the breasts is almost unheard of at this early age. In a very small percentage, some temporary swelling reactions may occur but they soon subside.

QUESTIONS FOR PERSONS CONSIDERING REDUCTION MAMMAPLASTY

Along with thorough physical examination and investigation, a plastic surgeon will probably cover questions like the following in discussing your individual problems. You might want to take pencil and paper and note your responses to these queries. If you really need reduction mammaplasty, you will answer "yes" to most questions:

1. Are you very self-conscious about the large size of your breasts?

2. Do you try to disguise their size by wearing very tight brassieres or binding yourself up?

3. Is your shopping for suitable clothing limited by the fact that your bust size is out of proportion to the rest of your measurements?

4. Are you hard to fit in general with standard clothing?

5. Do you experience neck pain, shoulder pain, or back pain after standing or walking for a long time?

6. Are the pains you get in your shoulders, neck or back either relieved by lying down, or gone after a good night's sleep?

7. Does the size of your breasts limit your working ability?

8. Does the size limit your sports activity?

9. Does it cause you to be constantly afraid of breast cancer?

10. Does it make you think there's something wrong with you . . . that you are "grotesque" . . . somehow almost inhuman?

11. Does it make you hesitate to dance with a man or have him embrace you?

12. Does the size of your breasts cause a rash or irritation on the under surface where your breasts and upper abdomen come in contact with one another?

13. Does your breast size stay about the same even though your overall body weight might fluctuate greatly as you gain and lose weight?

14. Do you feel that the weight of your breasts limits or seriously affects the extent of your physical activity?

15. Do you have a great deal of pain and discomfort in your breasts just before the onset of menstruation?

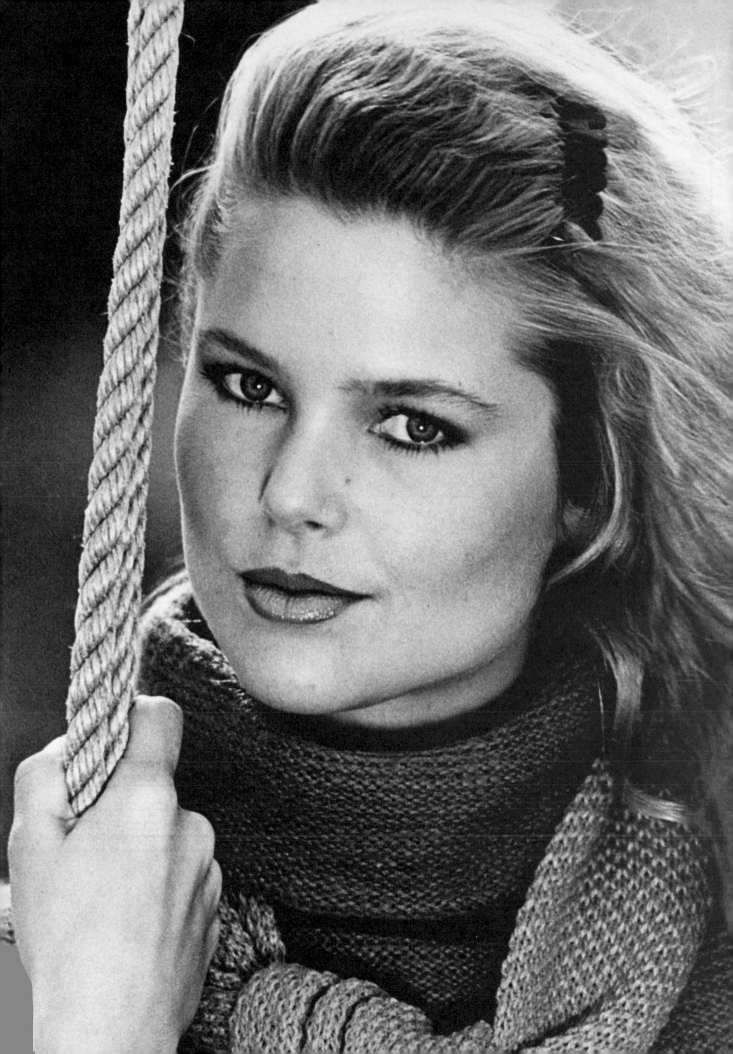

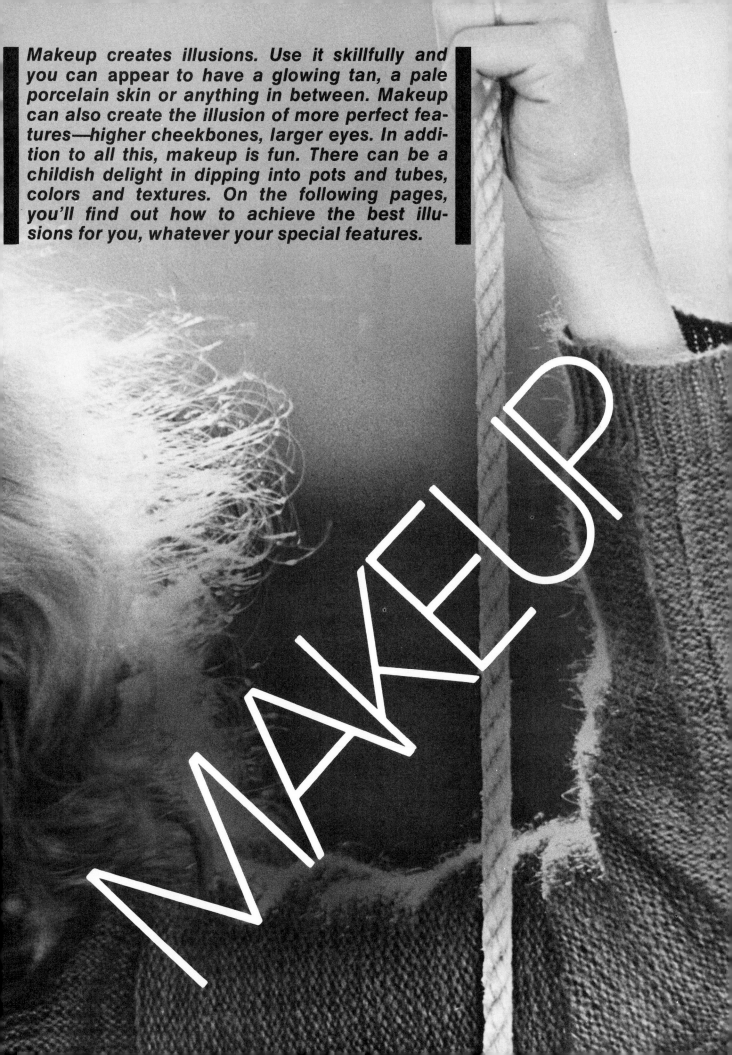

Makeup creates illusions. Use it skillfully and you can appear to have a glowing tan, a pale porcelain skin or anything in between. Makeup can also create the illusion of more perfect features—higher cheekbones, larger eyes. In addition to all this, makeup is fun. There can be a childish delight in dipping into pots and tubes, colors and textures. On the following pages, you'll find out how to achieve the best illusions for you, whatever your special features.

MAKEUP

How to be your own MAKEUP ARTIST

The one little thing that can make the most excitement and change in your look is a new makeup color— a new blusher, lipstick, eye shadow or whatever. There are dozens of choices, what you have to do is think of them as an artist would—in terms of your natural coloring and the colors of the clothes you like to wear. That doesn't mean a new makeup color for every piece of clothing, but it does mean choosing a color that fits beautifully with you and your clothes. Here you'll find ideas on how to do this for women with fair, medium or dark complexions, plus general rules to make the whole thing work beautifully.

1 Pick a blusher color that's close to what's worn near your face

The idea here is to pick up some clothes color with a blusher tone. The orange turtleneck, right, is a natural taking-off point for a peachy to tawny blusher.

2 Don't match eye shadow to clothes

Trying to match eye shadow to clothes color looks unspontaneous. Work within a color family instead of trying for a dead match. For example, the clear blue shadow with the mauvey scarf right is a good approach. Another idea might be teal blue shadow with a navy shirt.

3 Don't try to make your face out-color your clothes

Face and clothes aren't supposed to be in competition with each other. If you're choosing strongly colored clothes and are worried that they'll fade your face out, just be sure to pick fresh, clear, but naturally soft makeup colors. The green and pink, right, are good examples for the fashion look and the model's coloring.

4 Be aware that makeup colors can be either complementary or harmonious to fashion colors

All color experts know the beautiful effects you can get from working with either complementary or harmonious colors. Complementary colors are always opposite each other on an artist's color wheel (you can buy one in most art stores). Red and green are complementary colors. Harmonious colors are tones within the same family, red and orange, for example. Right, we show you complementary and harmonious colors for three basic fashion colors.

5 Apply blusher with face shape in mind

The sketches, right, show you where to apply blusher for different face shapes. Let blusher brush move in the direction and the angle that the arrows show you.

Any of the tawny to peachy tones here would turn on a glow above the orange turtleneck.

BLUSHER

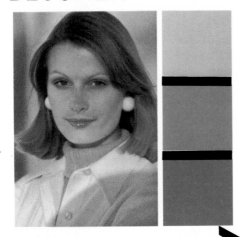

This clear blue shadow would work beautifully with any blue to mauve to plum color close to the face.

EYE SHADOW

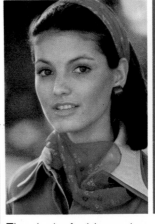

The dusky fashion colors, left, are great, but they need the strength of clear makeup colors like the ones below.

COLOR CLARITY

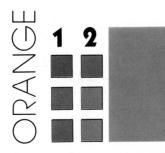

ORANGE 1 2

WINE 3 4

BEIGE 5 6

Large color swatches above are three basic fashion color families. Orange could encompass rusts and earth colors. Wine could encompass crimson, deep reds and mauvey tones; the beige, tans into browns. Smaller swatches complement and harmonize each group. Eye shadow is first, cheeks next, then lips.

One way to give your face more color and contour appeal is by shading blusher in specific areas. Sketches here show you how for your face shape.

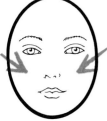
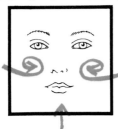
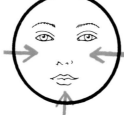
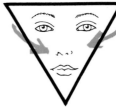

BLUSHER APPLICATION

Be your own makeup ARTIST

Here are makeup colors that give a nice lift to anyone with medium-toned skin and brown hair. There's a group for wine, for beiges and another for oranges— all wearable with medium complexions.

GENERAL TIPS

No matter what your coloring, your own psyche will respond to some fashion colors more than others. You may, in fact, find that you rarely wear certain colors. So here are a few basics to keep in mind no matter what colors you pick.

● Too much contrast—either light or dark—shouts "over madeup," so choose makeup tones in a range close to your complexion tone. The lighter your skin, the lighter your makeup application should be, too.

● If you adore a particular makeup but find the color just a bit strong, lighten your touch when applying it. The result will be the same color but in a subtler version.

● The new eye crayons and the consistencies of cream and gel shadows make them so easy to apply you can line lids with them, shadow, do just about anything you like for color effects. You might try some of the new eye shadows in wand form. Many have a sponge tip applicator that shades or lines beautifully. The consistency of the shadow also lends itself well to finger-blending.

● Remember that eye shadows are the one thing you may have to experiment with most to find a texture that works for you best. Some women find that powder shadows cake in the crease, others find creams bleed. Just keep trying different types until you find the one that works best on your lids.

● When you use a cheek crayon, try drawing an outline where you want color first, then blending to fill in. You'll get the most precise placement this way. You can, of course, make an outline with any kind of blusher, it's just easier to do with a cheek crayon.

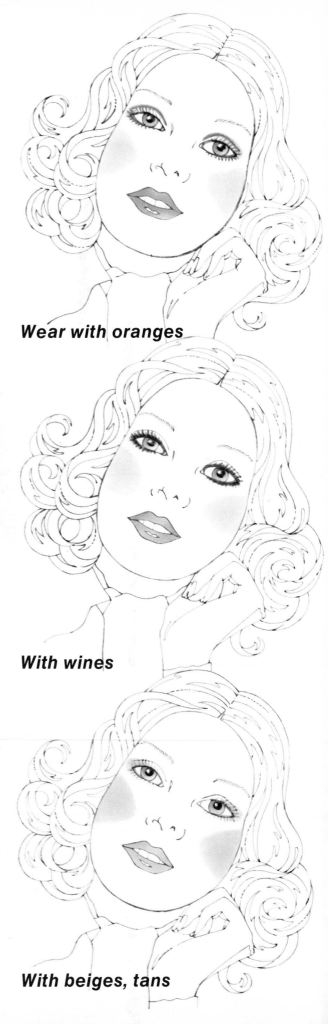

Wear with oranges

With wines

With beiges, tans

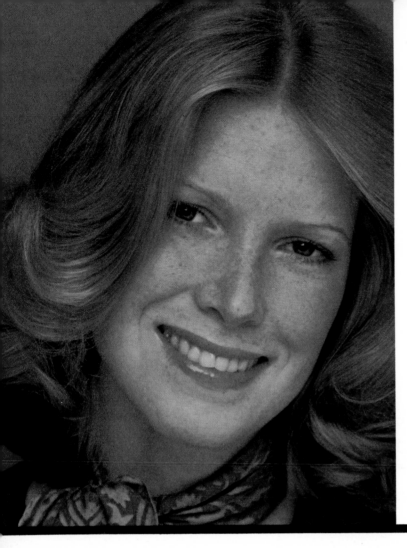

FAIR SKIN

Anyone with fair skin and blond to pale brown hair will find the makeup colors right and in photo left fabulous tonics for her kind of skin.

Wear with wine

For wine, crimsons or mauvey clothes, try deep to medium pink blushers, remembering to keep color contrast with your skin tone to a minimum. Soft peachy-pink colors work, too. Soft gray, mauve or smokey blue shadows work well, so would soft wine tones. For lips, soft wine, russets, burgundies.

With oranges

Peach or tawny blushers work best. Peach, coral, topaz, russets are good for lips. For eyes, mossy green, golden brown or smokey browns are good. For lips, try strong corals, russets.

With beiges, tans

Soft (not pastel) blues, golden brown, moss green are good choices for eyes. For cheeks, tawny corals, russets, peaches. For lips, soft russet, deep coral, soft browny colors (not the deepest tones).

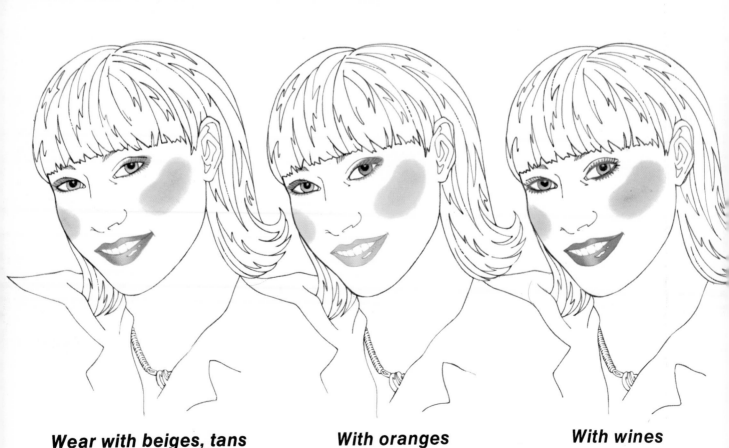

Wear with beiges, tans   **With oranges**   **With wines**

Wear with wines   **With oranges**   **With beiges, tans**

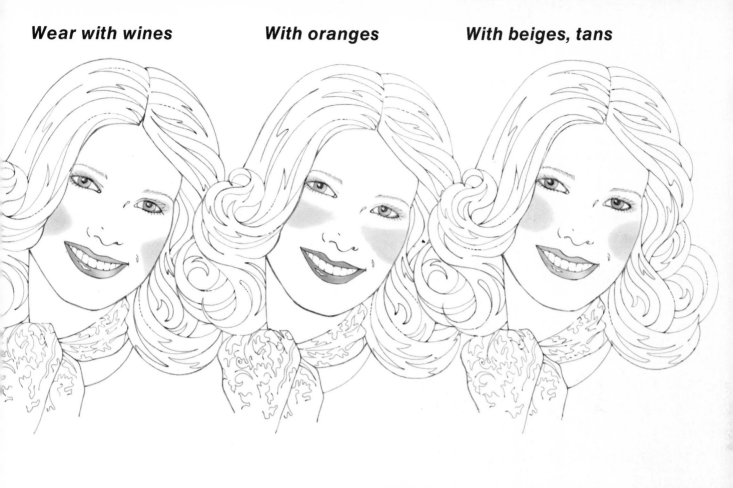

DARK SKIN

Any woman with a deep complexion and dark brown or black hair will find the makeups here give her a sensational beauty boost.

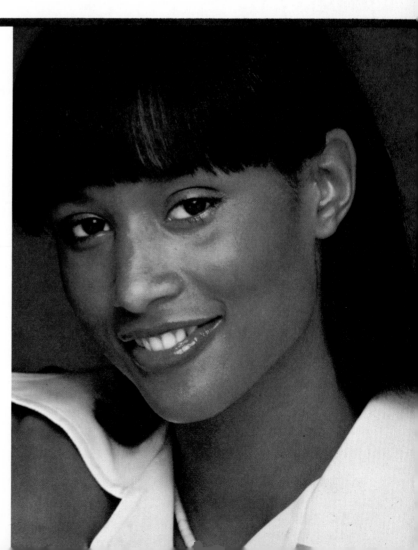

Wear with beiges, tans

Browned reds, deep russets, browned wines all look wonderful on cheeks. For lips, try browned reds, soft browns, deep rusts. For eyes, deep teal, deep or golden browns, rusty browns.

With oranges

For cheeks, try tawny tans, coppery or bronze tones. For lips, copper, brown-reds, chestnut. For eyes, rust-browns, copper, bronze, deep mossy green.

With wines

Deep red, browned or mauvey red or deep pink would be pretty on cheeks. For lips, try deep winey pinks, plums, deep rose. For eyes, violet, plum, deep blue, smokey gray.

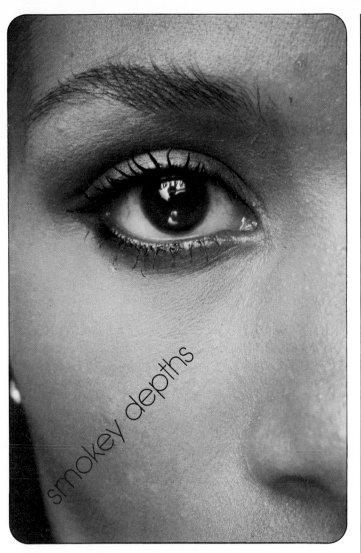

smokey depths

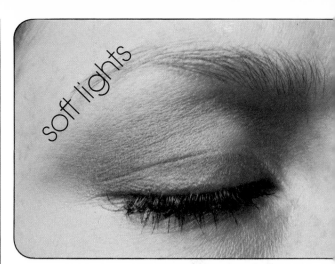

soft lights

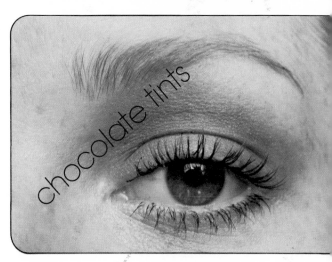

chocolate tints

Great colors for
EYES

The eye shadow colors here are fresh and contemporary. They work for most complexions, just remember to vary the color intensity depending on how fair or dark your complexion is. These eye shadows would be smashing with something in the same color family worn close to your face. Don't match, just keep colors in the same family.

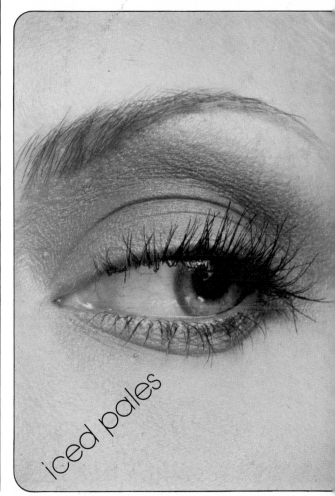

iced pales

APPLICATION TIPS

● Blend shadow well so that color never looks too dark or muddy.

● A cotton-tipped swab is excellent for blending color and getting contour emphasis. For example, color that's deep in inner corner and pale at the outer can be blended easily for this effect with a swab. It does a better job than your finger.

● A bit of moisturizer patted on lid will make shadows go on more smoothly.

● If you're using two shadow colors, the paler will usually look best above a deeper one. Another interesting effect is achieved by keeping color pale at inner corner, using a deeper one in the same color family on the outer corner.

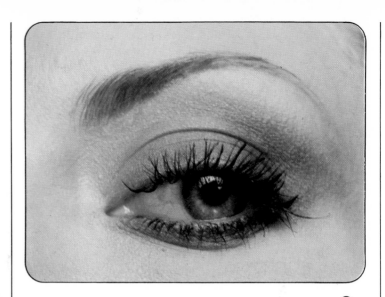

cool sheen

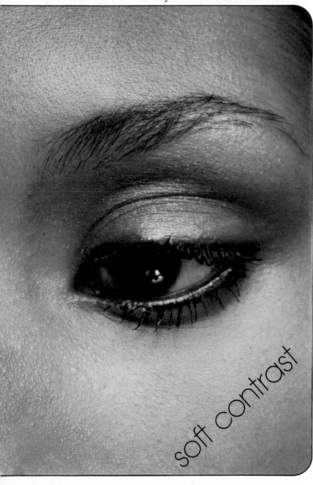

soft contrast

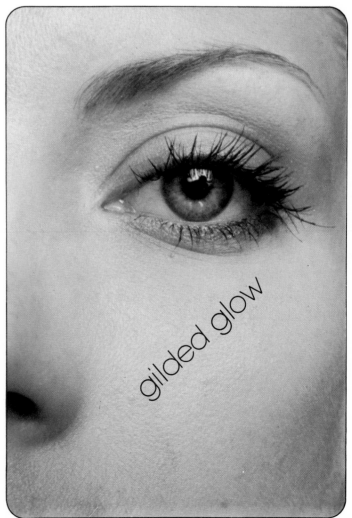

gilded glow

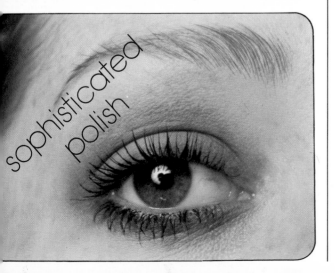

sophisticated polish

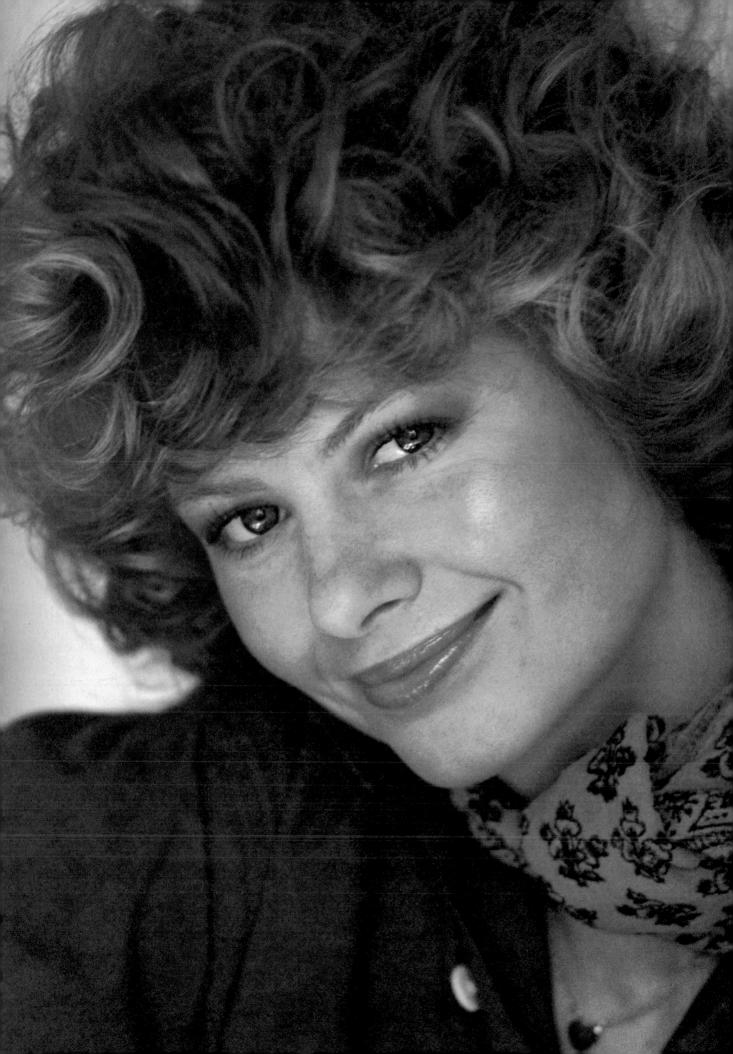

MAKEUP DO'S & DON'TS

If you're still wearing the same old makeup colors because they're safe and familiar, try something new and get more from all the pretty soft clothes colorings and styles around now. The DO'S and DON'TS here will help you pick something new without mistakes and also help you get the most flattery from your choice.

COLOR SENSE

DON'T wear much makeup when you're buying a new blusher, eye or lip color. Leave your face a blank sheet to try new colors on for effect. Try color on your hand first. When you've eliminated down to a couple, try them on your face, then buy. This way you won't spend money on things you won't like.

DON'T try to change your skin tone drastically with foundation. It will always look fake. One shade deeper or lighter is all you should try.
DO use a tinted moisturizer under foundation to help balance out skin tones. A green tint tends to tone down ruddiness, mauve to reduce sallowness, apricot to warm a too pale skin.
DON'T use a white highlighter under your brow. It's harsh and unflattering and too artificial with the soft makeups in focus now.

LIP PRINTS

DON'T judge a lipstick color by the way it looks in a tube. You'll be surprised at how different it looks against your skin coloring and the coloring your lips give it.
DO try the lip pencils to subtly outline your mouth and give lip color a nice clean line. In the photo, top right, a terra-cotta pencil gives coral lips a wonderful lively look. Use gloss for extra shine on top of the color.
DO try a tinted gloss, if your top lip is thinner than bottom, center picture, right.
DON'T be afraid of bright lip colors, especially if your lips are full. They look great as you can see from the picture, bottom, right.
DO remember to wear a blusher of equal color intensity with bright lip color.

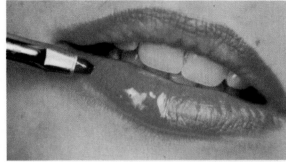
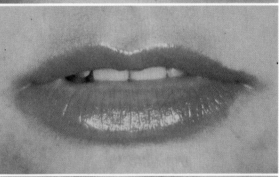
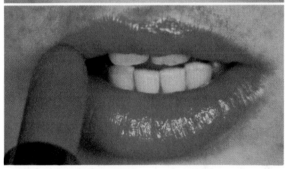

CHEEKS

DO try applying blush *after* dusting face with translucent powder. It makes blush last longer.
DON'T expect blush, or any makeup, to last all day. It will need to be retouched midday.
DO check that you've blended your blush well at hairline. You should see neither blush-colored hair nor a strip of pale, unblushed skin next to hairline.

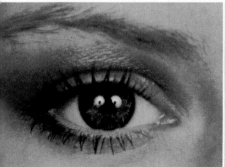
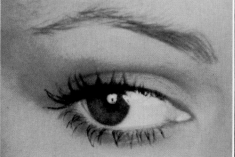
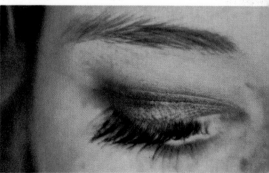

EYES

DO try applying lid color in one shade using a hint of contrasting color at the outer corners, see above, left. It's a great trick to make close-set eyes seem farther apart.
DO experiment with colors in different depths.

In the eye picture at center, a peach is used in inner corner, a deeper, golden peach in the outer corner.
DO try the softest colors for a natural look. The pewter shadow, above, is quite dramatic, and the color is so soft, it looks perfectly natural.

MAKEUP FOR YOUR BEST FACE

The colors you use, the way you use them and your skin all determine how your finished face will look. Here, four well-known New York makeup artists tell you how to polish the prettiest face you've worn yet.

Pablo of Elizabeth Arden talks about skin care

● Makeup is only as good as the skin it's going on. That's why Pablo stresses good care as the first and most basic makeup step. Ideally you should remove makeup with a tissue-off makeup remover, then wash with soap.
● A toner for dry or normal skin or an astringent for oily skin should be used after soap cleansing to remove last traces of soil. The last step is moisturizer applied to the dry areas of your face.
● For a long-lasting makeup job, Pablo suggests this: Use a bit of refrigerated astringent (cold helps make skin glow), then apply the tiniest bit of moisturizer while skin is still damp from astringent. Let dry and apply foundation, blot with tissue. The moisturizer forms a seal between your skin and the foundation and helps makeup stay smooth longer.

Benjamin Moss talks about color

● Think of color as a *mixture* of tones. Don't match lip color to cheeks or to a dress color. Aim for colors that blend and enhance each other and your skin, hair and eyes; not perfect matches.
● Don't try to change your natural skin tone, play it up. If it's dark, dramatize it with deep smokey colors. If it's pale, highlight it with soft rich colors like grays, plums.
● Don't try to match eye shadow to eyes. Contrasts bring more sparkle to eyes. Choose colors that flatter, maybe those that pick up a color you're wearing close to your face. Watch out for whitened shadow colors like pastel frosteds, especially in the blue family. They look unnatural and unflattering.
● Earth tones for lips and cheeks are generally natural-looking and flattering to many skin tones. Deeper, more dramatic ones work well for brunettes, softer ones for pale skins.

Way Bandy talks about application

● Makeup is being thought of more and more as a see-through glaze, *not* an opaque covering. Your natural coloring is what's important. Play up your best feature.
● Quick tip for pretty eyes: Powder lashes lightly. Use an eyelash curler to curl, making several firm, quick squeezes. Mascara tips of lashes.
● Blusher tip: To apply blusher in the most flattering way, use your fingers to locate your cheekbones, apply blusher just *above* and *on* bones. Blend *up* and into hairline so you have subtle halo of color.

Wendy Whitelaw talks about technique

● Knowing the right tools and how to use them is the secret of good technique. Brushes polish and soften colors, fingers are good tools for smudging and blending. Makeup crayons are great for applying color in a clearly defined area—around the eyelids or lipline. Creams can be glowy and pretty, especially on dry skins. Tip for blemishes: Apply a light shade of cover-up right over the blemish and gently pat, don't rub the cream into the skin. Tip for dark circles: Apply a light textured cover cream *under* the circle area and blend up and out. Pat, rather than rub.

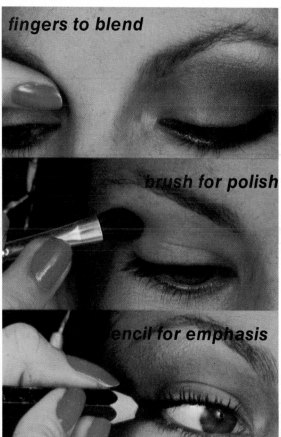

fingers to blend

brush for polish

pencil for emphasis

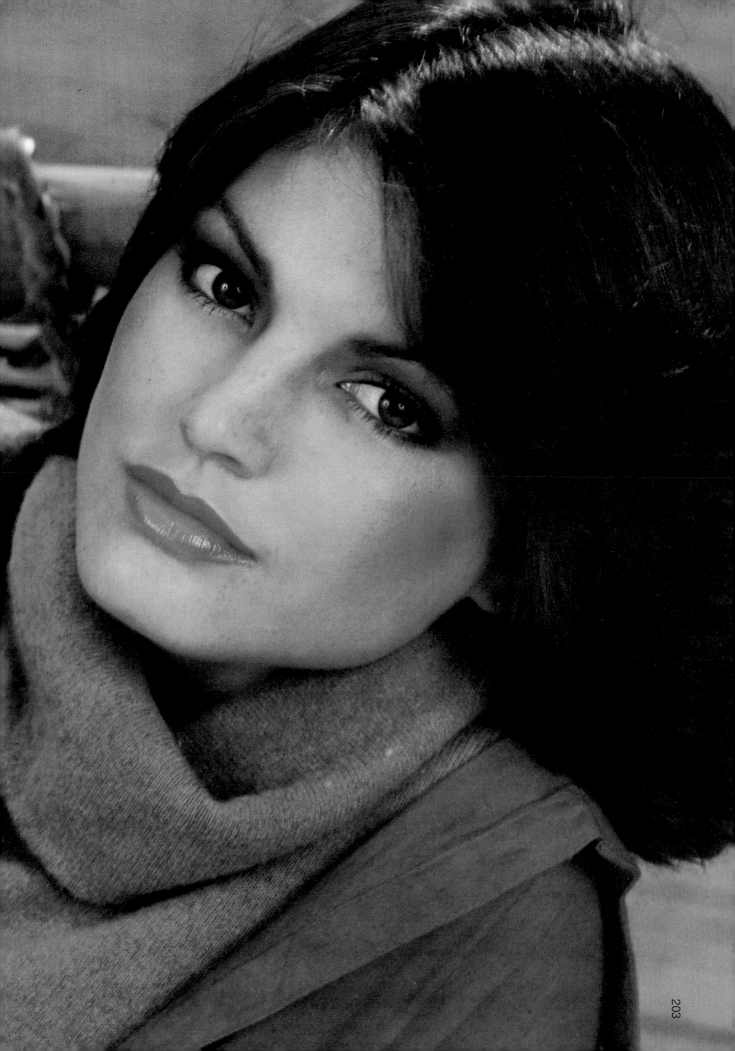

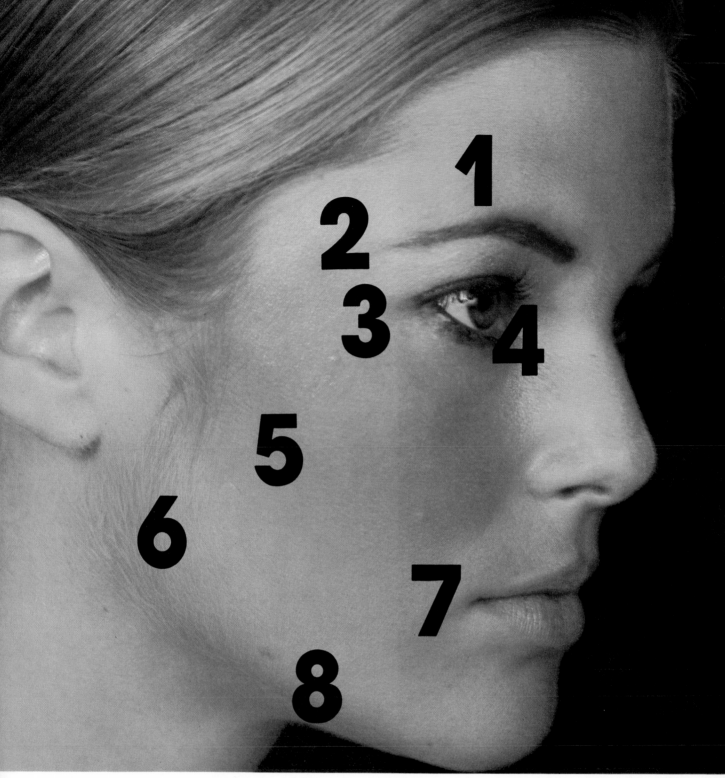

HOW TO AVOID THE 8 MOST

1. **Eyebrows**
2. **Brow highlighter**
3. **Eye Shadow**
4. **Mascara**
5. **Blusher**
6. **Powder**
7. **Lip color**
8. **Foundation**

1. Don't use eyebrow pencil as though you were drawing on canvas. If your brows are pale or uneven, use a pencil but pick a color *lighter* than brows and make short feathery strokes to fill in. You might also try some of the soft, brush-on powder brow products. Be certain you shape brows well by tweezing stray hairs. If they are well shaped, you may find brows look best natural, with no pencil.

2. Shiny, obvious brow highlighter spoils looks. Don't use stark white; try subtle pastels.

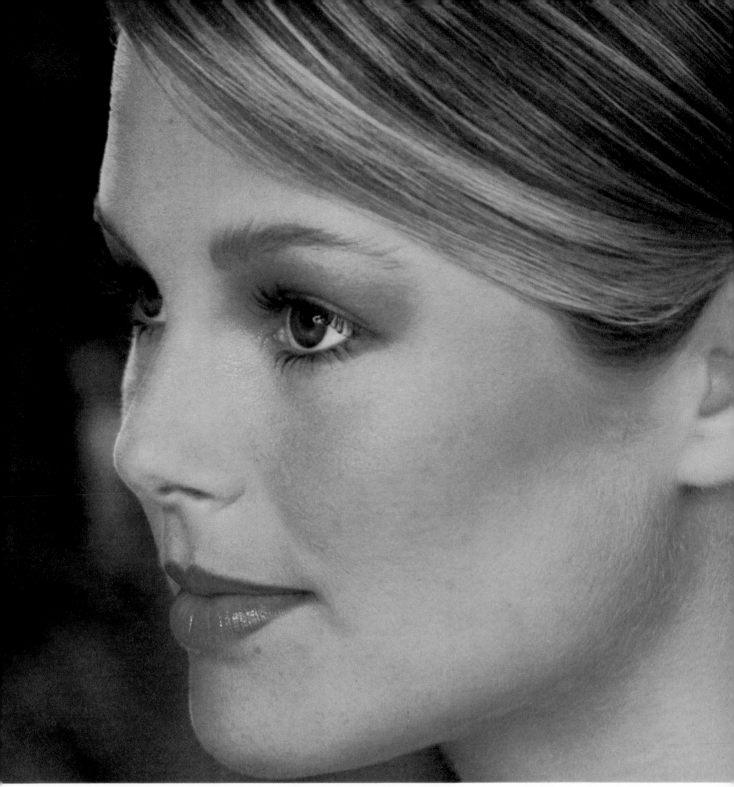

COMMON MAKEUP MISTAKES

3. Eye shadow should emphasize eyes, not the shadow. Blend carefully, pick transparent collors and don't overdo.

4. Mascara is to make lashes look long and lush, not glued together. Try this idea if you have this problem: Powder lashes lightly, then mascara lash tips first. Let dry, reapply mascara over entire lash. Then use a clean brush to go through lashes to separate.

5. Blusher is meant to make you look healthy, not feverish. Apply blush high on cheekbone, blend into hairline. Don't cover entire cheek.

6. Powder doesn't have to cling to facial hairs. Dust on lightly to prevent clinging; remove any excess with cotton.

7. Lip color that's too pale, dry and cakey has absolutely no sensuality. Use deep-colored gloss or deep, shiny transparent shades.

8. Foundation that's too heavy looks masklike. Apply lightly, blend well. Try using it only on problem breakout areas like chin, forehead or wherever you need cover.

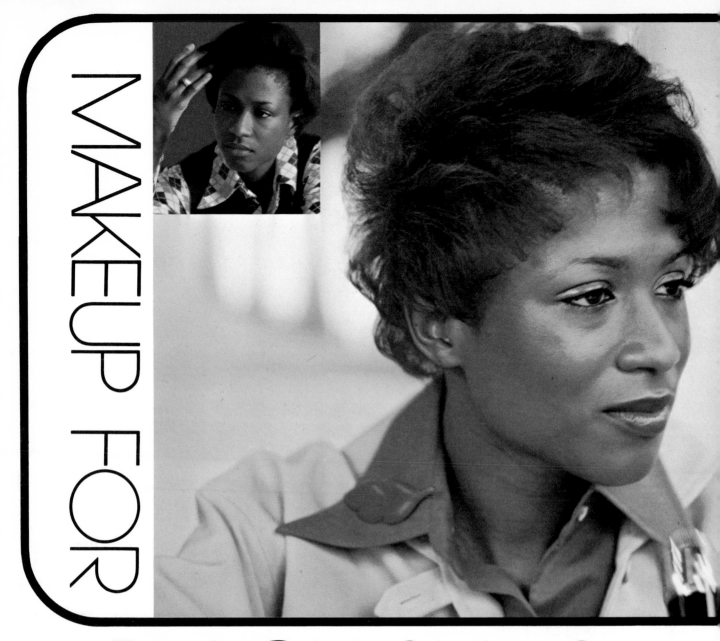

MAKEUP FOR BLACK SKINS

Some of the most lively makeup colors appearing now were designed especially to highlight black skins. The chart, opposite, will help you pick among them to find the most flattering for your skin tone. Keep these general tips in mind when you apply and select makeups.

TIPS

● It's especially important to try any cheek or lip color on your skin rather than by judging its color in the container. Black skin has many different colorings that are so vivid they show through the cosmetic and can alter its color.
● Since your skin has such good color and sheen, let it show through. Think of makeup as a see-through affair that highlights your own natural coloring.
● Makeups that shine, frequently those in gel form or with some subtle frosting, are particularly attractive on black skin.
● Stay away from muddy makeup colors of any kind. Look instead for clear, vivid color.
● Be adventuresome with some of the wonderful new transparent wine and brown colors for lips and cheeks. They look positively fantastic on black skin.
● Many black women are bothered by uneven pigmentation on their skin, especially as a temporary result of a blemish healing. A transparent foundation in a shade close to your natural skin tone will help to even out your coloring. If it's only a mark or two after a breakout, use a cover cream in a shade close to your skin tone. Black skin is very sensitive and should never be treated roughly by excessive rubbing or picking, which will often result in a skin trauma that leaves a temporary discoloration.

In the photo of the eyes, right, a transparent gel shadow is being applied to the eyelid. You can see how flattering the sheen and transparency are to black skin. Two different shadows in the same color family give a smashing effect. Try using one above the other and blend the colors so you can't see where one stops or the other stops. Experiment to see which you like best close to the lash line, the lighter or darker color. To some extent, it depends on your skin tone and the shape of your eyes. A little experimenting will give you a look you like.

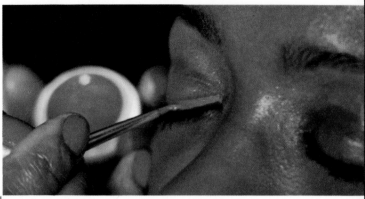

CHEEK FOCUS

Left, a transparent cheek gel was applied to give the cheek contour and a wonderful shine. The woman's own skin tone shows through imparting a special richness to the blusher. Coppery blush with a bit of frost would give a similar effect. Another wonderful color idea might be a deep wine blush that's very transparent.

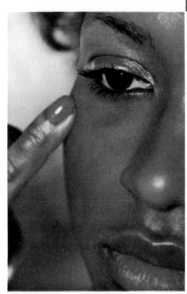

The chart, below, is designed to help you broaden your choice of flattering colors as well as choose the right tonalities to flatter the color intensity of your particular skin. You'll notice there is always a choice of more than one color so you won't get bored.

MAKEUP AND SKIN TONE

	EYES	CHEEKS	LIPS
light brown skin	rust apricot grayed sea green soft blueberry dusty amethyst	toffee melon rose pink peach	salmon browned coral brick deep apricot
medium brown skin	gold rich wheat burgundy evergreen charcoal gray	plum cherry browned wine dusty rose brick	plum brandy browned pink persimmon apple
dark brown skin	cinnamon burgundy deep rose carbon blue copper	wine mahogany dark red magenta	wine magenta dark red grape

EYEBROWS— MAKE THEM REAL EYE OPENERS

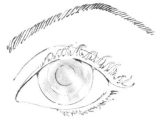

If you think a haircut is the only thing that will give your face a whole new look, glance over these before-and-after shots. Nothing's been changed on these women but their eyebrows—and the difference is amazing. Before you start on yours, here are some basics to consider. The first is shape. Never try to completely re-shape your brows, follow their natural line, giving a better, not new, shape. To find where brows should begin and end, try this: Hold a pencil up against nose so that it crosses the inside corner of your eye. The spot where the pencil hits brow area is where brows should begin. Then, slant pencil, crossing the outside corner of the eye with the bottom of the pencil still resting against your nose. This marks the stopping point. Although it's wise to tweeze mostly from the underpart of brows, a few stragglers on top can spoil an otherwise nice shape, so don't be afraid to pluck them, too. Following are some tips.

Thick brows with little arch

Creating an arch where there almost isn't one can really open up eyes. Start by cleaning up the area under brows, top right. Then tweeze from inner to outer corner to get a cleaner, more definite line, working the shape into a gentle arch as you do so. Pluck only a few hairs at a time, stopping every now and then to step back and check shape in mirror. Although there are no rules about where the arch should fall, it usually looks best a bit off-center from pupil, see above, but use your judgment as to what suits your face.

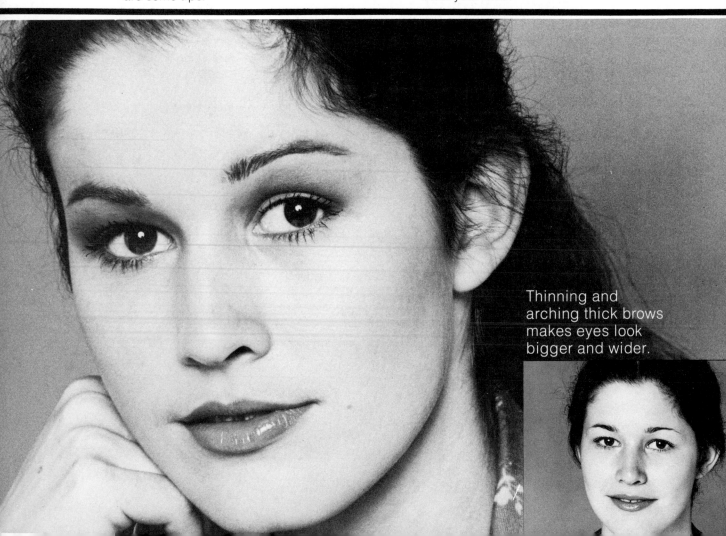

Thinning and arching thick brows makes eyes look bigger and wider.

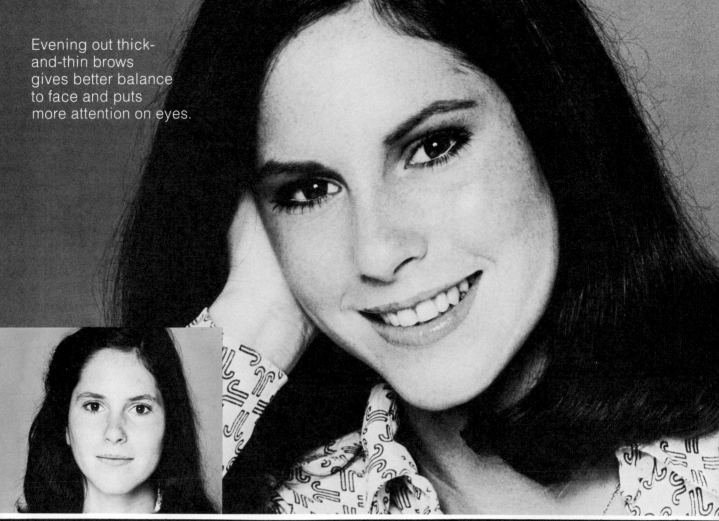

Evening out thick-
and-thin brows
gives better balance
to face and puts
more attention on eyes.

Unevenly shaped brows

This woman has a common problem—eyebrows that are unevenly shaped. They started
out fairly thick near her nose and narrowed to
almost nothing with hair sticking up in the center. To give brows like this a more pleasing,
well-balanced shape, lift brow hairs upward
with a small eyebrow brush (this makes it easier to see the misfits), tweeze strays and thin
out the thicker areas, removing one row of hairs
at a time (see photo top, right). Go slowly and
keep rechecking. Don't try to make the thick
parts equal in width to the thin parts or you'll
end up with overplucked brows. Instead, even
up the width by filling in thinner areas with a
soft pencil after you've plucked.

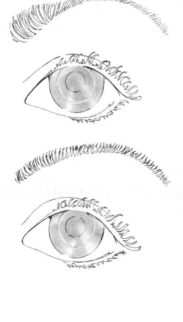

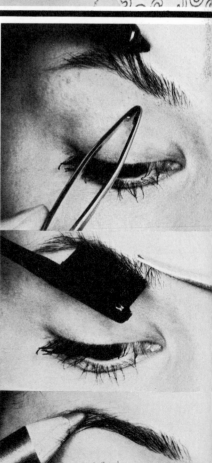

   If certain brow hairs are too long (which may
be adding to the thickness of the too-heavy
parts), you can trim them with cuticle scissors.
First, brush up and in direction they will lie with
an eyebrow brush, see photo right, and clip
carefully, making sure you don't cut off too
much.

   When filling in brows with color, choose an
eyebrow pencil in a shade a bit lighter than
your brows. Don't draw a continuous line, but
use short little strokes that resemble natural
hairs, bottom photo, right. Then blend with a tissue to remove excess and get a soft, natural
brow line.

EYE OPENERS

Straight, dark eyebrows like these can give a hard scowling appearance to even the friendliest face. The idea here is to thin out the brows and to give them more of a curve. If hairs are long, start by brushing the brows up and trimming off the very tips with cuticle scissors. This lets more skin show through so the brows look lighter. Then, after plucking stray hairs, and depending upon the thickness, pluck two to four rows of hairs from the underpart of brows. Do one row at a time and check in mirror. As you come to outer corners, pluck a few extra hairs so brows have more of an upward turn. And don't be disturbed if your brows don't match each other exactly; nobody's do.

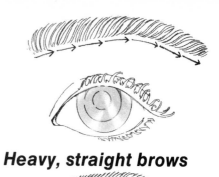

Heavy, straight brows

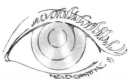

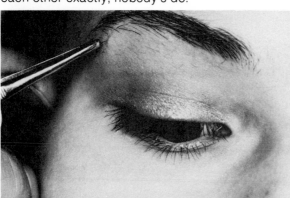

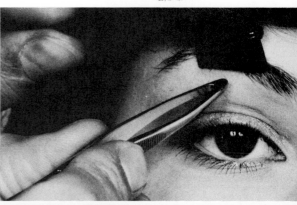

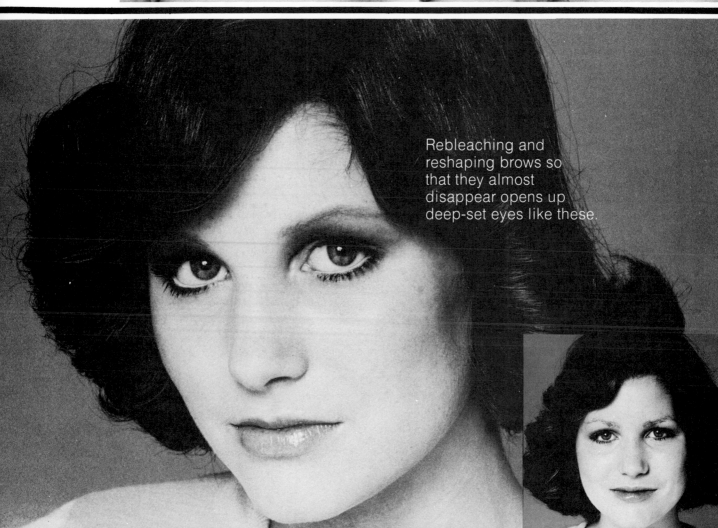

Rebleaching and reshaping brows so that they almost disappear opens up deep-set eyes like these.

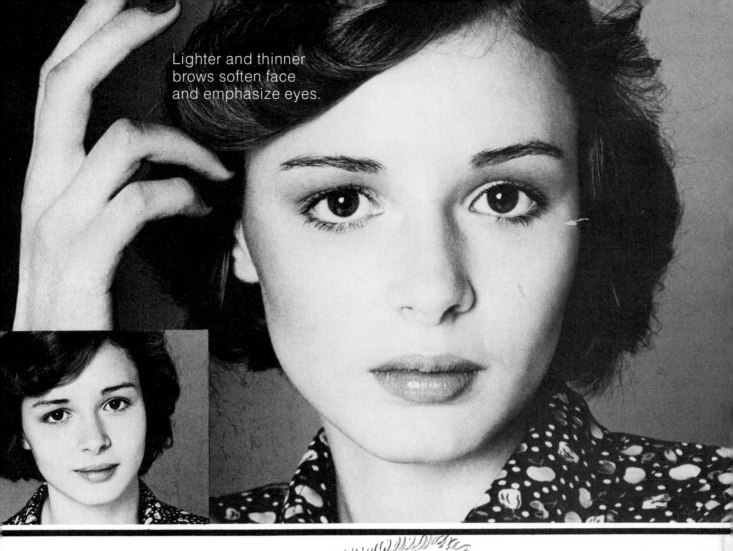

Lighter and thinner brows soften face and emphasize eyes.

Badly plucked, poorly bleached brows

Before you do anything to your brows, consider your eyes and the shape of your face. The woman here has deep-set eyes that almost got lost in her full face. To open them, she bleached and plucked her brows—the right idea, but the results were disappointing. Her brows weren't bleached properly and ended up a salt-and-pepper tone. Plucking left a straggly brow line. For such a definite brow change, you should probably see a professional and let her do the job.

To correct uneven brows like this, you have to tweeze very carefully and slowly. In fact, with brows that have been this badly plucked, you may find a magnifying mirror more helpful than a regular one in getting a clean, even line. Brush up individual hairs first, and pluck those that are out of line. Step back every so often to check the look in the mirror. Keep brushing and plucking till the entire brow has a clean shape, see photo, above, right. Fill in with brow color if necessary. Then check for new growth every few days and pluck regularly to maintain shape. If you want your brows bleached, see photo right, have it done by a professional. Even though at-home bleach preparations are available, the results you get at a salon are worth the money.

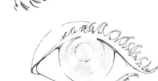

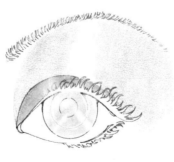

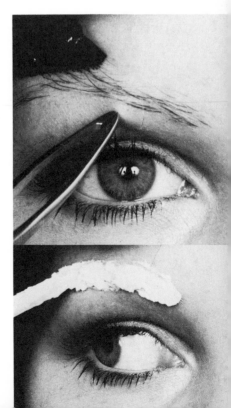

How to solve your biggest eye makeup
PROBLEMS

Practically no one argues with the idea that eyes are one of your most important beauty features. Luckily, their flaws are among the easiest to correct with makeup without it looking obvious. There's no need to blunder along with any of the following problems; here's how to solve them.

THIN LASHES

The obvious solution would seem to be lots of mascara, but unfortunately, thin lashes tend to stick together in spiky clumps when mascaraed. The solution: Powder lashes with baby powder, then apply cake mascara to lash tips only, top and bottom. Keep the cake as dry as possible by using very little water. This consistency won't tend to make thin lashes stick together as much as a thinner consistency would or as conventional wand-type mascaras. It takes a little longer to mascara lashes this way, but it's worth it.

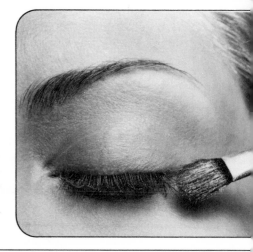

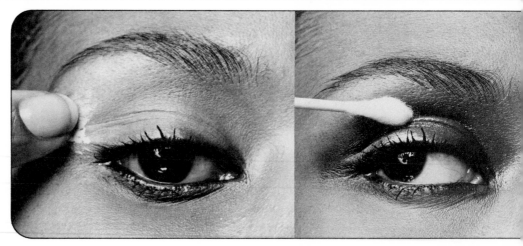

Near right: Use a paler shadow in crease of eye and on lid. This will bring the eye out more. Avoid deep shadow color in the crease, and don't highlight brow bone—it will only make eyes appear deeper.

Center: Use a deep-colored shadow under brows, concentrating color toward inner corner. Use a paler shadow in same tone on lid, finishing with deep color, blending slightly beyond outer corner of eye. This gives eye more interest and drama. Far right: Protruding eyes get shadowed near lash (pencils are good) with a shade close to eye color. This helps bring eye and lid on same plane, and eye seems to recede.

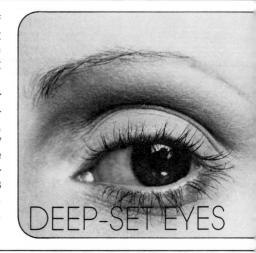

DEEP-SET EYES

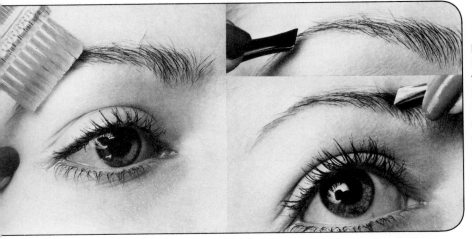

HEAVY BROWS

Full glossy brows are a definite beauty asset, but when they get *too* full, they can look grim and overbearing. Try this thinning technique: Brush brows straight up and pluck any hairs that straggle out of the general brow line. Then insert tweezers into the thickest part of brow and randomly pluck a few hairs here and there to lighten their look. Brush brows back into line and you'll be surprised at the difference.

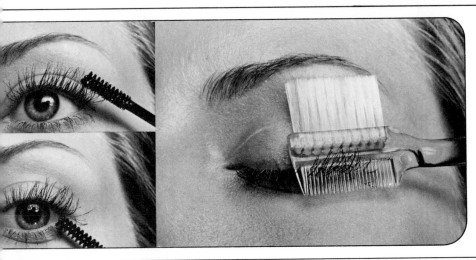

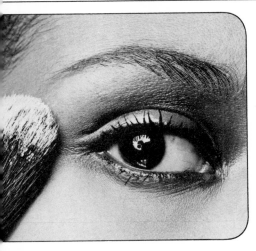

SHADOW CREASING

This is a problem for many women, especially those who have oily skin. Solve it by using a *little bit* of water-based foundation on lids (great for oily complexions, too), then follow with eye-coloring pencils or powder shadow (powders tend to crease less than creams). If you want the sheen of a cream, apply shadow, remove excess with cotton swab, then powder lid lightly with shimmering powder to set color.

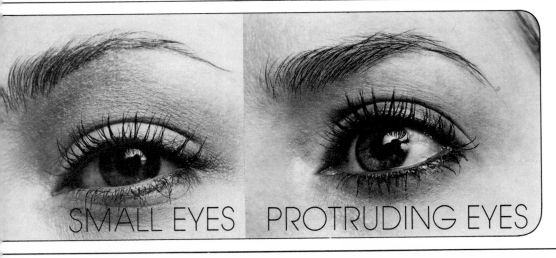

SMALL EYES PROTRUDING EYES

How to make the most of
YOUR EYES

Every eye shape is unique to its owner, but there are certain basic shapes that present small problems. Here are some solutions.

CHANGING SHAPES

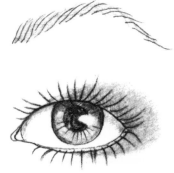

Close set

eyes can appear farther apart if you apply shadow at the corners, top sketch. The deeper, smokey tones of shadow will work best for this effect.

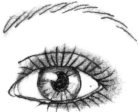

Narrow eyes

will take on a more oval appearance when shadow is applied all around the outer corner, center. Smudge the shadow for a soft effect and keep it close to lashes, blending past middle of eye.

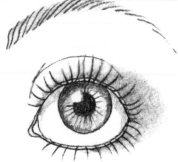

Too round eyes

can be softened with shadow spread across outer two-thirds of lid and brought in under lower lashes, just at the outside corner.

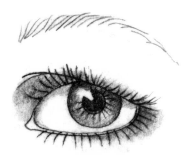

Overhanging brows

will perk up if you apply shadow from the inside corner of the eye over top lid and around under corner and bottom lid. Smudge the shadow to soften it.

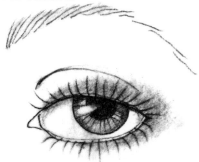

Droopy lids

will lose that sleepy look if you spread color up and out, following the natural shape of the eye, but widening the color band toward the outer corner and bringing color under eye to balance.

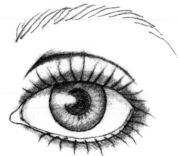

Protruding eyes

will seem less prominent if you smudge shadow almost like an eyeliner, going from inner corner to outer edge and around and under lower lid. Keep the band of color as narrow as the one you see in the sketch and use medium to deep colors. To experiment with these shadow techniques, treat yourself to some of the great new eye shadow colors.

EYEBROW SHAPING

The idea here is to neaten, but keep brows natural. When you pluck, you'll probably find a slant-edge tweezer easiest to work with. If you have long, fine brows that tend to droop, try cutting off the very tips, then lightly mascaraing them or use a bit of transparent mustache wax to keep them in line and add body. If you have scanty brows, fill in with a pencil in a lighter color than brows. Use your finger to smudge the lines slightly for a natural look. If you color your hair, don't forget to be sure brow color goes well with the new hair color. You may want to lighten or darken brows a bit to make them seem more appropriate for the new hair.

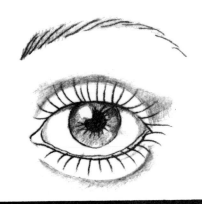

EYE CARE

Eyes are not only your most unique feature, they're probably your most sensitive one. They respond instantly to wind, dust, glare, lack of sleep, overindulging, even to your sleeping position. Here are some gentle ideas for their care:
● Protect eyes from dust and glare with sunglasses.
● Use soothing eyedrops when eyes are red and irritated.

● Moisturize well around eye area. There are fewer oil glands here than elsewhere on your face so this area tends to be especially dry. Moisturize at least a half-hour before going to bed so that the moisturizer doesn't contribute to the natural accumulation of fluids under the eye while you're sleeping.
● Be gentle when you remove eye makeup. It's best to remove it with a cotton ball saturated with eye makeup remover or use remover pads.
● Try not to get into the habit of sleeping on your tummy or side with eyes scrunched into your pillow. Doing it habitually can encourage lines around the eyes.

GREAT LASHES

To give lashes a silky and glistening look, try putting a bit of petroleum jelly or lash conditioner on a clean mascara brush and brush on lashes. This is a good idea for a natural daytime makeup look or as a conditioning idea for lashes at bedtime. Be sure to wash off mascara well.

EYE TECHNIQUES

A little color goes a long way toward turning on a really pretty look. A deep, smokey shadow in any color that flatters your eyes is a fantastic evening look. One of the metallic shadows, say a copper, pewter, silver or bronze, would be especially pretty. Blend these deep colors well to get a natural, unmadeup look.

For sensational-looking eyes, remember:
● Blend shadows well so you can't see a line where they start or end.
● If you're using a highlighter under the brow, blend it so that only the glow, not a real color remains.
● Be careful not to leave an unattractive gap between lashes and shadow. You can avoid this by starting shadow application just at lash line.
● Clean off any shadow that smudges on cheek or in eye corner. A cotton-tipped swab dipped in eye-makeup remover is good for doing this.

NAILS
that lead
beautiful lives

A manicure isn't just a "cosmetic" treatment for nails, it goes a long way toward protecting them from the harsh chemicals you use daily—cleaning products, detergents, etcetera. Here's the procedure for a good manicure. First, remove old polish with a gentle polish remover or remover pads. Then soak nails in mild soapy water, a couple of drops of mild dishwashing soap or shampoo in a small bowl of warm water is good. Dry nails, apply cuticle remover to one hand at a time and massage it in. Then, with the flat of an orangewood stick, gently push cuticle back to expose the white "half-moon" at cuticle edge. Don't use a metal instrument, it's too harsh; save this for scraping off any dead cuticle on the rest of the nail. Trim hangnails, don't trim cuticle. Rinse nails thoroughly to cleanse and create a good clean surface for polish to adhere to. Apply a base coat to bind polish to nails and to fill any ridges or ruts. Apply two coats of color, allowing drying time in between. Always apply polish in three strokes, the first down the center of the nail, then one on each side. Never go over the first coat to cover imperfections. The second coat of color will do a better job of covering than you can by patching. Apply a top coat if you like.

What causes irregularities?

From time to time, most nails get a few ridges, ruts or bumps; some you can control, others you can't. Horizontal ridges across the nail are usually caused by rough treatment around the cuticle. Using a sharp metal instrument to poke at cuticles will do it, as will a bang on your first knuckle. Treating nails gently will eliminate most horizontal ridges. Vertical ridges tend to be hereditary and there's little you can do to prevent them. They show up more in old age than youth. White spots are caused by air pockets forming in the nail as it grows. They're harmless, but you can't do much to stop them. Yellowing of the nail can be caused by smoking or from medications and sometimes by nail polish pigments.

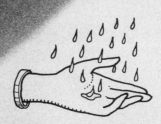

Weather changes nails

Since the part of the nail you see and manicure is no longer alive and growing, it has no potential to heal itself when you break, chip or expose it to a harsh environment. You can help by not using your nails as tools and by protecting them with polish and gloves when you put your hands in household cleaners, detergents and so forth.

Gloves can protect

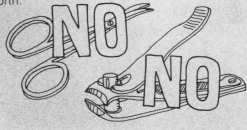

What's hard on nails?

Even too much exposure to sun, extreme cold and chlorine or saltwater can dry out nails and make them brittle. Cutting them with a nail clipper or scissors encourages splits and fractures. File away excess length.

How to shape a nail

The top three nail shapes in the sketch, left, are don'ts. The first is "balloon" shaped and tends to give your finger a stumpy, unattractive line. Center, the point, created when too much nail has been filed from the side, looks unattractive and also encourages breaks because the side support of the nail has been removed. The last nail hasn't been shaped at all. It gives an uncared for look. The bottom nail is an oval that's graceful and pretty and also leaves enough of the nail side area intact for support.

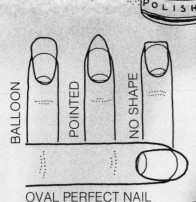

BALLOON
POINTED
NO SHAPE

OVAL PERFECT NAIL

How fast do nails grow?

Dermatologists tell us that the actual growing part of the nail is close to your first knuckle and as it grows, it forces its way into sight and down the base of the nailbed. Nails grow at a rate of about a quarter inch a month, so it takes about six months to grow a nail the length of the one sketched left. Toenails usually grow a bit more slowly.

APRIL
MAY
JUNE
JULY
AUG.
SEPT.

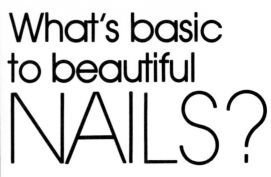

What's basic to beautiful NAILS?

Beautifully manicured nails are something any woman can have. All it takes is a little time—ten minutes for a manicure once a week, a few more minutes here and there for nail care—and some special tools to do the job right.

Basic tools to have on hand

Without the items, left, you can't do a first-rate manicure. Half the trick is the tools. *Emery boards* are essential for shaping nails, smoothing away the hardened skin at sides of nails. *Pumice stone* is necessary for softening cuticles or callouses. A *nail brush* is the best way to scrub nails really clean. *Cuticle cream* will help keep cuticles smooth and soft and help avoid future hangnails. A *cuticle crayon*, a stick of cuticle lubricant, is great because it's so easy to use. You could even carry it in your handbag in the winter when cuticles are so dry. A *nail white pencil* is invaluable for camouflaging stains under nails. *Orangewood sticks* are wonderful for gently pushing back cuticles and to clean up smudges of polish when you've finished your manicure.

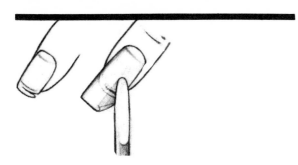

Help for splits and breaks

There's no reason to give up on a split or break in a nail. A good patching kit will mend it in minutes. There are several on the market. Most of them involve the use of a thin tissue that is glued to the nail with a special glue. You must polish over the patch. You see one being applied in the sketch above.

When to use scissors and clippers

It may come as a surprise, but you should *not* use scissors or clippers on fingernails. They tend to encourage splits and fractures; use an emery board instead. Save clippers for your toenails, which are harder and less apt to split. Start by soaking toenails in warm sudsy water to soften. Then, trim with clippers, leaving edges squared. Cut hangnails with scissors.

Manicure tips

● To get rid of dry or overgrown cuticles, use a cuticle remover. Apply it around cuticles, leave on a minute or so, according to instructions, then push back cuticles gently and rinse hands.
● Always use a basecoat. It gives your polish something to adhere to and prevents the deeper colors from staining nails.
● For the newest, freshest nail color look, you might like to try a transparent color. It "blushes" nails with see-through color.

For sensitive nails

If you have sensitive, easy-to-break nails, you might try a nail conditioner, a paint-on protein nail hardener that will help strengthen and harden nails. If you have delicate nails, be sure you use a gentle polish remover. One that has an oil base or that is labeled "gentle."

Is a nail "machine" good for you?

Electric or battery operated manicure machines are available. You can certainly get a good manicure without one, but if you're interested in doing the job fast, you might like to try one. Some take a bit of getting used to because they file nails much faster than you do with an ordinary emery board. Others also have attachments to smooth callouses on feet.

Quick-dry tip

Almost every woman has ten minutes to spare to give herself a manicure, but that's not really all that's involved. If you polish, you must allow about a half-hour for it to be hard enough to do anything with your nails. You might like to try one of the paint-on or spray-on quick dry products available. They speed up the drying time for the *surface* of the nail. They don't, however, harden the polish so you still can't open bobby pins or give hands a real work-out for a half-hour or more.

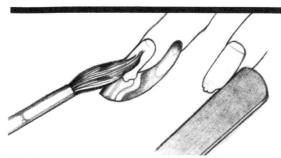

Make your own new nail?

You can, easily, with one of the nail-making kits available. You combine a special powder with a liquid and paint the mixture on your nail, using a form that fits around your fingertip. This is an excellent way to repair a badly broken nail. The new one lasts until it grows out and can be polished or not. Applying them does take some practice, though, so expect to try a couple before you become a pro.

Total nail care

Like any other part of your body, nails respond to regular treatment.
● Buff regularly to increase circulation.
● Give nails a rest from polish for a few days every few months. If they don't breathe, they may turn yellow.
● Take a few minutes to touch up chipped polish.

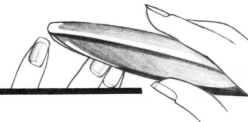

Special treat

● Consider having a professional manicure every four to six weeks. Besides the fact that it's so relaxing, it helps keep nails in excellent condition. The manicurist can establish a good nail shape for you, then you just have to follow it on subsequent manicures.

Massage treatment

Once of the nicest things you can do for your nails is to massage them with a rich cuticle or hand cream. Do this three or four times a week, especially in winter, and nails will be smooth and pliable. Massage lightly toward the cuticle and over the nail. You can also massage nails a bit with cuticle cream when you're giving yourself a manicure.

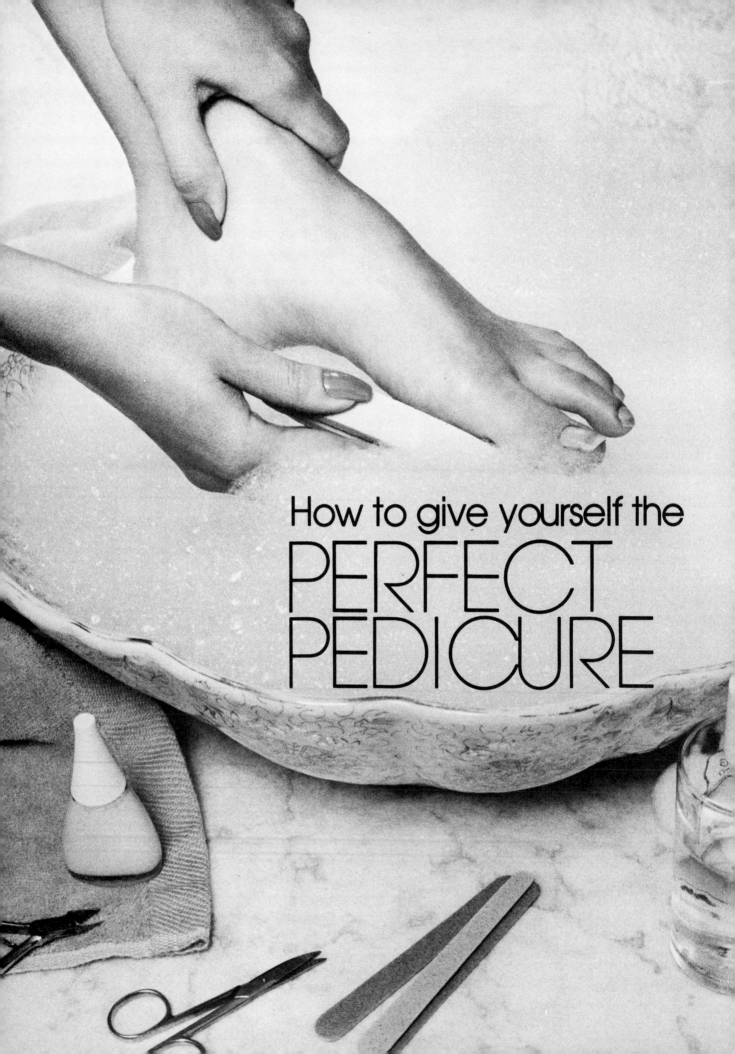

How to give yourself the
PERFECT
PEDICURE

A good pedicure is essential about once a month to keep feet and toenails in good shape. If you haven't given yourself one in quite a while, you'll find it worth your while to go to a professional, because a salon has more equipment and expertise to cope with neglected feet. Then follow-up yourself monthly.

Get equipment together

You'll find a pedicure easier if you gather all your tools together before you start. You'll also find that the bathroom or kitchen is the best place to work—this way if you spill some water on the floor, it's easily mopped up. You'll need a shallow basin large enough to immerse your feet in, a towel, facial tissues, cotton balls or pads, emery boards, clippers, cuticle snippers, pumice or callous remover, cuticle remover, polish remover and polish if you plan to polish toenails.

How to proceed

If you have polish on, remove it. Then fill basin about half-full with comfortably warm water and add several drops of shampoo or a mild dish-washing detergent. Soak both feet for about five minutes. Now that your skin is softened from the warm water, use the pumice stone on any rough or calloused spots. If you can find a callous remover (it looks like a small grater) in the dime- or drugstore, you'll find it very useful for removing dry, hardened skin on soles and at heels. Dry feet and apply cuticle remover around nail base, one foot at a time. Massage in. With an orangewood stick, gently push back cuticles. If nails are crusted with dry cuticle, gently scrape them clean with the edge of your cuticle snipper or a pair of cuticle scissors. Rinse feet and dry again. If toenails are long, clip with nail clippers, clipping so the nail is straight across. Don't clip into nail at the sides, it encourages ingrown toenails. File ends smooth with emery board. If you don't plan on polishing toenails, massage a good hand lotion into feet and you're finished. If you want to polish toenails, follow the procedure here.

Polish for gleam

The bright, vivid shine of polish is a nice finishing touch for toenails, especially in summer or whenever you plan to wear sandals. Pick a good, basic color that will go with many things so you won't have to change polish so often. Polish should last about two weeks. Now, separate toes with tissue woven in between them, or use cotton balls or rolled cotton pads. It will keep toes apart so polish doesn't smudge. Apply basecoat next. It's especially important for toenails because they tend to be rougher than fingernails and the base gives polish a smooth surface to adhere to. Now apply your colored polish by stroking down the center of the nail, then down each side. Let dry and apply a second coat. Finish with a top coat if you like. Allow plenty of time for toenails to dry—at least a half-hour—before putting on shoes. Massage a good hand lotion into feet when nails have dried.

Do's and Don'ts for feet

DO treat any corn or callous as soon as you notice it. If the corn is large and painful, see a podiatrist to have it removed. Some of the thicker callouses can also be professionally removed, then you can follow up with a callous remover or pumice at home.

DON'T ignore nails, especially a big toenail, that pulls away from the nail base at corners. You'll notice a dry, dusty accumulation of skin underneath. This is frequently caused by a fungus and although it isn't serious, it could, if neglected, cause you to lose the nail.

DON'T ignore the first signs of ingrown toenails—soreness and redness around nail corner. They infect easily and can be very painful. If you have the beginnings of one, gently lift the ingrown portion away from the skin and clip just enough to relieve the pressure. In the future, always be sure you cut toenails straight across. This keeps new growth from digging into nail sides.

DO get rid of any shoes that hurt your feet. They can cause corns and callouses that will take months to get rid of and it's just not worth it to try to wear them.

DO remember to apply hand lotion to your feet as well as your body after every bath or shower. Keeping skin supple and lubricated can discourage callouses and rough spots.

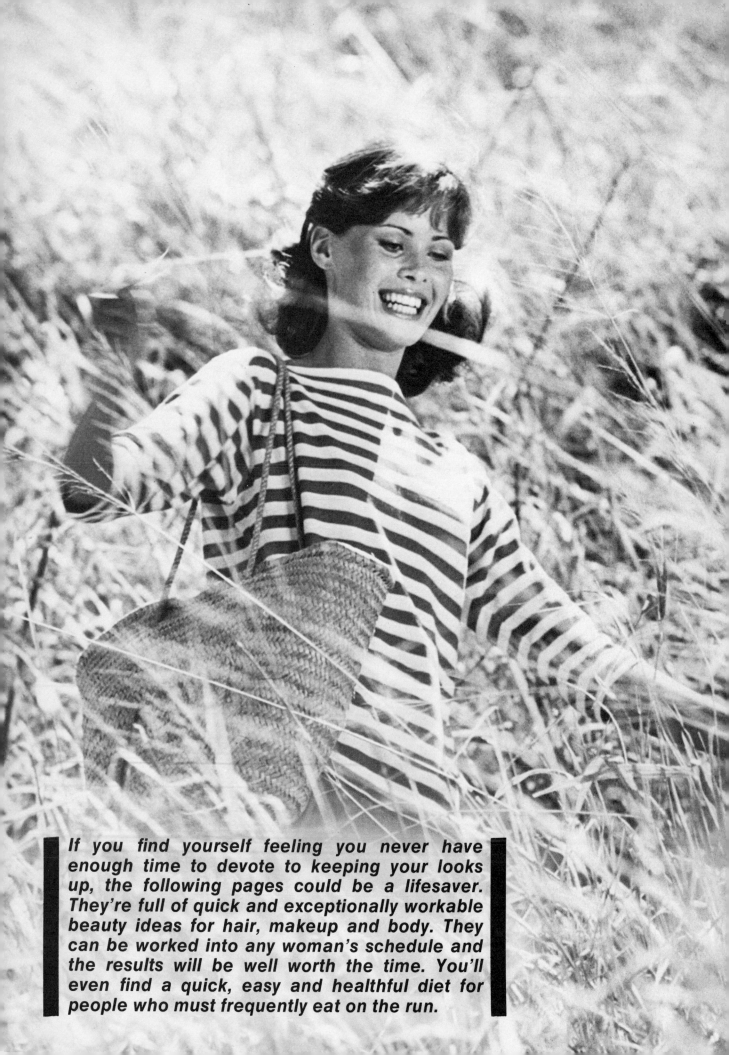

If you find yourself feeling you never have enough time to devote to keeping your looks up, the following pages could be a lifesaver. They're full of quick and exceptionally workable beauty ideas for hair, makeup and body. They can be worked into any woman's schedule and the results will be well worth the time. You'll even find a quick, easy and healthful diet for people who must frequently eat on the run.

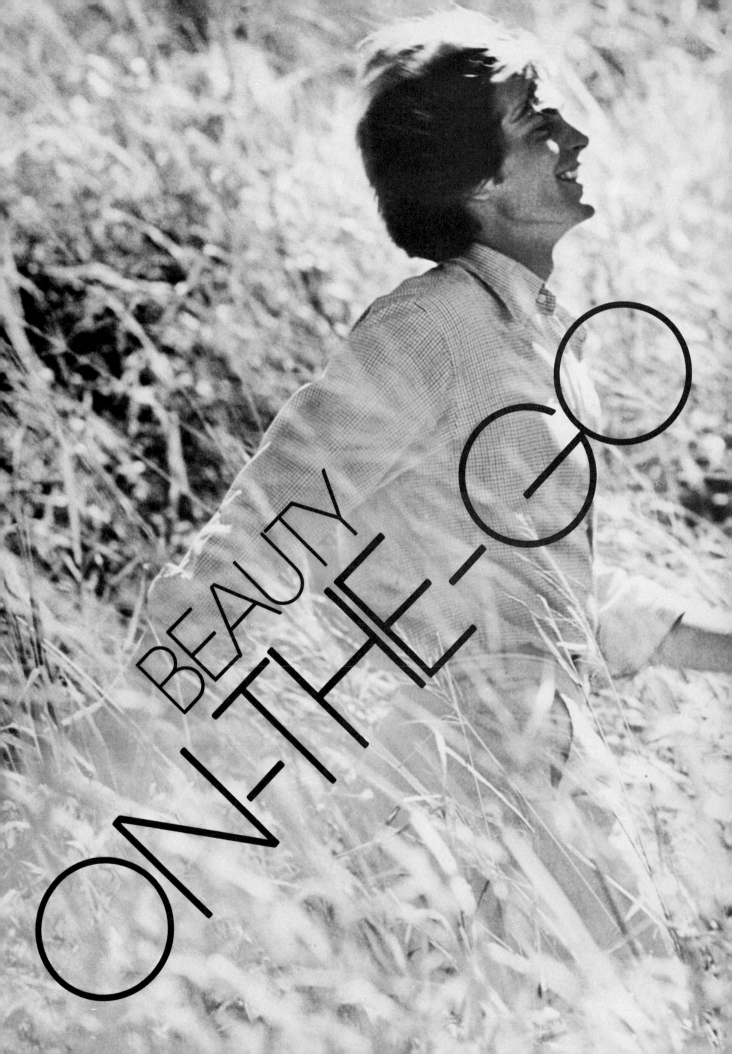

BEAUTY ON-THE-GO

12 minutes to a super new hairstyle

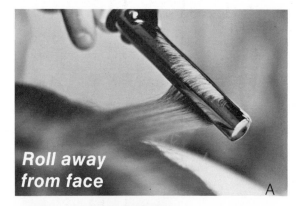

Roll away from face

A

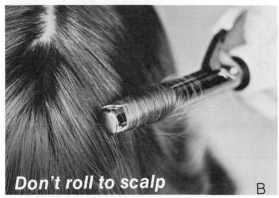

Don't roll to scalp

B

Clean dry hair, a good cut and a curling iron are all you need for the two looks here. For the finished look in E, start by rolling a section of hair in front, A (bangs, if you have them, are not curled). Roll hair away from your face and not all the way to the scalp. B shows you how close to roll it. Hold curl in place for a few seconds, then release, and without unwinding the curl, anchor it to your head with a bobby pin, C. Keep winding curls and pinning until you've finished both sides, D. If your hair doesn't hold a curl well, spray the pin-held curls lightly with hairspray. The back of the hair is left straight, but if you don't want an absolutely straight look, take big sections and roll loosely around the curling iron and pin. Let your hair stay pinned while you put on makeup. Remove pins and brush hair through lightly only once. Brush hair back, away from your face. For the look in F, follow exactly the same procedure, but make the sections you roll around the curling iron a bit smaller and roll them all the way to the scalp. Curl both the back of your hair and bangs, if you have them. When you're finished, brush through lightly. Don't aim for an "every hair in place" look. This is a casual, almost wind-blown look.

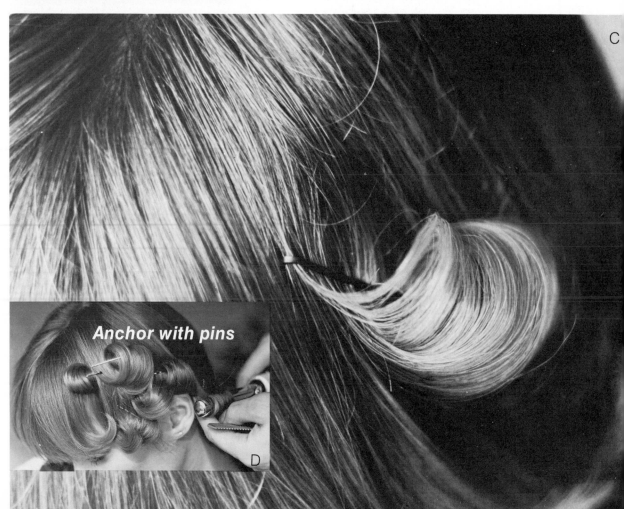

C

Anchor with pins

D

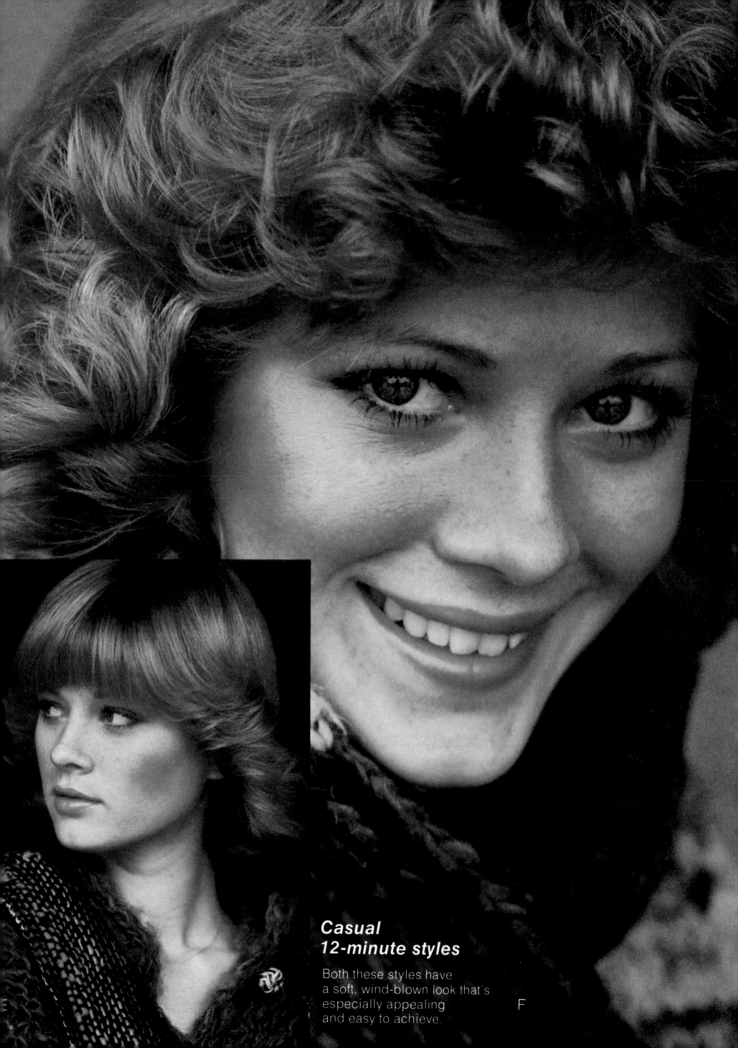

Casual
12-minute styles

Both these styles have
a soft, wind-blown look that's
especially appealing
and easy to achieve.

F

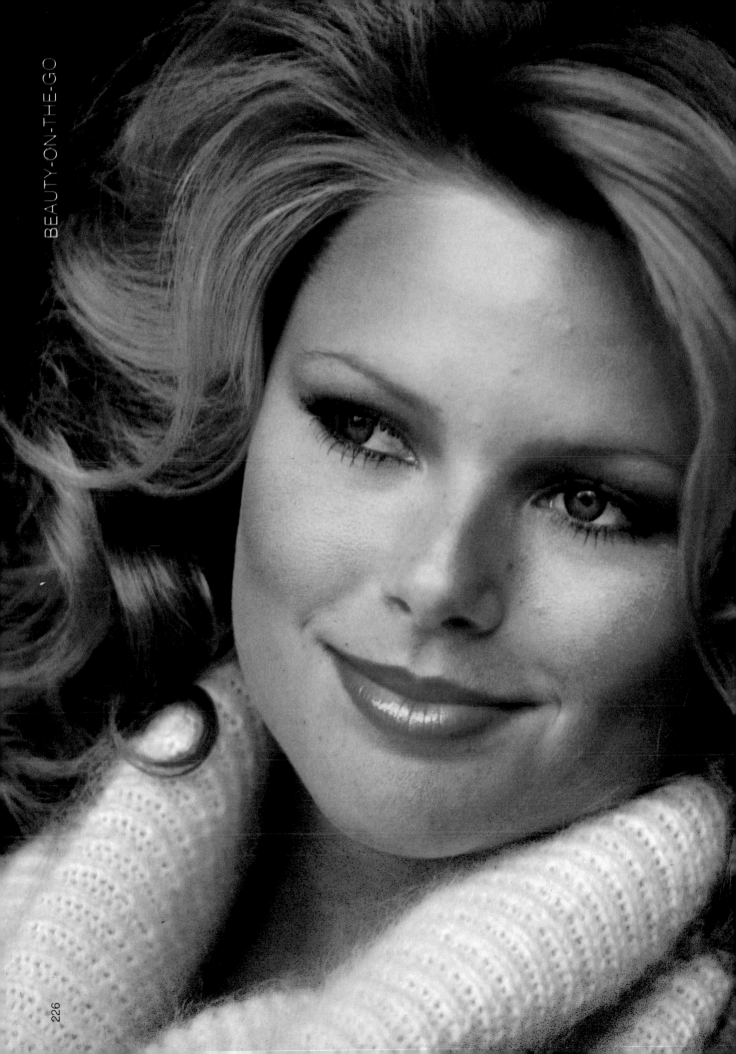

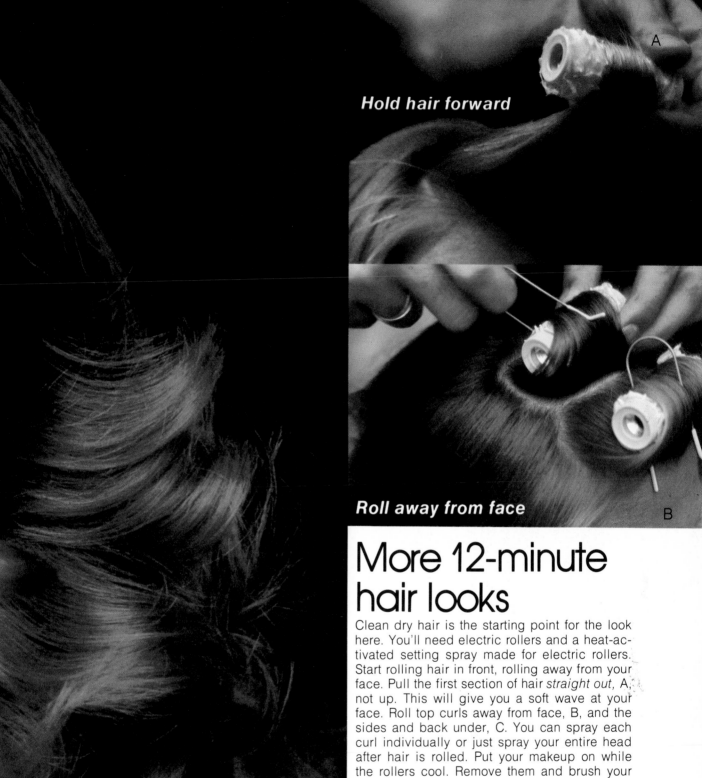

Hold hair forward

A

Roll away from face

B

More 12-minute hair looks

Clean dry hair is the starting point for the look here. You'll need electric rollers and a heat-activated setting spray made for electric rollers. Start rolling hair in front, rolling away from your face. Pull the first section of hair *straight out,* A, not up. This will give you a soft wave at your face. Roll top curls away from face, B, and the sides and back under, C. You can spray each curl individually or just spray your entire head after hair is rolled. Put your makeup on while the rollers cool. Remove them and brush your hair through only once to keep the curl as bouncy as possible.

Soft waves and curls— 12 minutes

The finished look, left, is as soft and pretty as you could want and it was done in just twelve minutes!

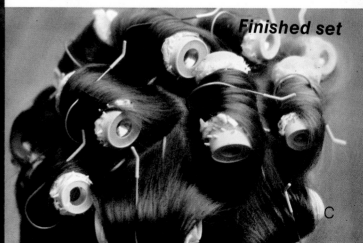

Finished set

C

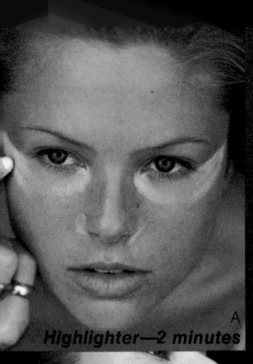

Highlighter—2 minutes A

This makeup puts the emphasis on defining facial features to give you an individual look without your seeming madeup. The colors are soft and easy to wear. Start with a creamy shadow-concealing base applied under the eye and blended carefully. It helps hide any discoloration and emphasizes the beginning of your cheekbone. Next blend a suntanned colored transparent foundation just under the cheekbone and under the jaw, B. The trick here is to blend very carefully. Next, high on the cheekbone, blend in a bright blush in a shade that's flattering to your skin tone. A tawny one would be pretty, especially when combined with the coppery shadow in C. Blend shadow over top lid so that it disappears beyond the crease in the lid. Finally add mascara to finish eyes. In this picture, D, the entire face, even the eyelids, is lightly dusted with baby powder to set makeup and add a subtle shine.

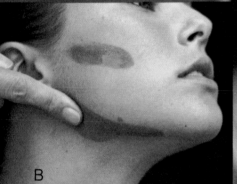

B

Blusher—3 minutes

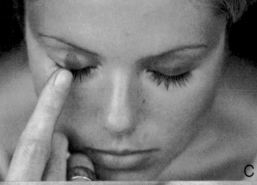

C

Shadow, mascara—6 minutes

12
minutes to a beautiful new makeup

You don't have to spend a fortune in time to get the beautiful, glowing look here. It's done with a minimum of makeup, but it looks polished and special enough for any occasion.

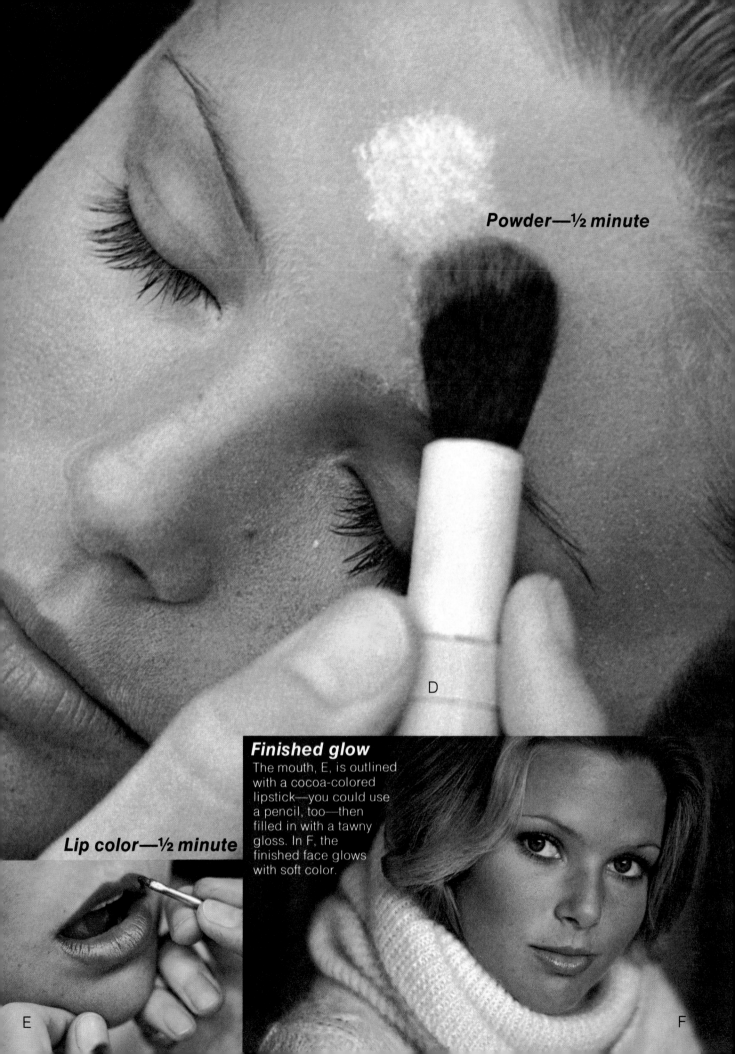

Powder—½ minute

D

Finished glow
The mouth, E, is outlined
with a cocoa-colored
lipstick—you could use
a pencil, too—then
filled in with a tawny
gloss. In F, the
finished face glows
with soft color.

Lip color—½ minute

E

F

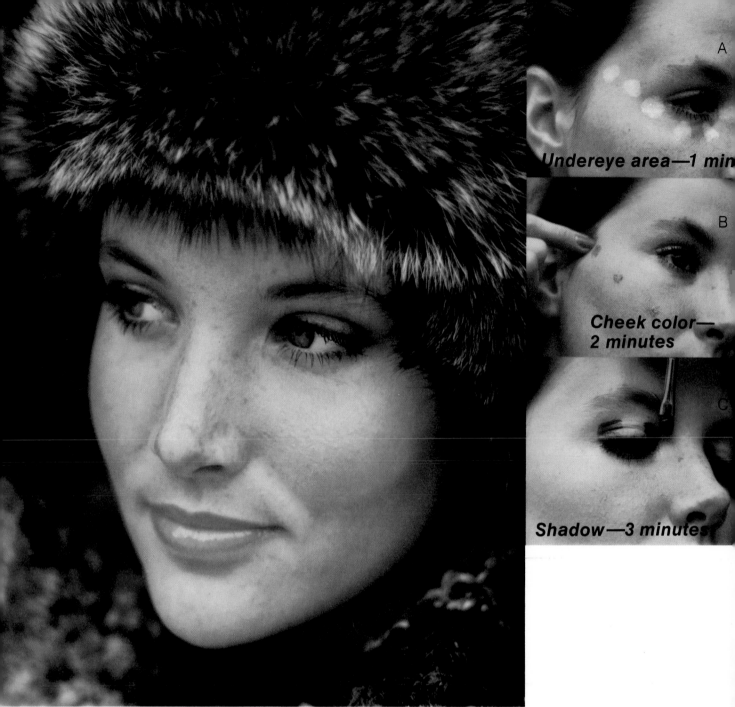

Undereye area—1 min

Cheek color—2 minutes

Shadow—3 minutes

Color gives polish

12 minutes to another beautiful makeup

This makeup puts the emphasis on color and how it can flatter and shape. Undereye concealer is dotted on and carried all the way to the hairline, A. With careful blending, this gives a wide-open setting for the eye. Blend a bit under brow bone, too. A warm peach-brown blusher is dotted on the line of the cheekbone and then blended for the most natural effect, B. Smooth a bit of blusher over the bridge of the nose and chin for a sunny look. A deep lilac shadow is applied to inner and outer corners of the lid with a brush, C. The shadow is blended with a cotton-tipped swab and smoothed slightly beyond the corners of the eye, D. A dot of peach cream shadow is applied in the middle of the lid to light and open the eye, E. For this makeup, a deep cobalt blue shadow was applied in a thin line just under the lower lashes. Skip this part if you're pressed for time. Several coats of mascara are brushed on with the wand tip to keep lashes nicely separated, F. A deep rose lip color is applied, G.

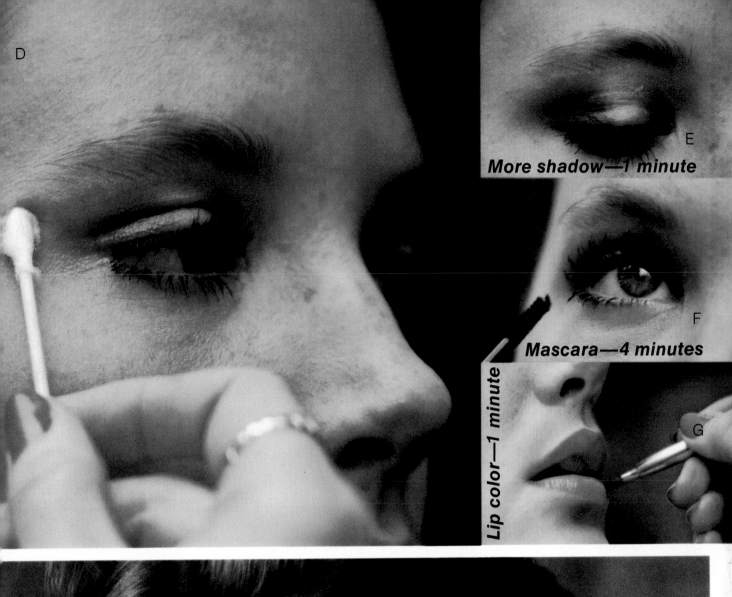

D

E

More shadow—1 minute

F

Mascara—4 minutes

G

Lip color—1 minute

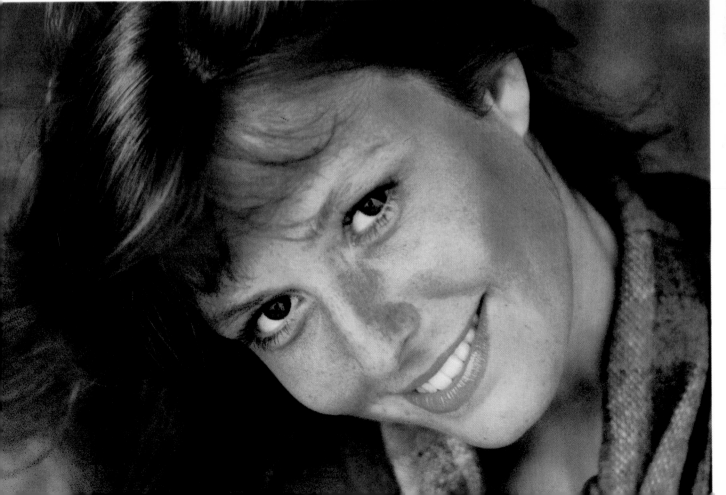

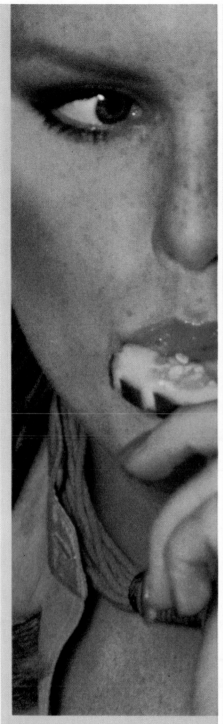

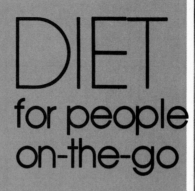

DIET
for people on-the-go

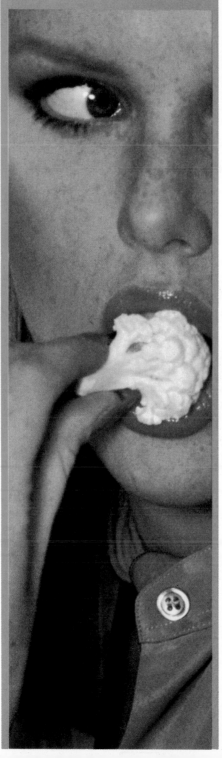

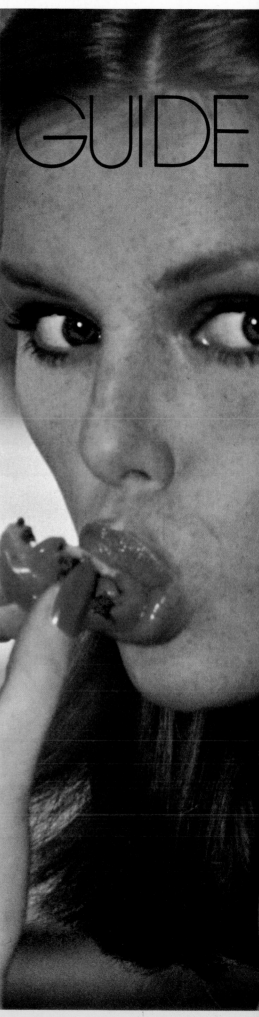

GUIDE

HOW DO YOU SHAPE UP AS A DIETER?

There's no reason why someone living alone or a busy couple eating on the run can't eat a very adequate diet, even if they almost never cook. "Someone eating a snack diet can still have a good nutritional profile," says Dr. Joan Gusso, Chairperson of the Program in Nutrition, Teachers College, Columbia University. There is also no reason why that same person can't lose weight. Compare yourself to the profile of an average American single or on-the-run eater by matching your eating habits against hers. Check off any habits, below, that match yours. If you have to check four or more out of a possible ten, read on, this is the diet for you.

- ☐ Cook? You can rarely be bothered.
- ☐ To you, the formal three meals a day are impossible on a regular basis.
- ☐ More often than not, you try to eat one good meal a day and the rest are broken up into minimeals or snacks, maybe six or so a day.
- ☐ You eat out more than you eat in.
- ☐ When you do eat in, it's mostly "heat and eat," "brown and serve," "shake and drink" type foods, canned or frozen, usually eaten while reading or watching TV.
- ☐ You wish there were more single-portion foods.
- ☐ You can't afford to but, nevertheless, you usually let leftovers spoil.
- ☐ You don't plan weekly food shopping sprees.
- ☐ You shop for food by need anywhere from three to seven times a week.
- ☐ You keep a few of the following staples on hand: canned tuna, soup in a packet or can, yogurt, cottage cheese, diet sodas, cheese and crackers.

EATING ALONE CAN BE HEALTHFUL AND THINNING

Single or on-the-run eating for a two-career couple is not determined by the clock or traditional habits. The most recent studies show that minimeals and snacks, anywhere from one to six a day, sometimes replace the traditional three. Dinner might be a hardy salad instead of meat, potatoes, vegetables, and salad; breakfast is sometimes a nutrition-fortified bar or a

canned nutritional drink or a Danish pastry. Convenience foods, frozen or packaged, frequently upstage cooking and cleaning up afterward. Eating out is sometimes preferable to eating home alone.

These are the facts and this eating guide is not going to try to change them. It will adapt them into a good sound healthful plan for eating that allows anyone to lose weight—without a lot of cooking, fussing or wasting food. Following are some alternatives and substitutes for the three traditional meals.

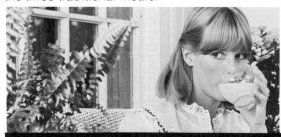

BREAKFAST
How to break the rules for success

Not all nutrition experts are convinced that starting off the day with a big breakfast is the soundest way of eating. But it is good common sense to eat something for breakfast, something that is nutritious and energizing enough to carry you through to lunchtime without such a ravenous or fatigued feeling that you eat double the lunch calories you would otherwise have eaten. All the breakfast food suggestions here are healthful and easy to fix, some you can even eat on the run if you must.

No-fuss ideas

AT HOME	ON-THE-RUN
slice of cheese	diet breakfast drink
slice of bread	yogurt, plain or
piece of fruit	with fresh fruit
black coffee or tea	chopped into it

How nutritious is it?

Breakfast is the one meal you're most likely to consume empty calories at—that Danish you grab on the way to the office, the stale doughnut you forage at home. A healthful breakfast should include protein. Eggs, hard cheeses, yogurt and skimmed milk are good low-calorie protein sources. Breakfast is traditionally the time for your daily dose of Vitamin C. Grapefruit and tomato juice are good low-calorie sources. The instant breakfast drinks and nutrition squares are also fortified with C. Vitamin fortified cereals plus skim milk give you protein with reasonable calorie counts. Beware of the unfortified cereals. They can be empty calories, too. Check the box for nutritional information.

How caloric is it?

slice of Swiss cheese 104*
slice white bread 75
peach 35
grapefruit, 6 oz. 75
tomato juice, 6 oz. 38
instant breakfast drink, 10 oz. 225
breakfast nutrition square, 1 185
yogurt, 8 oz. plain 130
soft-boiled or poached egg 80
nutrition fortified cereal, 1 cup . . . (no milk) 110

*All calorie values are approximate.

IN A COFFEE SHOP	AT YOUR DESK
soft-boiled or poached egg slice of toast tomato or grapefruit juice or vitamin fortified cereal with skim milk tomato or grapefruit juice	vitamin-fortified snack bar or square skim milk, 8 oz. coffee or tea

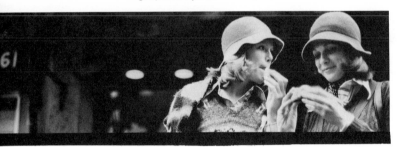

LUNCH
Brown-bagging it

AT YOUR DESK
● Fill little plastic bags with fresh vegetable sticks and eat them with cottage cheese or a hard-boiled egg.
● Pack frozen shrimp or crab cocktail in the morning and by lunch it will be thawed, but cool and delicious. Eat with saltines, finish up with a piece of fruit.
● Drink: Coffee, tea or diet soda.

BROWN-BAG PICNIC
● Try the classic picnic of cheese and fruit. A few saltines with your cheese adds texture interest.
● Cold roast chicken and fruit make another good quick lunch picnic idea.
● Drink: Bring a container of homemade lemonade with as little sugar as possible added.

Diet ideas

Make lunch your big meal of the day if you don't like eating alone in restaurants at night any better than dining at home alone.
● Avoid the post-lunch candy bar or coffee cart snack by having a box of raisins handy.

They're nutritious, supply quick energy and are only thirty-one calories a satisfying tablespoonful.
● If you're a sandwich addict, try eating only *one* slice of bread. Avoid the salad mixes like chicken or egg, they're loaded with mayonnaise calories, one hundred per tablespoon. Substitute mustard, only twenty-four calories a tablespoon. ● Give yourself the illusion of eating a whole sandwich using two slices of thin or diet-sliced bread—only fifty-two as compared with seventy-five or eighty for regular bread. ● Walk off your lunch by taking a half-hour walk after eating. You'll walk off about one hundred sixty calories in a half-hour.

When the brown bag is ordered in:

● Hot dog with only half the bun and a cool tomato or grapefruit juice to drink. Add a piece of fruit if you're still hungry.
● Hamburger with only one side of the bun *or* open-face turkey sandwich. Drink tomato or grapefruit juice or add a piece of fruit.

Low calorie

carrot 21	Cottage cheese, ½ cup 120
celery, per stalk 6	Frozen crab cocktail,
cucumber, average size 29	(4 oz. jar) 110
radish, 4 small 7	Frozen shrimp cocktail 110
apple, average . . . 80	roast chicken, 4
apricot 18	oz. 208
banana, medium . . 87	hamburger, with ½ bun 187
grapes, ½ cup 33	hot dog, with ½
cantaloupe, ½ 58	bun 226
cheese: 1 oz. Muenster, Camembert or Swiss 104	saltine 12

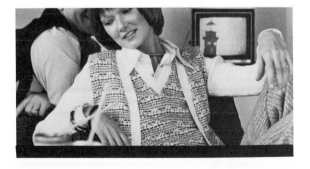

DINNER
Diet dinner salads

Try some of the low-calorie, quick-fix meals here. You'll cut calories two ways: first from their low-calorie content, and second from the satisfaction you'll derive from enjoying your meal enough not to be tempted to snack an hour or so later.

CRISP DIET SPINACH SALAD
Make a salad of crisp raw spinach leaves, sliced raw mushrooms, imitation bacon bits and diet blue cheese dressing. You can even splurge with a four-ounce glass of wine because the salad is so low in calories.

TUNA SALAD WITH COLD VEGETABLES
Mix one small water-packed can tuna, drained, with one small onion, finely chopped and a teaspoon of capers. Add several squeezes of lemon juice or 1 teaspoon diet mayonnaise. (The tuna will taste tangier if you let it stand a half-hour or so, but it's good eaten right away.) A dash of curry powder is another good addition. Eat this with a salad of cold vegetables. Bean sprouts are great with a squeeze of lemon juice or a dash of celery salt.

MIXED VEGETABLE SALAD
A nondiet version of this is a staple of French and Italian cuisines and it's delicious; so is this diet version. Mix cold leftover peas and carrots—the canned version will do—with diet mayonnaise. Add a little chopped onion for more tang. Eat with melba toast and a small wedge of any hard cheese.

Convenience foods, low-calorie substitutes

Nothing makes a better case for eating low-calorie substitutes than this comparative chart. We've also included some of the substitute ingredients you need to dress things up a bit.

regular margarine, 1 T.	100
diet margarine, 1 T.	50
slice whole wheat bread	65
slice-thin diet type	44
American cheese, 1 oz.	104
diet American cheese	50
cottage cheese, creamed, 1 cup	213
low-fat cottage cheese, 1 cup	155
regular cream cheese, 1 oz.	104
imitation cream cheese, 1 oz.	52
regular vanilla ice cream (¼ pt.)	132
ice milk (¼ pt.)	97
French dressing, 1 T.	65
low-calorie French, 1 T.	21
tuna in oil, 3¼ oz.	268
tuna in water, 3¼ oz.	105

DIET SALAD CALORIES

string beans, 1 cup	34	grated Parmesan	
broccoli, 1 cup	50	cheese, 1 T.	27
carrots, 1 cup	64	imitation mayon-	
peas, 1 cup	120	naise	40
spinach, 1 cup	9	diet blue cheese	
mushrooms, 1 cup	20	dressing, 1 T.	13
bean sprouts, ½ cup	8	imitation bacon bits,	
capers, 1 T.	6	1 T.	29

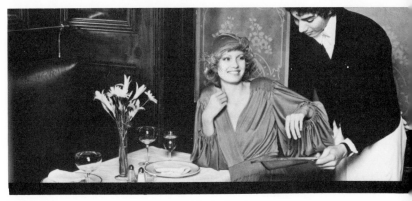

EATING OUT

How to judge portions

Meat: Base your meat judgment on a hamburger. The standard in this country fits perfectly into the top of a medium-size mayonnaise jar and weighs about 3 oz. The average steak portion served in a restaurant is at least twice this, maybe more. One medium-lean lamb chop or chicken thigh weighs about 3 oz. Sandwiches: Most coffee shops serve 3 oz. of meat in their sandwiches. Big deli specials contain about 4. Vegetables: Practice measuring out half-cup servings at home until you're able to judge. This size serving is ideal for dieters.

Best bets/Worst bets

● Have a light appetizer like tomato juice to stave off hunger.
● Order lean, unsauced broiled meat.
● A steaming cup of espresso will make the end of your meal something special.
● Beware the hot hors d'oeuvres and peanuts served in bars.
● Don't order fried foods, cream sauces or cream soups.
● If you must succumb to the rich dessert, remember the second half tastes just like the first, so don't eat it.

DRINKS			
daiquiri, 4 oz.	252	coq au vin	400
martini, 4 oz.	236	mussels à la mari-	
whiskey sour, 4 oz.,		nière	270
80-proof	260	French pastry	250
any 86-proof		**ITALIAN**	
whiskey and water,		veal piccata	430
2 oz.	140	sausage and pep-	
wine, 4 oz. red or		pers	550
white	100	shrimp scampi	270
beer, 8 oz.	100	fettucini Alfredo	650
		lasagna	515
FRENCH FOOD		spaghetti and	
beef Burgundy	450*	meatballs	370
duckling à		cheesecake	300
l'orange	650	rum cake	540

*Calories for French, Italian and Chinese are approximate since portions vary with restaurants. These are for average servings.

235

CHINESE

Chinese foods are a best-bet when you eat out. Ingredients and sauces are relatively low-calorie.

pork chow mein . . 400
chicken chow
   mein 385
shrimp fried rice 200
egg roll 45
fried rice, ½ cup 135
fried noodles, ½
   cup 135
fortune cookie 30

FAST FOOD

Jumbo hamburger
   with all the
   trimmings 500
Regular ham-
   burger 250
Fried chicken,
   drumstick 220
Frozen custard,
   small cone 113
Hot dog with trim-
   mings 265

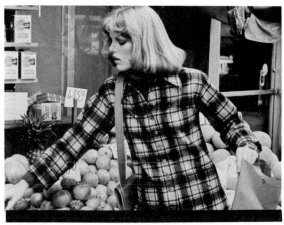

DIET AND HEALTH

Shop healthfully

What young on-the-go people eat is often determined by what's on hand, so make sure your stockpile includes some healthful low-calorie staples:

REFRIGERATOR
cottage cheese, yogurt (both keep about a week)

hard cheese, fresh fruit, such as oranges, apples or grapefruit, all keep well.

CUPBOARD
water-packed tuna or crab

soup (canned or packets, not creamed)

bouillon cubes, vitamin-fortified cereals, diet breakfast and snack bars, canned or bottled fruit and vegetable juices, canned low-calorie vegetables for quick salads, raisins, canned fruits, diet sodas

Tip sheet for healthful diet eating

As a nation, we eat about twice as much protein as we need. We'd all have more healthful diets if we ate raw fruits and vegetables plus whole grain or whole wheat bread (when you eat bread). Remember that grain has protein, too; you don't always have to get it from meat. Grain also has the big advantage of providing

necessary fiber or bulk. Be careful to check calorie counts on whole-grain products, though; some of the health food cereals can be very high in calories.

● Try sautéing with chicken broth, soy sauce or wine instead of butter or oil. You can assume that 85 percent of the calories in wine will evaporate in the cooking process. Chicken broth and soy sauce are both low in calories.

● If you do sometimes cook, bone up on East Indian or Turkish cuisine. Both use lots of yogurt and fresh vegetables, much more slimming than cream sauces.

● Try to be more aware of how much and what you've eaten during the day—keep a little pocket calendar for the first week of your diet. It will help you learn to count calories and change your eating habits.

HAPPY IDEAS FOR EATING ALONE

"Eating is a social act," says Dr. Joan Gusso. The sociability of eating is deeply ingrained as Dr. Gusso points out, even "the infant is socialized while being fed. . . . The whole notion of eating alone—separating eating and sociability—is very destructive." Dr. Gusso suggests that single people who live in large apartment complexes form "eating co-ops." Members could take turns cooking, then eat in groups once, twice, or as many times a week as they agree on. You might also form an eating co-op especially for dieters and let the sociability and communal desire to lose weight reinforce your own diet ambitions.

Here are more ideas for making eating alone a happier experience:

● If you're bored with the usual tuna, hard-boiled eggs or broiled hamburger, keep a paperback cookbook in your desk at work and leaf through it for dinner ideas. This way you know just what to shop for and can pick it up on the way home.

● If you shy away from eating alone in restaurants, especially the nicer, more interesting ones, try to conquer that feeling. Loads of women have. Take along a newspaper or paperback book to read, too. It may make you feel more at ease.

● Once a week, cook something really delicious, just for you. Here are two recipes to start you off. Both are thinning as well as tasty.

BAKED LEMON CHICKEN

½ chicken breast, boned and skinned
1 clove garlic, peeled and halved
Coarse salt
Juice of ½ lemon or lime
2 tsps. chutney

Preheat oven to 400°. Pound chicken lightly to flatten. Sprinkle all over with 1 teaspoon coarse salt and rub well with garlic clove. Place chicken on a piece of heavy-duty aluminum foil. Pour juice over it and spread chutney on top. Fold foil up and enclose chicken tightly in it. Bake for twelve to fifteen minutes. Serve garnished with lemon or lime wedges.

SESAME STEAK

1 club or shell steak (or other small steak)
* no more than one-inch thick*
Seasoned salt
Black pepper
1½ tsps. sesame seeds
1 T. diet margarine
1 or 2 thinly sliced scallions
½ tsp. Dijon-style mustard
½ tsp. Worcestershire sauce

Toast the sesame seeds by shaking them in a skillet over high heat until lightly browned. Remove seeds from skillet and reserve. Make small gashes in the fat of steak and sprinkle with seasoned salt and pepper. Rub the skillet with a little of the steak fat and fry the steak on both sides until done to your taste (about three minutes per side for rare). Remove steak to a warm plate. Sauté scallions in diet margarine for one minute. Stir in sesame seeds, mustard, Worcestershire sauce and pour over steak.

HOW MANY CALORIES MAKE A REDUCING DIET?

Obviously, it's not just *what* you eat, but also *how much* that makes any diet successful. We've given you lots of suggestions and calorie counts; now here's a guide to help you know just what will make it all work for you.

PRESENT WEIGHT	CALORIES TO MAINTAIN	CALORIES TO LOSE
105–109	1920	1200
110–114	2000	1300
115–119	2100	1400
120–124	2190	1450
125–129	2250	1500
130–134	2300	1550
135–139	2400	1600
140–144	2500	1650
145–149	2600	1700
150–154	2700	1750
155–159	2800	1800
160–164	2900	1900
165 and over	3000	2000

Many things will influence how fast you'll lose weight—primarily your metabolism and your activity; the more exercise you get, the faster the weight comes off. But regardless, most dieters find they lose most the first week of dieting, begin to level off the second and reach a plateau the third. You may find you won't lose at all the third week. Don't be discouraged. Your body is just getting used to new eating habits and you'll start to lose weight again at a steady rate if you keep your calories down.

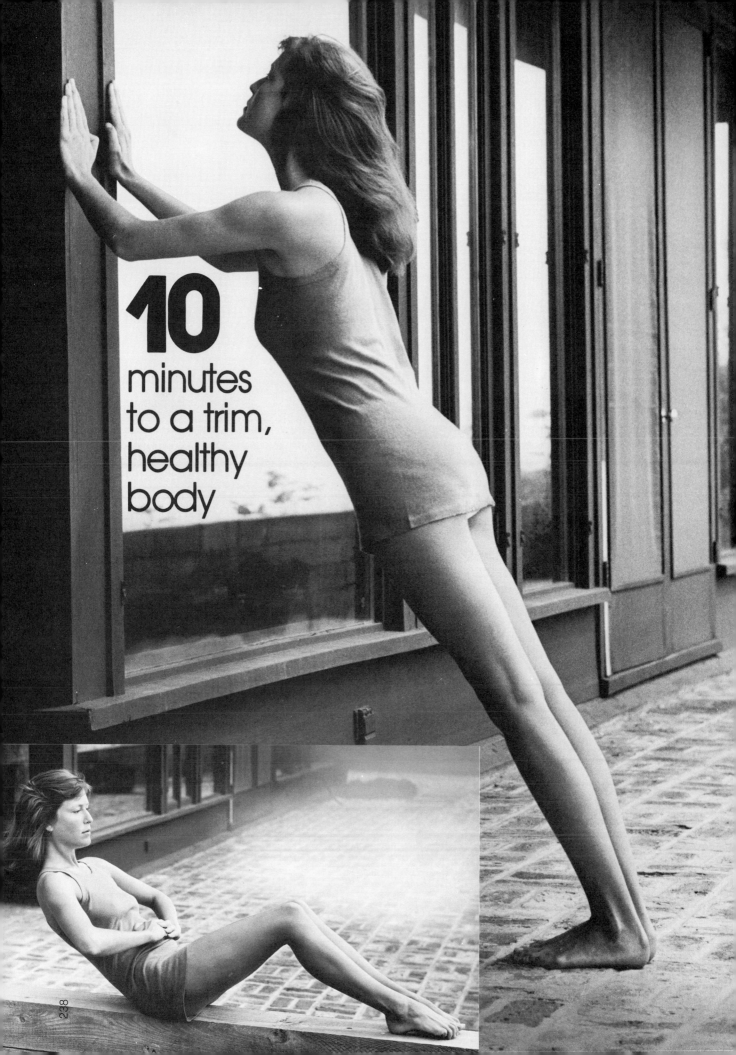

10
minutes to a trim, healthy body

Just ten minutes, three times a week can make the difference between a limber, fit body and one that's soft and poorly conditioned. This kind of thirty-minute weekly program was what got—and kept—the astronauts in such good shape and it can do the same for you. The basic idea is to lower your calorie intake just a little—no starvation diet, really—and to raise your activity level through a ten-minute workout three times a week. The workout should include a minute's worth of gentle stretching, say reaching toward the ceiling with one hand, then the other; next, four minutes of the following fitness exercises on this page and finally a five-minute period of aerobic exercise (any activity that substantially increases your heart rate). The hopping exercise, right, is one idea. The exercises here are all adapted from the book *Total Fitness in 30 Minutes a Week** by Laurence E. Morehouse, Ph.D., and Leonard Gross.

* Laurence E. Morehouse, Ph.D., and Leonard Gross, *Total Fitness in 30 Minutes a Week,* Simon and Schuster, New York, 1975.

Fitness push-aways

Stand a little beyond arm's reach from a wall. Put your hands against the wall at shoulder height. Lean forward until your chest nears the wall, then push away until you're back in the starting position. Repeat about fifteen times, then gradually increase to twenty. As you get better, move farther and farther away from wall and gradually lower hands to breast level.

Aerobic exercise

Hop up and down from one foot to the other, bringing your knees up high as you do it. Do it at a steady, even pace, increasing the speed as you build up endurance. You must do this exercise continuously for five minutes to get the endurance benefits. If you're tired when you first start, stop. Day by day you'll build up enough endurance to get up to a continuous five minutes' worth.

Fitness sitbacks

Sit on floor with your knees bent. Hook your feet under a piece of furniture when you first start doing this exercise—it forces you to use the correct muscles. Now move your chest forward to your knees, or as close as you can get. Place hands on stomach so you feel the muscle action. Now move back away from your knees until you feel your stomach muscles begin to tense. If they quiver, that's as far back as you should go. Lean forward again and repeat exercise until you're tired. As you become more and more fit, you'll be able to lean back farther and farther.

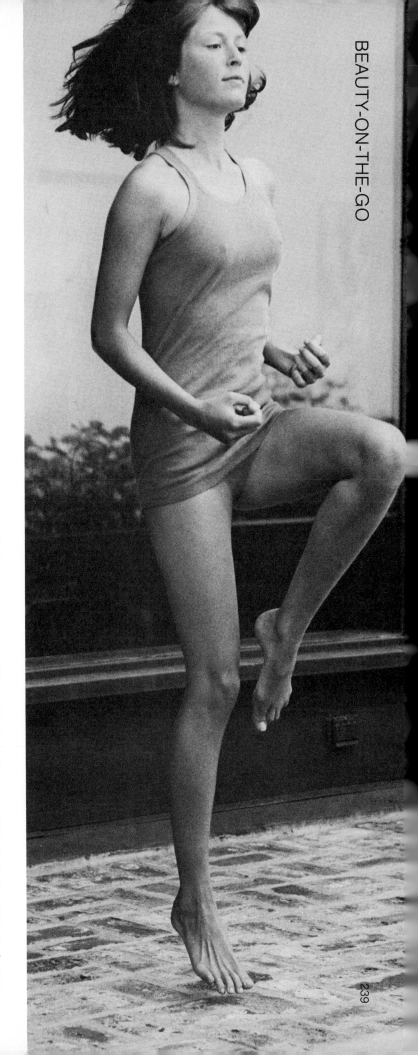

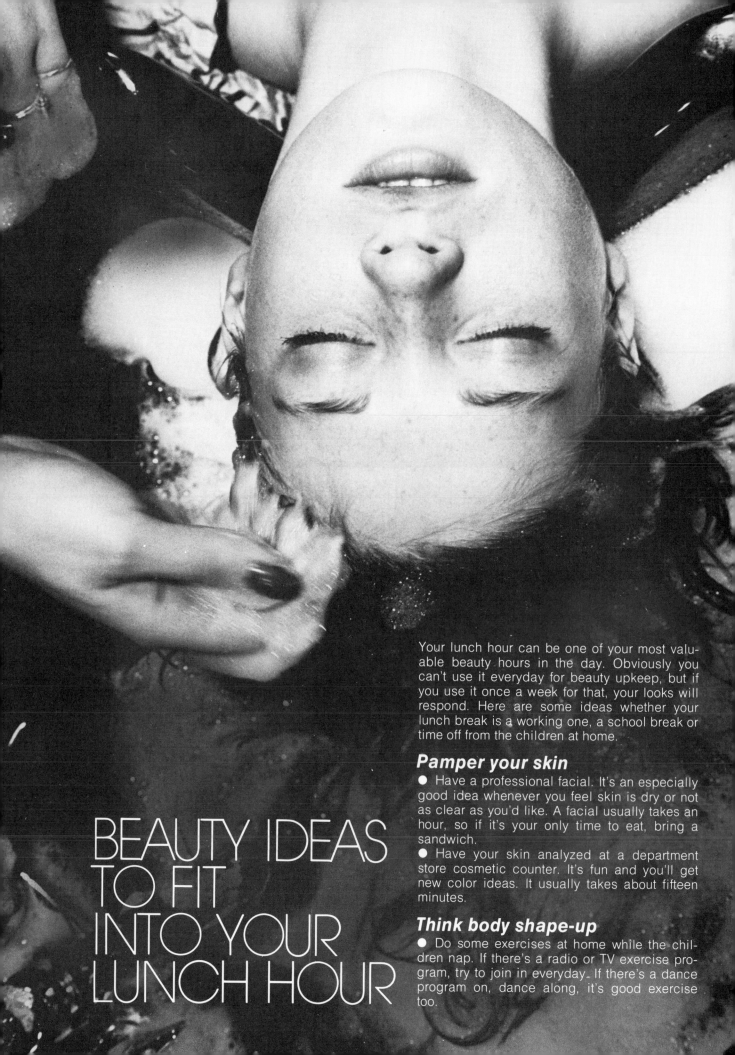

Your lunch hour can be one of your most valuable beauty hours in the day. Obviously you can't use it everyday for beauty upkeep, but if you use it once a week for that, your looks will respond. Here are some ideas whether your lunch break is a working one, a school break or time off from the children at home.

Pamper your skin

● Have a professional facial. It's an especially good idea whenever you feel skin is dry or not as clear as you'd like. A facial usually takes an hour, so if it's your only time to eat, bring a sandwich.

● Have your skin analyzed at a department store cosmetic counter. It's fun and you'll get new color ideas. It usually takes about fifteen minutes.

Think body shape-up

● Do some exercises at home while the children nap. If there's a radio or TV exercise program, try to join in everyday. If there's a dance program on, dance along, it's good exercise too.

BEAUTY IDEAS TO FIT INTO YOUR LUNCH HOUR

At-home beauty lifts

● Give yourself a facial at home and include some kind of mask to help get rid of the dry outer layer of skin that has been building up since the last time you used one. This should take about twenty minutes.
● Shave your legs and use a callous remover on heels and knees or wherever there are rough spots. Takes about fifteen minutes.
● Take a long, relaxing bath with the works—bubble bath or bath oil, a body loofah, pumice for your feet and elbows. Then, if you have time, give yourself a manicure. Takes about an hour for both.
● Shape and pluck your eyebrows in ten minutes.
● Get a book on calories and food, and bone up on low-calorie, high-nutrition eating.

Get a new hairdo

● Have your hair washed and blown dry, just for the pleasure of pampering yourself for a special date or to pick up some blowdry techniques from a pro. This should take from forty to fifty minutes.

Brighten your eyes

● Have your lashes dyed professionally, or if you've lightened your hair, have your brows lightened professionally. This takes only about twenty minutes.
● Have your brows plucked and shaped professionally. It will give you a good shape to follow at home. This will take about twenty minutes.

Learn something new

● Investigate yoga, judo or some other form of exercise. Most Y's offer inexpensive lunchtime classes. The exercise will do your mind and body good.
● Take a course in another language. Many adult schools and some Y's offer them at lunchtime. Takes about an hour.
● If you're already involved in a foreign language, organize a weekly lunch with other people who speak the same language. You can practice with each other.
● Take tennis lessons and improve your game.
● If you're at home all day, make it a point to get out for at least twenty minutes, preferably after lunch to exercise off a few calories. You can walk, ride your bike, jog.

Become more informed

● Pick a book you've been meaning to read and set aside at least ten minutes everyday for a week to get into it.
● Make a point of remembering at least one item from the daily paper that you can add to a conversation. You'll be more interesting, feel more stimulated.

Get some inspiration

● Go to a museum or an art gallery to revive your spirits on a "down" day.
● Check the paper to see if there are any noon lectures or discussion groups you'd be interested in.
● Check out short movies at museums or galleries; some churches sponsor noontime films of interest.

Pamper your body

● Go and have a relaxing massage at lunch hour; it's especially good if you're having a frantic day or you've had one the day before.
● If you're home with children and can't get out for a massage, buy a book on how to give one.

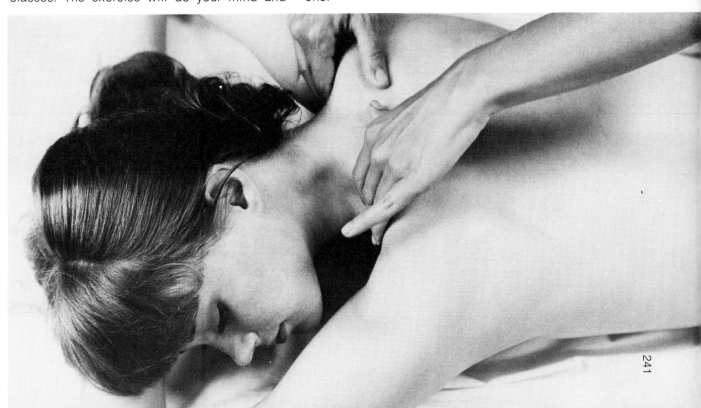

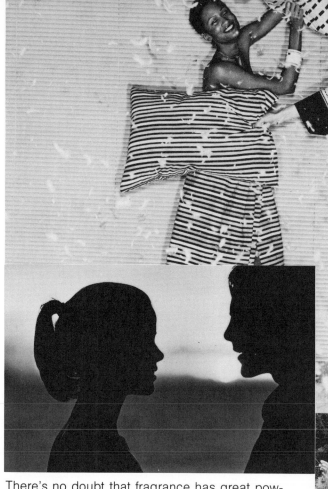

There's no doubt that fragrance has great powers to evoke and intensify moods. It can bring back memories you thought you'd forgotten, set the scene for new ones—and it can do it in a hurry. It takes just a few seconds to surround yourself in a mood-evoking scent and you can carry its potence wherever you go—tucked into your handbag or a pocket. Here are some ideas to help you make the most of fragrance.

Set a mood

Fragrance can enhance your mood, whatever it may be, from the fun-and-full-of-surprises mood, right, to a deeply romantic one. Tip: Don't limit yourself to just one scent. Accumulate a "wardrobe" and let your natural sense of association help you pick the right one for the right moment.

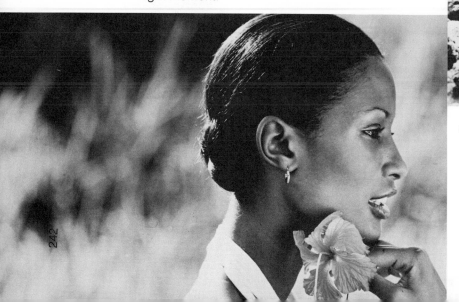

Be subtle

The usual way with fragrance is a dab behind your ear or on your wrist. That's fine, but try being subtle, too. Put empty scent bottles in drawers or closets to gently scent clothes. Put a little cologne in your final rinse water when you wash your hair. Spray your hair with cologne.

Be a romantic

Just about nothing says "romance" better than a soft gentle fragrance. If you've just met a new man or you want to make a lingering impression on one already in your life, try wearing your favorite fragrance whenever the two of you do something special together. He'll soon associate the scent with you.

Treat yourself

Don't save fragrance for just those times when you're with other people. Treat *yourself* to the pleasures of fragrance, too. Tip: Alternate between two or more fragrances from day to day so that your nose doesn't get accustomed to the scent and you no longer smell it.

Scent for sport

Don't save fragrance for "special" times only. These days there are so many wonderful sporty or casual fragrances around that there's one for almost every kind of day—on the courts, on the road, whatever. Tip: Don't apply fragrance to any skin that will be directly exposed to sun. It can cause a bad sunburn.

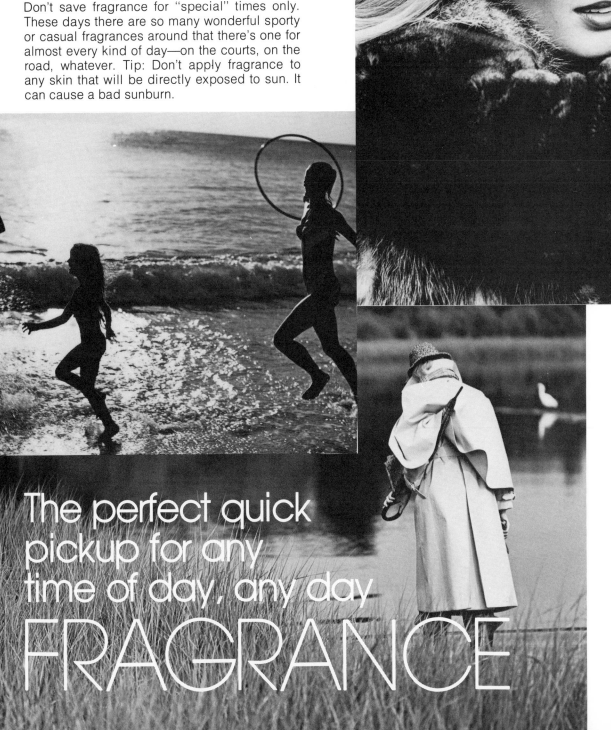

The perfect quick pickup for any time of day, any day
FRAGRANCE